THE POLITICAL ECONOMY OF HEALTH CARE

Where the NHS came from and where it could lead

Second edition

Julian Tudor Hart

This edition published in Great Britain in 2010 by

The Policy Press
University of Bristol
Fourth Floor
Beacon House
Queen's Road
Bristol BS8 1QU
UK

Tel +44 (0)117 331 4054
Fax +44 (0)117 331 4093
e-mail tpp-info@bristol.ac.uk
www.policypress.co.uk

North American office:
The Policy Press
c/o International Specialized Books Services (ISBS)
920 NE 58th Avenue, Suite 300
Portland, OR 97213-3786, USA
Tel +1 503 287 3093
Fax +1 503 280 8832
e-mail info@isbs.com

British Library Cataloguing in Publication Data
A catalogue record for this book is available from the British Library.

Library of Congress Cataloging-in-Publication Data
A catalog record for this book has been requested.

ISBN 978 1 84742 782 3 paperback
ISBN 978 1 84742 783 0 hardcover

Cover design by Qube Design Associates, Bristol
Front cover: image kindly supplied by Science Photo Library

REVIEWS OF FIRST EDITION

"... cries out against a world in which people are valued by what they acquire and consume not by what they create and produce ... passion for service, and the NHS, spills out of every page. The book is a spirited defence of a social institution which embodies what is best about society, against what he sees as the rise of rampant consumerism and free market values ...

This committed book is the *curriculum sua vitae* of a life well lived in the service of others. More than that, the book is a call to defend a noble institution ... To miss this book would be to miss the acquaintance of a remarkable man.

Sir Michael Marmot, Lancet

"This altogether splendid book provides an incisive critique of the politics and economics of health care – the major determinants of who gets what kind of care and how much of it. What makes this book unique is that none of the 'usual suspects' have written it... Julian Tudor Hart is a clinician, a British general practitioner who served for 30 years in Glyncorrwg, a Welsh mining town ... Although his principal focus is the United Kingdom's National Health Service, he extensively references the United States as its counterpoint ... I wish I could persuade our presidential candidates to read it."

New England Journal of Medicine

"[Julian Tudor Hart] analyses the relationship between patients and health care staff and sets this in an economic context, arguing that patients should be co-producers of health, not consumers ... the basis of the argument in good models of clinical care (which are increasingly seen as optimal but still not universally practised) is enticing ... this health partnership model is quite different from the current mantra of a patient-led NHS, derided by former Labour Health Secretary Frank Dobson as the equivalent of a passenger-led jumbo jet."

Sociology of Health & Illness

"At last, a coherent alternative to the healthcare agenda promoted by all political parties! This is a short but hugely challenging book ... if you care about healthcare, read it!"

Gut 2006, BMJ Group

"A contemporary, pioneering general practitioner, John Coope of Bollington, commented that one of Julian's talents is his nose for what matters in the published literature, and in this book it is on display – an amazing range of pertinent references, collated over a professional lifetime, as general practitioner, epidemiologist, researcher, social advocate and polymath, committed to the appliance of science in the National Health Service. It is inconceivable that Google could assemble such a mix. The book is worth reading for its footnotes alone, a glorious mixter maxter of sources, illustrations, anecdotes and asides – an NHS miscellany, that leaves 174 pages of text and argument, 'as slanted as a mountain slope, and exhilarating as a ski run down it'."

International Journal of Epidemiology

"*The Political Economy of Health Care* throws out a challenge to its readers, doctors, teachers, public servants and everyone else, to steer the NHS away from the marketplace to which it has been led by politicians ... [This] book should be read by all who want to understand why we must never take the NHS for granted or be complacent about its future."
    The Herald

" ... an intellectually challenging volume. Reading it can only enhance one's view of where we could be going dramatically wrong in changing the ethos of a much-loved organisation."
    John McGarry FRCOG

"The book is a blast ... as usual, the author has his finger on the pulse of what is happening in the NHS."
    British Journal of General Practice

"One of the most important works in the area of health economics. It is well researched and the style of writing is very readable.... This book is for everyone to read not just members of the healthcare profession."
    A reader on www.amazon.co.uk

"This is a remarkable book by a remarkable man. In an era when politicians of all parties are cynically destroying the NHS, this book offers a real alternative vision of how people should be treated."
    A reader on www.amazon.co.uk

"Health care shaped by market forces and 'commodification' does not deliver services efficiently, let alone equitably. For those who support the principal of universal, equitable access to cost-effective health care, Julian Tudor Hart's radical vision of what is needed will come as a breath of inspiring fresh air."
    Sir Iain Chalmers, Editor, James Lind Library, UK

"This is an important publication for North American readers – both Canadian and US. *The Political Economy of Health Care* prompts us to look at the historical and political origins of different national health systems ... a very valuable resource for those who want to develop health as a universal public good."
    Dr Bob Frankford, retired GP, former elected member of the Ontario Provincial Legislature and Parliamentary Assistant to the Minister of Health

"Lucid, informative and persuasive. The contrast between reductionist-fragmented and more dialectical-holistic approaches is brilliant. I hope that this book influences a new generation."
    Dr Helena Sheehan, School of Communications, Dublin City University, Ireland

To Mary, for everything

About the author

Dr Julian Tudor Hart was born of medical parents in 1927. His teenage ambition was to become a general practitioner serving a coal mining community developing practical ideas for a future socialist society. After five years as a GP in North Kensington he worked under two famous epidemiologists, Richard Doll and Archie Cochrane. Returning to general practice in a South Wales valley community, he combined clinical work with epidemiological research led by his wife Mary and supported by the Medical Research Council. He has published four previous books and many papers in peer-reviewed journals, visited many countries as a lecturer or visiting professor, and served as an elected member of the Council of the Royal College of General Practitioners. He is an Honorary Fellow of four Universities, a former President of the UK Socialist Health Association, and now President of the SHA in Wales.

Contents

Abbreviations and acronyms

ADHD attention-deficit hyperactivity disorder
A&E   accident and emergency
BBC   British Broadcasting Corporation
BMA   British Medical Association
BMJ   *British Medical Journal*
EBM   evidence-based medicine
EU   European Union
FDA   Federal Drugs Administration
FSA   Farm Security Administration (US)
FSA   Financial Services Authority (UK)
GP   general practitioner
HCA   health care assistant
ICC   International Cochrane Collaboration
IMF   International Monetary Fund
ISTC Independent Sector Treatment Centre
IT   information technology
JAMA *Journal of the American Medical Association*
MRC   Medical Research Council
MRSA methicillin resistant *Staphylococcus aureus*
NHS   National Health Service
NICE National Institute for Clinical Excellence
OECD Organisation for Economic Co-operation and Development
PBR   payment by results
PCT   Primary Care Trust
PFI   Private Finance Initiative
QOF   Quality and Outcomes Framework
RCGP Royal College of General Practitioners
TUC   Trades Union Congress
UN   United Nations
WB   World Bank
WHO   World Health Organization
WTO   World Trade Organization

Foreword

Julian Tudor Hart's book addresses in a scholarly and thoroughly empirical way what has happened to the NHS since its inception. He traces its history, and examines the successive reforms particularly in relation to the management of the NHS and to increased specialisation which threaten the original conception and intentions of its founders.

The recent 'industrialisation' of health workers is likened to the processes that occurred in England in the 18th century, whereby the workforce competes in a health market. He concludes that the consumerism affecting the health industry – every man for himself and every woman for herself – stands in opposition to the public belief in the solidarity of health, a belief which remains steadfast today.

His analysis of the reasons why the NHS came into being – in particular the anticipation of major civilian casualties during the Second World War which led to a fundamental re-evaluation of the country's needs – is a fascinating insight into how social, political and military factors interrelated to produce one of our most enduring and much-loved social institutions. It is a book not just about the National Health Service, but also about the conflicting principles and ideals to which the service has been subject over its 60-plus years of existence.

Tony Benn
Former Labour MP and Cabinet Minister

Preface to the
second edition

Events have confirmed all the main trends suggested in the first edition
of this book, published in 2006. The worldwide drive to reshape
health care away from public service towards commercial models,
with varying support from the state and participation by for-profit
corporate providers, has become a dominant government strategy
virtually throughout the world.

The US has been the prime mover, but as its own commercial health
care market becomes an ever more spectacular failure, its salesmen
have had to look elsewhere for evidence to support their claims.
UK governments, first Conservative, then New Labour, offered our
National Health Service (NHS) as the most influential site for their
experiment. This would, they believed, surely demonstrate the immense
gains, in quality of service, value for money and staff productivity, to be
expected from market competition, consumer choice, industrialisation
and motivation by profit. Unfortunately commercial secrecy, and the
natural reluctance of governments to admit even the possibility of
error, precluded any systematic collection of data to provide conclusive
evidence either way.[1] So we must judge as best we can, from the
medical, public health and administrative literature, from the more
responsible parts of our news media, and from colleagues we know and
trust. Judging from these, spending money on health care by putting
it into the pockets of commercial providers has at best not improved
care any more than we might have expected from spending the same
money directly on previously existing public service. At worst, it has
inflicted serious damage on staff morale, and on patients' understanding
of care processes. Commercialised, competitive, marketed care still has
powerful advocates, who assure us that their medicine will eventually
work, if only we would swallow a bit more of it. They hold political
power which they will continue to use as long as they can.

Early in 2008 deregulated financial markets collapsed, starting
in the US and the UK, the countries whose rulers had been most
devoted to solving all problems through market competition. Blind
faith in the profit motive, which sets simple personal greed as proxy
for complex social wisdom, caused that collapse. At that elementary
level, millions of people all over the world are already approaching a
consensus view, learned from their own experience. They now know
that experts accepting millions a year in exchange for their integrity

and devotion to public duty no longer possess these qualities. People have rediscovered that they must think for themselves – above all, those with least power in society.

The world has entered a period of crisis unprecedented in history. We have a conjunction of three simultaneous global crises: a crisis in the global trading economy, a crisis in the climate and resources of the natural world, and a crisis in ideas that have subordinated every human activity to the single supreme aim of accumulating wealth in a small dominant fraction of society, measuring our worth not by what we are able to do, but by what we are able to consume. Much of the crisis in health care arose from this context, so from change in this context we should look for solutions.

The four years since the first edition have confirmed my belief that from study of the NHS when it operated as a gift economy from 1948 to the early 1980s, and of the first shoots of new relationships between staff and patients which developed over that time, we may find the beginnings of economic, political and cultural alternatives to the state we are now in – not just for health care, but for society as a whole.

Changes in this edition

As in the previous edition, this book is designed to be readable at two different gear speeds. The main text tries to present a coherent argument, with empirical data to support and illustrate this restricted to a (fairly generous) minimum. The notes and references provide a lot more empirical evidence and discursive argument and opinion.

I have never worked from a full-time academic base, so my analysis could draw on personal experience of actually providing primary health care, in relatively difficult circumstances, over a lifetime spent mostly in one place, with the same population, and reading some of the main English-language journals every week. From these I took evidence that seemed relevant to my own work, as a generalist with responsibility for primary care, and referral to specialist care, for a community of around 2,000 people, mostly coal miners and their families. The aim of medical care for a population is to change its experience of illness. We have more than enough books derived chiefly from other books, but we are desperately short of new ideas derived from real experience of planned social change of any kind.

However, though high theory can start from low practice, to be generally useful, it can't end there. Real economists and real sociologists must develop the theme of co-production in a gift economy as I think it deserves. Perhaps this process has already begun.[2] Equally, I cannot write with authority about specialist areas of care, or about reintegration of generalist and specialist care, an important issue badly in need of development not in the heads of academics, but, combining theory with experimental practice on the ground, by a younger generation of innovators. All I can do is to indicate some examples of the sorts of development such reintegration might need.

Mine is a view from below, from the coal-face, not from the boardroom. That has some great advantages, but also some serious weaknesses. I am ashamed to admit that I only got round to reading Charles Webster's splendid short history of the NHS in the last weeks of writing this second edition.[3] His masterful overview, together with the more recent work of John Lister bringing it up to date, is more competent than anything I could achieve, but these are views from above, albeit from an essentially socialist perspective. I was working at what was then the base of society. There, at the point of production, I then believed was the main source of power for fundamental social change in a forward, civilising direction. However, a view from below is in important ways incomplete. Webster's book made me re-read everything I had written, and already revised many times.

Finally, I must apologise for being a very old man, now 83, writing on a subject that needs a much younger author, more familiar than I can possibly be about recent practical developments in clinical medicine and the organisations, reorganisations and re-disorganisations of the NHS, and still working inside it at some typically overworked and under-resourced point of production. No such paragon seems to be currently available, so I have done the best I can. To compensate for not being able to provide as much up-to-date empirical data as I think my argument deserves, I have given readers a lot of interesting older stuff with which few are likely to be familiar. It is often useful to look at the beginnings of new ideas, and not always easy to find them, even with the internet.

Why political economy?

Political economy is not normally an attractive subject for students of health care, or for most people concerned with the NHS as users, though both are my intended readers. In fact quite the opposite: at least since the late 1970s, whenever most economists have commented on health care, it has been to explain what cannot be done. Alan Maynard actually defined health economics as the study of choices in conditions of scarcity. The founders of economics, William Petty and Adam Smith, took a more positive view, never detaching economics from politics.[4]

Smith's *Wealth of Nations* started from analysis of contemporary production. He was more concerned with expanding productivity than with defining its limits, and had no illusion that economics could ever become a socially neutral, apolitical technology.

Students find applied human biology hard enough by itself. Adding political economy may seem only to make this study even more difficult, and even less human. They are unlikely to face any overtly political or economic questions in their examinations, and in their subsequent professional lives most of them plan to stay as far as possible from both. I understand how they feel, but people who turn in disgust from either politics or economics leave the field clear for careerists who see little wrong with either of these two corrupted fields as they now are. Events are revealing the consequences of this abdication from the responsibilities of citizenship. If we want our children to lead civilised lives, the world will have to change course, away from competition toward cooperation. We know already who will resist that change, but who will promote it, and how? The first step must be to understand where we are, how we got here, and where else we might go, using available empirical evidence. We have to start not from where we might like to be, but from where we are. And we must start not with the people we might prefer, but with those we have.

Media discussion, and much professional discussion, has long deplored the apparent dehumanisation of care, 'getting better but feeling worse'. This unease seems to have grown alongside the exponential growth of science-based care over the past 50 years or so. Assumptions that science is somehow itself a dehumanising force are now commonplace. Analysis of functional relationships between staff and patients in the continuing processes of care show that this perception is false. Where these relationships are allowed to escape from a provider–consumer model to cooperation in a gift economy, where health care functions as cooperative production of real wealth rather than as competitive production and consumption of commodities, long-standing traditions of mutual trust can be recovered, expanded and sustained. Such beginnings could be developed as foci for rebirth of community and social solidarity in otherwise disintegrating societies.

My central argument is that commerce (and the forms of industrialisation produced by commerce) is inappropriate to this area of wealth production. For production of almost all objects, and many if not most simple services, profit motivation, extreme division of labour, and eventually replacement of human labour by machines, has led to order-of-magnitude gains in productivity, even though these processes have in many ways dehumanised labour, misdirected investment and degraded our planet. However, for production of objects and some personal services, it can still be claimed that human and environmental losses may be outweighed by gains in productivity, at least if pursuit of profit is strictly limited by state regulation. Production of health gain through medical care presents an entirely different picture. In this field, commercialising and industrialising processes are a confusing and destructive force. They deflect, deform and ultimately demoralise staff motivation and imagination; they shift the directions of investment from what is most needed by people to what is most profitable for business executives and impatient investors; they limit the imaginations of researchers in medical science; and they invite corruption and fraud.

Why Wales?

Wales is a small country, with fewer than three million inhabitants. And so is Great Britain, centre of a once mighty world empire, but now barely even a second-rate power, its manufacturing base largely eliminated through investment elsewhere, its financial sector inflated beyond all reason, making us more vulnerable to speculation than any other major economy. From experience of so small and atypical a base, it may seem impertinent to write a book about global principles. And so it may seem to write about the whole of medical care from experience limited almost entirely to a small coal-mining community in the course of losing its main justification for existence.

One has to start somewhere. Why not from experience of organising innovative care for real people in a real place, for most of a real life, which fortunately coincided with the birth of the NHS, the death of coal-based industry and the first signs of a new, knowledge-based economy? I entered practice in 1952, when the new service was just beginning to find its feet and when conditions and methods of work had hardly changed since the late 19th century. I have therefore experienced virtually the whole life of the NHS so far, both its advances and its retreats, as well as the expansion of applied medical science from a small fraction of practice at the beginning, to almost total dominance today. That perspective is a useful safeguard against over-confident assumptions about the future, and as good a way as any to look at reality as wider views from further above. We need both.

I realise that experience in countries exposed to the full force of privatisation of all public services – including experience of state and civic violence, for example in Argentina, Chile, Russia, Poland, Greece and many parts of Africa and Asia where the International Monetary Fund, the World Trade Organization and the World Bank have imposed the beliefs of the Chicago school of economists without regard to local history or opinion – might provide a more compelling narrative. In some of these countries, this process has been a matter of life and death, not just in hospital beds, but in streets, prisons and torture chambers. I have not shared those experiences, so I can't write those books, and excellent ones already exist.[5] On the other hand, Wales is where the ideas underlying the NHS first began. For several decades after the Second World War, the NHS provided the main model for state-funded and state-owned free health care services in other industrially developed economies. Because the frankly commercial health care system in the US is regarded by most people in other countries as a market failure, the authority of the NHS has been used as the main platform for export of ideas for so-called 'reform' of public health care services throughout the world since the 1980s. Britain was the birthplace of industrial capitalism, where privatisation of common land first created an industrial working class, entirely dependent on employment by owners of industry. The iron- and copper-smelting and coal-mining valleys of South Wales were its cradle. These valleys were the first to give birth to prepaid health care as a locally controlled public service, funded collectively according to ability and provided free according to need – the first step on a road leading ultimately to the NHS.

Coal mining in Wales is now virtually extinct, and even steel production faces an uncertain future. We are now well into what seems to be the next, and possibly final, stage of capitalism – post-industrial society, in which people are losing their pride as producers. They are sinking into a humiliating social role as passive consumers, compelled either to rediscover a new basis for social solidarity or to perish in attempts to retrieve an illusory imperial status they have already lost. In Wales we have endured every phase of this apparently universal sequence. We may provide as good a place as any to look for whatever comes next.

Wales has a rich tradition of radical thought and action, barely visible today, but not wholly forgotten. The partially autonomous Welsh Assembly government, together with the regional governments of Scotland and Northern Ireland, has taken first steps towards reversing the policy of commercialising health care, in which central government, always obedient to the commands of transnational wealth, still stubbornly persisted through three New Labour adminstrations. Their successor, the Conservative-Liberal coalition, is now going full tilt down the same road.

Wales was the birthplace of the NHS. If the Labour-Plaid Cymru coalition in the Assembly holds its nerve, Wales could be the battleground for its future. The labour movement in Wales can still distance itself from the fraudulent 'New Labour' experiment, get back on track towards democratic socialism, and discover what this slogan could mean in practice, through an NHS within a truly plural post-industrial economy, with a strong culture of public service, and renewed commitment to solidarity. I am not trying to see beyond that.

Truth is concrete. I suspect that the very elementary conclusions drawn from a small base in this small country can mostly be applied in outline elsewhere, at least for a start, and providing that huge international differences in history and culture are always borne in mind. For this last reason, I have presented the early history of primary medical care in Wales in some detail, to demonstrate the sort of evidence needed anywhere to understand what is locally possible, and to encourage others to find their own path from their own origins.

The many friends and colleagues who helped me with constructive criticism of the first edition were thanked when it appeared in 2006. I am extremely grateful to Tony Benn, Graham Watt, Ben Hart, Tony Beddow, Stevie Stevenson and Andy Tate for their generous and tolerant help with this one.

Julian Tudor Hart
July 2010
julian@tudorhart.freeserve.co.uk
www.juliantudorhart.org

ONE

The NHS as wealth production

All health care systems, even including those so unsystematic that they are hardly worthy of that name, claim to produce something. So one way of looking at them is as production systems, with measurable inputs, outputs and social relationships within their processes, so that different ways of organising them can be compared.

From 1948, when the British NHS began, until the early 1980s, when successive governments began to re-introduce most of the features of industrial commodity production and competitive distribution, the NHS was much simpler than any other national public care system.[1] It included every person living in, or even visiting, any part of the country who found themselves in need of medical or nursing care. All contacts between patients and staff, all diagnostic investigations, and all medical or surgical treatments, either at home or in hospital, were entirely free. So were all dental care (including orthodontics), spectacles, hearing aids and a wide range of simple appliances like crutches, sticks and surgical footwear.[2] Direct patient charges (in health economists' jargon 'co-payments') were introduced for the first time in 1952, four years after the service began, starting small but ending very big indeed for some services, most notably for dentistry – but even today, compared with almost all other countries, the NHS is still a universally available service for UK citizens, free at the time of use for more than 80% of users.

Virtually all the wide variety of British hospitals were nationalised in 1948, by a single Act of Parliament, making elected government responsible for the employment and distribution of what soon became, and has since remained as, the largest single workforce in the world after the Red Army. For complex reasons explained in Chapter Four, general practitioners (GPs) were left as independent self-employed contractors, paid by the state to provide a public service, but initially, at least, left free to define for themselves what they actually did. Private practice remained legal and, for about half of all consultant-level specialists, provided significant (sometimes colossal) added income. For most GPs, private practice either vanished, or became a marginal activity.

Originally, all NHS funding was intended to come from taxation, which in those days mainly meant income tax. Aneurin Bevan, the Minister of Health in the 1945 Labour government which introduced the NHS, was a real socialist; his socialism was defined by what he did, not just by what he said.[3] On the insistence of Cabinet colleagues of lesser faith, a small part of funding (less than 5%) was made to come from contributory state insurance, but even so, entitlement to care did not depend on these payments. Everyone could register with a personal doctor of their own choice for primary care.[4] Everyone could be referred by this personal doctor for specialist care at a hospital without charge, even if they had never contributed to state insurance. In effect, if somebody – anybody – walked into a GP's office needing treatment, we could initiate care, without worrying about entitlement or who would pay for it. In my entire working life of 40 years in the NHS, I never had to ask a patient to pay me a fee, or worry about whether any patient could afford the care they needed, either from me or from a hospital-based specialist.

The NHS created an extraordinary and unprecedented economy more or less independent of the surrounding marketplace, in which health care, previously a highly valued commodity, was suddenly made available to everyone at zero price. Economists told us then that, at zero price, demand would be infinite. The new NHS economy was utopian, against human nature and bound to fail. Well, it did not fail. Despite great initial difficulties – a rationally distributed service of adequate size was bound to take several years to develop – it was a huge popular success.[5]

Private or commercial medical practice, though still legal, rapidly declined after 1948, to less than 5% of all spending on health care. Even after UK governments began to encourage commercial competition in the 1980s, almost all students of health sciences, none of whom then had to pay any university fees, wanted and expected to work all their lives within the NHS, with a secure pension at the end, linked to inflation. For at least 30 years, health care professionals expected to pursue secure careers either as specialists or generalists, in secure patterns of work determined partly by their own interests, but chiefly by patterns of state investment directed toward the perceived health needs of the entire population, so that necessary but unfashionable specialties like psychiatry, geriatric medicine, control and treatment of sexually transmitted disease, or care for people with early learning difficulties, and unpopular places like areas of heavy industry or remote agriculture, could all be developed according to need rather than the relative wealth and power of these communities. More or less equal distribution of GPs was achieved by the 1960s, by allowing GPs to set up new practices in poor, previously under-served areas, but forbidding them to do so in rich, over-served areas. This was not the balance needed, because workloads were much higher in poor than in rich areas, so they needed higher than average ratios of staff to population, but the gross inequalities of the past were ended. Equal distribution of specialists was achieved throughout the UK by the 1970s, at least in terms of population (though, as with GPs, not in terms of workload), by creating more posts in under-served areas. Long before the US, all surgery and other highly skilled technical tasks in the NHS were being performed by fully trained full-time specialists, and all population centres had such specialists.

For 35 years the NHS operated as a nationalised industry with its own gift economy.[6] Commercial activities were pushed to the edge, the boundary between gift economy and commerce. The NHS was protected from the surrounding commercial economy, developing its own independent culture of public service, away from traditions of condescending charity, towards relationships of co-operation and trust.

On 5 July 1948 health care, valued everywhere more highly than any other consumer good except food or shelter,[7] ceased to be a commodity sold for profit, except for luxury trade at the fringes of practice. Despite frequent assertions that no such economy could survive,[8] in fact it flourished, though not without difficulties (above all, the low priority for funding[9] conceded by political parties compelled to accept responsibility for a costly institution too popular to get rid of).

Until the 1980s, virtually all health economists accepted that the NHS had become an extremely cost-effective system by world standards, particularly when compared with the marketed system of care in the US.[10] That reputation persisted until the worldwide retreat from Keynesian economics in the 1980s. This retreat started in Ronald Reagan and Margaret Thatcher's strongholds of unregulated capitalism. It was soon exported to more socially responsible states in Europe, and imposed on developing economies as a precondition for continued loans from the World Bank, the International Monetary Fund and similar agencies under similar influence.[11] The success of the NHS gift economy was achieved despite the facts that hardly any NHS clinical staff knew the cash value of anything they did or used, and that nobody working in NHS hospitals could be motivated by profit.

Throughout that time, the NHS seemed politically unassailable, despite its many powerful opponents. In 1946, the Conservative Party had voted against the NHS Act at every stage of its passage into law. From then until July 1948, when the Act came into force, the party and its newspapers did nothing to discourage the British Medical Association's (BMA's) threats, right up to the eve of its birth, to organise a professional boycott of the new service by GPs. Eighty per cent of GPs promised to support such a boycott (they had threatened the same in 1912, against Lloyd George's Insurance Act, but never carried it out; both the BMA and the government remembered that). Three months before the launch, the BMA finally understood that without support from the hospital specialists, and with GPs unlikely in fact to pursue their threatened boycott, it would have to retreat.[12] Within weeks of the start, virtually all doctors were participating, and over 95% of the British population were registered with NHS GPs. From its birth, the NHS was immensely popular, creating a profound and apparently permanent place in public affection that precluded any direct assault by any political party concerned to win the next election. No other nationalised industry achieved anything like this success. Of all the state industries created after 1945 (coal, steel, railways, road transport, ports, telephone communications, gas, water and other public utilities) only the NHS now survives intact, as visible evidence that a gift economy can flourish in practice outside the commodity market, its staff motivated by the outcomes of care rather than by exceptional staff earnings or profit for their employers.

It is this experience of roughly three decades of relatively efficient, non-commercial health care for every citizen as a human right, funded from progressive taxation, planned to meet human needs, which provides the initial basis for the theory of political economy presented in this book.

'Reform'

Managed care,[13] developed in the US and adopted as a policy goal by every British government since 1979, sought to escape this apparently anomalous gift economy and return to a model of health care as a commodity transaction between providers and consumers, albeit still funded by the state, and accessible to the whole UK population. This reorientation was described by its authors as 'reform', a term soon universally and uncritically adopted by news media and the commentariat, as though its implied claim to represent social advance rather than retreat required neither discussion nor evidence. This was part of a general worldwide offensive by dominant transnational corporate interests to shift public services from provision by non-profit state agencies, to provision by corporate providers working for profit.[14]

This began in the early 1980s as the Cold War, the ideological contest between capitalist and socialist command economies, approached its end. Welfare agencies were no longer necessary in the West to maintain popular consent, and could provide new opportunities for profitable investment. Liberal and Social-Democrat parties, and most academic and managerial sources of expert opinion, adapted to and mostly adopted the new message.[15]

Managed care sees the state as a proxy collective purchaser of a wide range of care processes from competing commercial providers. Public health services are reduced, at whatever pace electorates will tolerate, to a basic function as purchasers of services now provided not by state agencies, but by private or corporate entrepreneurs, working for profit. Their target population is individual consumers, but as the principle of a service free at time of use must be preserved (once conceded, this becomes irretrievable as long as governments still depend on votes), the state pays all or most of their fees.[16] In Europe, the extent of this proxy payment varies from one country to another, with more or less extensive co-payments by patients, usually for prescribed treatments, and often for consultations,[17] generally imposed for ideological rather than empirical reasons.[18]

As I shall argue throughout this book, this transactional model conflicts fundamentally with growing clinical realities. It can (though I don't believe it should) be applied with some success to virtually all separate clinical tasks in isolation, for example hip joint replacements or cataract surgery, but it cannot be applied to any system of health care as an integrated whole, either for individuals, for communities or for nations, without fragmenting care and dividing short-term processes from long-term outcomes, so that nobody has a clear view of the aims or effects of care over lifetimes. It is a crude model, applicable without glaringly obvious immediate damage to most of the fragments of the health care process, but visibly false for any coherent health care system trying to maximise health gain for its whole population, including mobilisation of people to participate collectively in development of a healthier and happier society.

The fundamental reason for this is that effective health care, whose product is health gain and in which clinical processes are means to that end rather than ends in themselves, always and increasingly demands an active role from patients and communities, beyond passive consumption. Effective health care has to be built around real continuing personal stories, not episodic fragments of standardised process.[19] This centrally important theme will be explored in detail in later chapters. Patients cannot help to produce health gain efficiently as episodic consumers. An affordable service requires active, sceptical citizens, continuing co-producers of health, assisted by sceptical health care professionals able to make decisions independently of any commercial loss or gain, either for themselves, for corporate employers or for the purveyors of medications. This is so for entirely practical reasons. Patients who understand what is happening to them and can participate intelligently in their own care are essential for efficient delivery of medical science, particularly at the earlier stages of impairment, when appropriate care may be simplest and most cost-effective, and inappropriate care (on the gigantic scale implied by mass anticipatory care) can be extremely wasteful and counterproductive for health.

Patients as consumers, rightly distrustful of professional providers in a commercial relationship but desperate to believe in them, inevitably swing about between credulity and nihilism in a market sustained by uncritical hopes, unlimited by scepticism, with consumers' decisions prompted by symptoms and fears, rather than by reason and evidence.

Rational application of medical science requires development of a non-commercial, post-industrial mode of production in a gift economy. Intuitively, this already has overwhelming support from our general population,[20] so much so that even now, no political party has dared openly to oppose it, or make frank reversion to the marketplace an election issue. Every step back toward commercialised care has been taken by duplicity and stealth.[21] Elements of this new gift economy are already latent within every health care system, even those whose health professionals still believe they can act only within the constraints of commodity production and sales, and that specialised fragmentation and crude industrialisation are inevitable. An organised gift economy could release medical science and imagination from these constraints, so that its advances could be applied rationally according to need, and imaginatively to deal with problems as they actually are, rather than as they have to be understood to maximise market opportunities. A co-operative gift economy would not of itself solve any health problems, but it could greatly simplify their solution by clearing commercial interests out of the way, allowing health workers to tackle ill health and unhappiness directly, according to rational rather than commercial priorities, and to imagine wider solutions than those most obviously divisible into commodity tasks.

Profit motivation and job satisfaction

Health care is a field in which Adam Smith's invisible hand cannot operate without introducing a potentially lethal infection, the profit motive. We may learn to cope with this from car salesmen, but from doctors or nurses it is surely intolerable, both for them and for their patients. In all countries, we still have politicians who do not understand that effective health care needs no other motive. Granted a sufficient but not obscene salary, confident in a well-funded educational system for their children and relieved from the huge costs of their own education, the satisfaction of having done their work well, with visible and tangible gains in the health and happiness of real people, is far more powerful for most professionals than adding more riches to the generally good incomes they already receive in mature economies. People who don't understand that should not be in charge of health care systems.[22] The NHS should produce wealth, but not in commodity form or according to commercial priorities.

I therefore do not pretend to present any of the currently accepted versions of health economics, all of which offer at best only modified versions of classical economics, modifying its crudest assumptions by elaborate exceptions. University libraries have plenty of these books for those who want them. They may be useful for making rational choices about some particular tasks, but they fail to address the irrationalities of care systems as a whole, or provide even outlines of more rational alternatives. Classical economics are simply irrelevant to health care as a rational mode of production for health gain. They are designed to serve trade for profit, not the rational application of science in an advancing civilisation.

Nor do I pretend political neutrality. William Petty and Adam Smith, the founders of classical economics, and the late John Kenneth Galbraith, its most experienced and internationally respected recent exponent, all accepted that no economy could ever be understood outside its political context – and, Galbraith would have added, no economist claiming political neutrality should ever be trusted. No such animal has ever existed. Economies, and theories of how they operate, are human constructs derived from human choices. Economic laws are not laws of nature. Though they can't be changed simply by mighty exertions of will, they can be, and have been, changed by global shifts in human behaviour, particularly by modifying their expression through changing laws of property. These have occurred time and again at critical turns in history. We have now entered such a critical turn. As I write, most people still seem willing to wait for our bankers and top business executives to find sufficiently profitable ways to save our societies and our planet, to make a serious start in doing so. But probably not for much longer.

All economy is political economy. The two words should be inseparable – as they always were, until the late 19th century when Alfred Marshall introduced the idea that economists were somehow above the battle, technical experts making value-free judgements dealing only in numbers, detached from the material world they were supposed to measure and represent. In 1999, after damning evidence appeared in the *New England Journal of Medicine* against profit motivation in health care, battle raged in its correspondence columns. None of the angry defenders of profit offered any countervailing empirical evidence to support their case, their beliefs having reached religious intensity. The following passage comes from one of these letters:

> To claim ... that free market principles do not apply to health care is akin to believing that the law of gravity does not apply to certain objects on this planet. Upholding this myth can only be compared to clinging to a pre-Copernican view of the universe. ... When money is the mission, everyone wins.[23]

The physician who wrote this was, like most of his generation, an orthodox disciple of Friedrich Hayek, Milton Friedman and the Chicago school of economists. Like many others then doing well out of the global market,[24] he had blind confidence in his own rectitude, wherever it might lead. As always, leaders of society say hard choices have to be made – by which they mean hard, not for themselves or their friends, but for everyone else. To make economic progress they must harden their hearts without regard to immediate results such as mass unemployment or rubbishing of skills, because in the long run this will create more wealth. Though this will of course accrue to those who live from what they already own, some of it will eventually trickle down to those who live only from what someone finds it profitable to employ them to do. There is, and can be, no other way.

Such faith in a profit-motivated universe, where economic theory is not tested against empirical experience, not tested for its predictive power and not asked to explain or solve obvious, gigantic, exponentially growing problems in the real world, is itself our main problem. The pre-Copernican universe failed when it was compelled to explain and predict real observations and real events in the real world, being made by growing numbers of new people who were seeing more of the world and acting upon it in new ways. In health care it is becoming every day more obvious that when money is the mission, everyone loses. The poor lose all but emergency care, the rich lose their peace of mind and the doctors lose their integrity.[25] The wealth flows up, not down, and in a flood, not a trickle. By 1996, 358 billionaires (US$) held wealth equal to the combined incomes of the poorest 45% of the world population, 2.3 billion people,[26] a process of polarisation which has continued ever since at an accelerating pace. Almost everywhere, wealth is increasingly concentrated in the tiny minority who own and control the global economy.

It need not be so. The following chapters look at health care in this new way – as a system that produces not commodities bought or sold, but more and better life, for everyone in a collectively advancing global civilisation. It has already been shown to work, even in its most elementary form. Even readers in the US can be reassured that no doctors or nurses have consequently been enslaved, nobody has been denied choice of their family doctor, GPs still make house calls without charge when they are needed, and no committees select people too sick or too old to qualify for free treatment.[27] The British Medical Association now supports the principles of the NHS with almost as much energy as it opposed its birth 60 years ago.[28] People do, after all, learn from experience.

TWO

What does it produce?

Wealth is not a simple concept, as King Midas discovered when his food turned to gold. Gold, or money, represents wealth as a means for exchange, but as we rediscover in times of crisis or war, money is not itself a useful resource. Nothing is more useful for life than life itself, and health through which to enjoy it. This is not the only sort of wealth which the NHS produces, but like all health care systems, whether for fees, profit or public service, this purports to be its principal product.

For commercial health care, for professional or corporate trade, health gain is in fact a byproduct. It is necessarily subordinated to the profit required to justify the business of either entrepreneur professionals or corporate providers. Only through public service is it possible to set health gain as a planned social goal and a direct objective. However, even if this possibility is pursued in practice, health gain is not the only product.

Health gain can be measured as the aggregate of healthier births, healthier lives and healthier deaths.[1] All public care systems have other social products, the most important of which is stabilisation of society by legitimising the state (or the power of other corporate providers), but any system depends on this central promise of health gain for its credibility, whether this promise is real or illusory.

Healthier births are easily measured by maternal, perinatal and infant mortality rates, but in fully industrialised economies these are generally too low to provide more than a crude measure of output.[2] Measuring healthier lives is difficult.[3] To include all the possible impairments of life which health care tries to address, useful measures of healthier lives can only be essentially subjective measures of happiness and contentment, supplemented by measures of function – what people can or cannot do, not only individually, but as families, communities, nations and (as we are at last being compelled by events to recognise) as our entire human species, trying to survive on this planet. Measuring scales exist for all of these, but are not much used, because we still underestimate the value of subjective measurements, and overestimate the value of objective measurements such as X-rays, blood tests and so on.[4] Measuring healthier deaths is also difficult, because even the concept of healthy death is not yet universally accepted. Where doctors have to compete with each other to defy nature in all circumstances, every death may seem a professional failure. Even in our most humane societies, where premature deaths are already exceptional, we are only beginning to accept timely deaths as natural, inevitable and eventually desirable events, where the rational aim of treatment should be palliation rather than salvage.

Process and outcome

NHS outputs are therefore rarely discussed by leading politicians or news media in any but the simplest terms. For the most part, they prefer to consider output of process, not outcome. Since the early 1990s there have been two chief measures of success: waiting times between first contact with the NHS for an episode of illness, usually through a GP, and receiving definitive specialist treatment; and economic viability of provider units, mainly hospitals. More recently, starting in 2004, targets for waiting times have been joined by targets for performance of a rapidly increasing list of clinical tasks, defined by expert committees at the National Institute for Clinical Excellence (NICE) as indicators of quality of care. As each designated task is performed, a box can be ticked and funding can be claimed, either for GPs as contracted entrepreneurs, or for hospitals as competing providers of specialist care. This whole bundle is generally referred to as 'tick-boxing', an important concept to which we shall return. Where output targets are unmet over substantial periods of time, provider units earn less state funding and may eventually be allowed to fail. As the work they do must be done by somebody, it should, in a fully operative market, pass to another competing provider. In practice, it has rarely been allowed to do so.[5]

Output of health gain is affected not only by how care is organised, funded, rewarded or controlled, but also by progress in medical and nursing knowledge and culture. Almost unremarked by politicians or media, there has been rapid progress over the past few decades not only towards new, more effective forms of diagnosis and treatment, but also towards their more rational selection and use.[6] However, we are still far from the point where we can assume that just because a clinical task has been performed, a patient's health has improved, or its further deterioration has been delayed.[7] Despite this, efficiency is still measured almost entirely by process, not outcome.

Less than 10% of consultations with GPs entail referral to any other agency: about 4% are referrals for possible surgery and 6% to other specialists. When these figures were obtained, virtually all NHS hospital work originated from consultations with GPs, little of whose work could be easily classified.[8]

The aims of, for example, prescribing, giving injections, turning an unconscious patient every 30 minutes, removing a uterus or gallbladder, or organising a programme for protecting old people with pneumococcal vaccine, are not just to perform these tasks competently, but to produce better health or delay its loss, and to do so with reasonable expectation of doing more good than harm. Health includes happiness. Unhappy people are not in optimal health (though this doesn't mean it is useful to regard everything short of happiness as disease).

If, in these terms, we assume that a familiar procedure will be productive, we are flying on autopilot (which, be it remembered, works well enough most of the time). Meaning well does not assure doing well.[9] Intervention processes can never completely assure their outcomes. Paradoxically, to intervene safely we must learn procedures so thoroughly and repeat them so often that they become second nature, like walking or driving. This autopilot state bypasses conscience. Here is what George Bernard Shaw, an Irishman, had to say about English medical conscience:

> Doctors are just like other Englishmen: most of them have
> no honor and no conscience: what they commonly mistake
> for these is sentimentality, and an intense dread of doing
> anything that everybody else does not do, or omitting to
> do anything that everyone else does.[10]

In my experience this applies to all nationalities and professions, not just Englishmen or doctors. Without conscious effort to think critically about what they are doing, sentimentality plus doing what everyone else does is the way most people work most of the time, unless prompted actively to think critically.[11] Critical thought is most effectively achieved through participation in teaching or other kinds of innovation and discovery.[12] Because every clinical problem occurs in a real person with a unique personal history, all problems are in fact different, so all clinical care needs to be innovatory, all clinical decisions need to be judged critically and all that we do is in some sense experimental. I had hands-on responsibility for patients for more than 40 years, but the time when I would feel completely competent, a totally safe pair of hands for other people's lives, never arrived. Right up to my last week in practice I still feared making potentially serious mistakes, and with good reason.[13] Any attempt to apply knowledge from human biology to specific real lives entails a significant margin of error. Though my mistakes rarely had lethal consequences, that was just good luck. Clinical processes are in fact increasingly well (or decreasingly badly) selected and performed, but suggestions that any more than a few technical procedures can reach the virtual certainty we take for granted in, for example, air travel or engine design, are unrealistic.

The chief source of error in medicine is not the quality of performance of processes (though this can never be taken for granted), but the quality of decisions to initiate those processes, taking into account their full personal, social, economic and historical context.[14] Doubt, and recognition of error, are the foundations of science, but have yet to be made the foundations for all medical practice. For nursing, such recognition seems even more remote. Aggressive NHS managers, contingency lawyers and self-righteously ignorant media editors and journalists make this transition to constructive scepticism even more difficult.

Does health care produce net health gain?

Even assuming full technical competence, we have to keep worrying about whether decisions we take and procedures we perform actually lead to net health gain.[15] We need evidence that the probable good we do exceeds probable harm by a substantial margin, justifiable in simple terms to our patients. If such evidence is lacking, we need to remember the often surprising capacity of bodies and minds to recover health through their own capacities, neither assisted nor impeded by clinical tinkering.

Why worry? Is it not self-evident that, on the whole, medical care has done well? In Britain, average expected lifetimes have increased by 40 years since 1840. They still show no sign of reaching a finite span, assuming that any such limit will ever be reached, which seems increasingly doubtful. Globally, expected lifetimes have doubled over the past two centuries.[16] In Britain, average lifetimes expected at birth have risen from under 50 years in 1901 to about 80 for women and 75 for men in 2001. On present trends, they will continue to rise steadily, with no end in sight.

One reason for this gain is health care. It is not the only or even the main reason, but because availability of care is closely associated with quality and availability of education, food, shelter, regulated labour, rising personal incomes, increasing equality of incomes and other social factors supporting health, it is difficult and perhaps impossible to separate all these causes and measure their 'independent' contributions to health.

How can we measure an 'independent' effect if all relevant social factors are in fact always interdependent? For example, better educated people make more effective and efficient use of health care, simply because they know more. At least in the US, they are also richer and have better access. It is hard to conceive any real situation in which availability of health care could actually be independent of other categories like income, nutrition, education or housing, on a sufficient scale to reach any useful conclusion. If so, this is not a scientific question, since it can be neither confirmed nor refuted either experimentally, or by continued observation of statistical trends.

There are a few examples suggesting that once basic levels of material subsistence are assured, availability of health care may become a major determinant of health. After its revolution in 1959, Cuba soon attained infant and adult mortality rates at roughly the same levels as the US, despite vastly lower average income and health care spending per head of population. Annual cost of health care in the year 2000 in the British NHS was £750 per head, less than half that in the US, despite similar mortality rates. This compared with £7 per head in Cuba, where 45% even of this small sum was spent on primary care, compared with 16%–18% in the NHS.[17] Low personal incomes in Cuba were combined with high social incomes (facilities of many kinds available free, or at very low cost, and shared by the whole population). As a consequence of this high shared social income, Cuban rates for literacy (a major associate with all health indicators) were probably better than those in either Britain or the US,[18] and health indices reached West European levels.[19]

Cuban experience confirms that a well-organised health care system including the whole population can help to sustain good mortality indices despite a low GNP, low average personal incomes per head, and demoralisingly low professional incomes, providing that society as a whole remains stable and cohesive, with a strong and shared sense of social and historical direction, and that the health care system is participative at primary care level and open to change.[20] Cuban experience has an interesting historical parallel in Sweden, albeit before clinical decisions for individual patients could have any positive net product, and everything depended on local public health measures.[21] Though Sweden was one of the poorest European countries in the late 19th century, it then attained, and has maintained ever since, the world's best public health indices in virtually all dimensions. This was achieved through universally accessible and inclusive health care and education systems used by all of the people, a high social wage, and a strong and increasingly successful reformist socialist movement which set a path towards a much more equal society. This development preceded, and to some extent enabled, development of a modern industrial economy. Through a lifetime of rigorous research, Richard Wilkinson and his colleagues have established beyond reasonable doubt a close, positive and consistent association between indices of social equality and indices of morbidity, mortality and many other indicators of social success – high literacy, low criminality, indeed virtually any mark of civilised living.[22]

At least until the US economic blockade forced it to accept a dual economy (a burgeoning dollar economy of hotels and revived prostitution, alongside an extremely austere socialised economy of rationing), Cuban society had achieved many other features known to favour good population health: universal literacy, vigorous traditions of local solidarity and community, virtually no unemployment, high average energy expenditure and participation in sport, low indices of social inequality, and very low levels of crime, alcohol and narcotic dependence and sexually transmitted disease. The state of siege imposed upon it ever since Cuba dared to take this independent path, and consequent intolerance of dissent, have impaired development of Cuban society (as its enemies intended), but its positive achievements provide unique evidence that if care systems are planned to maximise whole-population health gain and community participation, they can achieve high productivity and make a huge contribution to public health.

Can we measure health gain?

Counting interventions, such as doctor-visits, operations or hospital admissions is easy, but these measure clinical process, not outcome. Measures of personal health do exist, most of them complicated and impractical to use except as research tools on small samples of people. An underused alternative is simply to ask people to rate their own health, and do so repeatedly over time. For middle-aged men, even a simple one item self-report of health status ('Would you say your health is excellent, very good, good, fair, or poor?') is as powerful a predictor of mortality over the next 4 to 9 years as more detailed clinical indicators, confirmed by the NHANES-I study of 6,440 adults aged 25–74 over 12 years. The simple question proved less useful for older people or women.[23] Validated instruments of this kind have been developed and should be more widely used, not as aids to personal care, but as tools to measure NHS productivity in personal terms.[24]

The alternative, instinctively preferred by management and most professionals, is to measure intervention processes, as proxies for health gain.[25] These are usually presented with warnings that they do not necessarily represent health gain or loss accurately, but this advice seems usually to be ignored when it comes to policy decisions and media comment. Policy makers like to have some information to justify their decisions, even if in fact these decisions usually precede the evidence on which they claim to be based. To such policy makers, the quality of information is less important than just having some. Don Berwick has drawn attention to a report from the UK Office for National Statistics which concluded that between 1995 and 2003 overall NHS productivity declined by 3%–8%, depending on different methods of calculation.[26] As he rightly asks, 'Production of what?'. It turns out that in this case the 'product' was a weighted average of 16 different NHS activities, all processes rather than outcomes. The weighting was supposed to reflect the relative burden incurred by each activity so that, for example, episodes of inpatient treatment weighed 14 times as much as episodes of outpatient treatment. This could lead to the absurd conclusion that a general shift away from inpatient hernia repairs or varicose vein stripping through hospital day care (which is government policy, and everyone agrees would be a more efficient use of both staff and patient time and hospital resources) represented a fall in efficiency.

With 96% coverage and completeness of coding for inpatient episodes in NHS hospitals and little less for consultations in primary care, outcome measurements that truly reflect personal health gain attributable to clinical decisions are certainly possible,[27] but their design would have to include critically important decisions on weighting. These will in turn depend on experience of caring and its long-term outcomes in terms of health gain. Such understanding is not just a technical matter, at every point it entails experienced social judgements.[28] The general shift away from clinical judgements towards algorithmic decisions following centrally devised guidelines is a diverse bag of both dangers and opportunities. Neither conservative nor radical approaches can provide simple answers across the board. There might eventually be a clinical and scientific consensus in favour of such measurement systems, for research if not for day-to-day management. But even if this were so, they would differ fundamentally from the present management consensus, which seems to be derived from Japanese concepts of 'total quality control' devised for car production in the 1970s.[29]

Collective health, at local, national or global level, is usually represented by maternal mortality (pregnancy-related deaths per 1,000 births), infant mortality (deaths under one year of age per 1,000 live births), perinatal mortality (stillbirths plus deaths under six weeks of age per 1,000 live births) and life expectancy at birth (calculated from survival tables). A simple modification which has proved useful for measuring significant differences in quality of medical care between localities and between social classes is mortality under 65 years of age (normal retirement age in the UK) – premature mortality.

All these measure the existence of life, but not its quality. To measure quality of life in medical terms requires measures of morbidity (perceived illness or disability). These generally follow much the same pattern as mortality – where there is more sickness there tends to be earlier death. Great advantages of mortality data are that they are now available for almost all countries, that they are simple (even the least competent doctors can usually tell whether a person is alive or dead), that they can be readily understood by everybody (providing they take account of the age structure of the population) and that, compared with most measures of morbidity, they are much less susceptible to government manipulation.

Negative outputs?

Despite daily experience that health care systems can and mostly do contribute powerfully to net health gain for individual patients, there have been repeated attempts to discount the net value of clinical interventions as a whole, or even to suggest that on balance they are counterproductive. Paradoxically, these doubts seem to have had more influence on political and academic thought in the last quarter of the 20th century (when there was far more convincing evidence of net benefit than ever before in history) than in previous centuries when there was little evidence that more than two or three clinical interventions ever did more good than harm. Starting in the 1970s, extreme scepticism got intellectual support from a new literature of professional defeatism and populist nihilism, best exemplified by McKeown[30] and Illich[31] respectively, who both denied that clinical interventions as a whole made any significant net contribution to health gain. That this nihilist trend is alive and well, despite even larger recent advances in applied medical science, was shown by republication of Illich's *Medical Nemesis* by the *British Medical Journal* (*BMJ*), with enthusiastic editorial endorsement,[32] and by McKeown's continued influence on orthodox public health teaching and thought, despite damaging expert criticism of his original demographic evidence[33] and serious questions raised by other expert critics to which he gave no answer in the second edition of his book.[34]

Health care systems can themselves become engines of social change on a much broader front than their central tasks imply. They can promote professional and public hopes of social progress, and may then be opposed philosophically by people who think such expectations are misleading. Up to the 1970s, public respect for the power of health care seemed generally reassuring to rulers. In Europe at least, with strong socialist and communist movements after the Second World War, it may have seemed cheaper and less dangerous to concede demands for personal health care than collective demands for higher wages or more socially regulated pursuit of profit. Social progress was still conventionally conceived in the frame of the 18th-century Enlightenment, a beneficent state supplementing and containing the competitive greed otherwise necessary for material progress. McKeown and Illich fanned the first flames of a scepticism which prepared the ground for retreat. My mentor Archie Cochrane almost, but not quite, joined in this nihilism, but his seminal book, *Effectiveness and Efficiency*, also cleared away much traditional rubbish obstructing progress towards more humane and effective care, a most necessary task.[35]

All three authors implicitly accepted that health care systems must be judged by their product in net health gain. McKeown's and Illich's arguments were almost wholly negative. Essentially they claimed that all systematic attempts to prevent illness, or to change its natural course, other than through less specific social measures, had an aggregate net product of zero or less, in terms of health outcomes.

Cochrane's critique of care systems was more constructive, and opened possibilities in two entirely different and ultimately opposed directions.[36] Influenced by Alan Williams and other pioneers of the York University School of Health Economics, he looked at the NHS as a production system. Cochrane found it gravely deficient in effectiveness, efficiency and humanity, an item he unfortunately omitted from his title but developed as an important theme. His book appeared in the right place at the right time. It persuaded an entire generation of senior clinicians and health policy experts to accept health economics as essential for policy formation.

Cochrane was mischievously attracted to the idea that doctors not only might do more harm than good, but on balance actually did so. In informal discussion he was not seriously interested in the many other possible explanations for his finding that after standardising data for differences in GNP per head, countries with more doctors (or paediatricians) per head of population had higher infant mortality rates.[37] Though never biased in statistical handling of data, in discussion, he was systematically biased against the effectiveness of clinical medicine, perhaps because he was irritated by the smug assumptions of so many clinicians.

Legitimation of the state

Cochrane left out of account legitimation of the existing order of society, which had for centuries been at least as important a product of public care systems as health gain. He wanted the NHS to become more rational, entirely in terms of its contribution to health gain, rather than measured process. Health he rightly conceived in the broadest possible terms to include happiness, although this was harder to measure. He drew particular attention to disgracefully low NHS spending on 'hotel' functions for care of sick elderly people (feeding, housing and generally looking after them as guests rather than inmates or prisoners). Encouraged by the York School economists, he analysed (not very systematically, as his subtitle admitted) the NHS as an industry, with inputs, processes of manufacture and measurable outputs. However, he paid little attention to what we might lose by evaluating health care only as production of proven health gain, using the crude measuring instruments then available. He also ignored the political and historical context in which all his questions were posed. This was in the 1970s, when the social optimism of 1945 was already in decline, and defeatism and retreat were already becoming fashionable among Western intelligentsia, disillusioned by command socialism in the USSR and disturbed by the sometimes infantile leftism of their children and grandchildren after 1968.

Cochrane was thinking at the level of grand social and political strategy, required at times of historic transition. Writing a century earlier in 1867, when Benjamin Disraeli launched his bold gamble to extend the vote to men with no property except the houses they lived in, the conservative journalist Walter Bagehot gave the following useful advice to rulers in such times:

> As yet, the few rule by their hold, not over the reason of the multitude, but over their imagination and habits; over their fancies as to distant things they do not know at all, over their customs as to near things which they know very well.[38]

Bagehot ignored medical care, because at that time it played a far smaller part in securing public consent than it does today. To governments of, by and for the rich, continuing to rule in their own interest but now compelled to obtain consent from ever wider electorates, Bagehot taught three fundamental principles, as relevant today as in 1867, particularly to strategies for health care.

First, such rulers must learn to respect the brains of their voters. The poor could reason just as well as the rich. The old adage of the advertising industry is still apt: never underestimate public intelligence, never overestimate public knowledge.

Second, rulers should so far as possible control and contain the imagination of the multitude about 'distant things they do not know at all', meaning the whole world outside the familiar experience of their daily lives. The agenda for public information is still dominated by very rich men who own newspapers not only to make money, but to exert power, above all by shaping public imagination in the ways they want. Interest in football or in celebrity singers is to be encouraged, but interest in trade union organisation or politics is unhealthy and boring. Liberal news media and public service broadcasters may modify this agenda, but they seem rarely to appreciate how far their own imaginations may be guided by self-interest. Even in the age of mass tourism, multitudes at home fear and remain ignorant of multitudes abroad. This ignorance is not an empty vacuum. It is filled with crude, stereotyped and divisive images which limit brains and maximise stomachs and genitalia.

Thirdly, the rich should prudently respect the people's 'customs as to near things which they know very well'. So far as possible, they should make themselves appear sponsors of these popular near things. In the UK, but not in the US, free access to doctors, nurses, hospitals through the NHS became such customs, deeply entrenched within the first months of its existence, and impossible to delete thereafter. Nothing, not even the Royal soap opera, is more precious to ordinary people than these NHS rights to care 'from the cradle to the grave', as everyone came to believe soon after 1948.[39]

Limits to liberalism

McKeown, Illich and Cochrane all philosophised within the assumptions of liberalism. All three questioned whether clinical medicine really had any positive net product in terms of health gain, and the first two doubted if it ever could. The NHS shifted processes of health care in the UK from functioning as quasi-commodities, in a market whose failures were erratically modified by charity and the state, to a human right in a gift economy, but if these gifts had no product in net health gain, the whole thing was fraudulent.

If the net NHS product is real, this is a decisive step beyond liberalism. The term 'liberal' is ambiguous and rarely defined. It rightly combines two opposed yet inseparably associated meanings: freedom of thought and tolerance of dissent on the one hand, and freedom of property on the other, united by free trade in both. This dual meaning was originally opposed to conservative ideas of monarchy, aristocracy, and inherited ownership of land as foundations for stratified and immobile societies. The dual meaning is inherent in the concept. In May 2010, the convergence between neoliberal policies of all three main parties, Conservative, Liberal Democrat and New Labour, had its inevitable result. No party had a working majority on its own. With 36% voting Conservative, 29% Labour, 23% Liberal Democrat and 12% for Scottish and Welsh nationalists and independents, the ruling class got what it wanted, fundamental revision of the welfare state created in 1945. The most serious global crisis of capitalism since the Wall Street crash of 1929 and a decade of privatising 'reform' by New Labour governments have created a window of opportunity of which full advantage will be taken. The first coalition budget starts a redivision of national wealth and power, restoring pre-war social polarities. The entire public sector of employment is to be cut by 25%, and the entire NHS budget in England is to be handed to GPs as independent contractors. GPs are clinicians, not strategists or administrators. Few will see any alternative to inviting some commercial provider to accept this responsibility, and make as much profit as they can from what was hitherto public service.

This coalition perfectly illustrates both these aspects of liberalism: one party to make the rich richer and more powerful, the other to deplore the consequences, providing just enough hope of moderation to retain public consent. As a gift economy dealing in real needs for everyone, the NHS went beyond the limits of liberalism.

In Wales, the only part of the UK where the Labour Party still has power in government, the NHS rock still stands. Rejecting commercialisng 'reforms' pursued by New Labour in England, the Labour-Plaid Cymru coalition in Wales is a potential fortress, where hard-learned principles can be used to develop a better future, the next time we emerge from the tunnel. For the second time in history, Wales could build foundations for progressive society.

Analysis of health care as a production system

Health economists adapting to neoliberal agendas welcomed Cochrane's *Effectiveness and Efficiency* as an important step towards more rational care, freed from what they saw as utopian aims. Had they not accepted this, had they stayed loyal to the socialising path on which Bevan had set their feet, *Effectiveness and Efficiency* could have served progress. Instead, economists assumed that, as a production system, health care must function in essentially the same way as the industrial commodity production and trade with which they were familiar and comfortable, albeit with numerous qualifications. Cochrane would probably have endorsed that view, had he lived longer. Despite his fondness for mischief, he was ultimately an Establishment man, moving a little ahead of his times. On the other hand, I think he would have had more respect than many of his readers for Bagehot's Machiavellian advice. Social stability is indeed an important part of the NHS product, an important contributor to health in its own right.

Historically, analysis of health care as a production system reaches back to the first birth of health economics and its companion science, epidemiology, through the work of Sir William Petty. Petty was a prominent actor in the English Revolution in the 17th century.[40] The next notable quantifier of evidence was Pierre Louis, who lived through the series of French revolutions from 1789 to 1848.[41] Since then, objective analysis of social health and health care has endured repeated cycles of birth, decline and rediscovery, always related to contemporary political and economic climates of democratic advance or oligarchic retreat.

Every rebirth of health care economics met majority professional resistance, mainly because any rational measurement and analysis endangered trade in a then extremely doubtful product. In 1914, Codman presented an objective analysis of measured inputs and outputs of surgery in a Boston hospital. He was scorned thereafter by his professional colleagues for the rest of his life.[42] In the first months of the NHS, Ferguson and McPhail[43] analysed the consequences of UK hospital medical care, as it was when hospitals were first nationalised. Two years after discharge from hospital, 57% of patients were either no better, worse or dead – a shocking statistic at that time, and therefore generally ignored and quickly forgotten. News media then saw doctors as bastions of social authority, not as promoters of (to them) irrational public demands for free care in an otherwise entrepreneurial society. Few professionals had enough faith in the effectiveness of their work to welcome a challenge to measure their outputs, so for the next 30 years, nobody dared to do so.

Withdrawals of medical labour in trade disputes or strikes created natural experiments. If doctors really did something useful, when they stopped doing it, there should have been measurable falls in output. In 1976 a slowdown of medical labour in protest at high malpractice insurance rates in Los Angeles County was convincingly associated with reduced population death rates: when doctors stopped working, more people survived. This paradoxical result probably occurred because of a reduction in planned surgery.[44] Most of this surgery was probably done not to prolong life, but to improve its quality, but this inevitably entailed some operative risk, so more operations meant more risk.[45] In 1983 a GPs' strike in Jerusalem lasted 27 weeks, during which all public sector care ceased except emergency hospital admissions (which rose by over 20%). Mortality was exactly the same during the strike weeks as during the two weeks preceding the strike, and as in the previous year, when there was no strike.[46] Similar conclusions were reached by a remarkable study of operations for abdominal pains attributed to appendicitis in Germany in the 1960s: more operations were associated with substantially more deaths, even though when appropriately used for acute appendicitis, appendectomy was certainly life saving.[47]

Evidently the nihilists had a case good enough at least to deserve an answer. This raises the issue of whether shifts in life expectancy are in any case a valid measure of NHS production. If most NHS processes concern not saving life, but making it happier and less painful, then gains in happiness and reductions in pain are necessary additional measures of output. They are much harder to measure, but certainly not impossible, each having its own substantial research literature. On the other hand, reliable data on deaths, and ages at which they occur, are far easier to obtain and interpret, and they have immediate intuitive meaning for everyone. The most serious negative byproducts of medical and surgical interventions designed to improve life rather than extend it are fatal events. Though almost all surgery is now associated with less than 1% consequent mortality, except in very old people, this still means that more surgery implies more deaths. Mass medication also implies negative as well as positive outputs. As even positive gains are usually small, positive balance of quality-of-life gains against length-of-life losses should still begin from comparisons between treated and untreated people, and in terms of all causes rather than disease-specific mortality. Mortality is a crude measure, but still provides the most convincing foundation for argument and action. We also need measures of morbidity and, perhaps even more, measures of self-rated well-being, but these almost always follow the same patterns as mortality, and lessons from them are usually much the same.

Closing the gap between possibilities and realities

John Bunker's classic review *Costs, Risks and Benefits of Surgery*[48] repeated Codman's work in a more critical but also more confident and therefore less defensive era. Later, in 2001, he estimated the overall contribution of medical and surgical care to prolonging life over the 50 years since the Second World War, when he entered practice as an anaesthetist. He concluded that possibly half these years of life added in the second half of the 20th century might be attributable to medical intervention.[49] In a masterly review of the entire English-language literature on the actual and potential contribution of medicine to reduced mortality, Nolte and McKee[50] found Bunker's assumptions too optimistic, mainly because he had more or less ignored the gap between what had been proved possible in research trials and what was actually achieved in practice. Routine care in whole populations does not match research practice, even in populations selected as representative of the whole. In my time, even routine practice failed to reach a high proportion of people who needed it, despite universal free access to NHS care. This is now changing, but slowly, and progress could easily come to a halt if the NHS again suffers systematic underfunding.

Nolte and McKee compared mortality rates for disorders amenable to treatment in 19 developed economies in 1998. Sweden held first place, with the best mortality figures. The US ranked 15th for disability-adjusted life expectancy and 16th for premature mortality from treatable causes. The UK ranked 10th for disability-adjusted life expectancy and 18th for premature mortality from treatable causes.[51] So neither country had much to boast about.

Ever since pioneers began searching proactively for treatable chronic ill health in whole populations, we have known that roughly half of most common chronic disorders in the English-speaking world are undetected, half those detected are not treated and half those treated are not controlled – the 'rule of halves'.[52] This approximation was originally derived from community studies of high blood pressure,[53] but similar whole-population studies of many other problems have indicated a similar order of magnitude for under-diagnosis, under-treatment and loss from follow-up. These have included type 2 diabetes,[54] deafness,[55] visual impairment[56] and incontinence in the elderly,[57] glaucoma,[58] coeliac disease,[59] asthma in children[60] and adults,[61] kidney failure,[62] vertebral fractures from osteoporosis,[63] suicidal depression,[64] domestic violence,[65] prostatic obstruction,[66] heart failure,[67] atrial fibrillation,[68] schizophrenia,[69] follow-up after strokes[70] and coronary heart attacks,[71] and psychosocial problems in children.[72] Institutionalised patients, nominally under regular skilled supervision, fare no better, with roughly half of all their treatable needs not recognised.[73] This list is incomplete, just evidence I have come across while reading a few journals of general medicine over the past decade or so. 'Halves' is only an order of magnitude, but in many of these studies the proportion of people with unmet needs was much more than half. In Britain during the past three decades, presented, identified and treated health problems together represent about half the real problems of which they are a part, often less. For whole populations, US figures seem similar: higher rates of ascertainment, more aggressive attitudes to treatment and higher expectations from patients with access to personal care all combine to reduce unmet need, but the 15%–20% with access only to emergency care often have gross unmet needs which are now rarely seen in the NHS. *Per contra*, through operation of perverse market incentives, many more patients in the US probably endure treatments they do not need, incurring risk without probable benefit.

Eliminating the rule of halves

Where health care is free, and primary care teams have registered patients whose names, addresses, telephone numbers (and soon e-mail addresses) are known, we don't have to wait for people to feel ill to search systematically for important avoidable risks to their health, on a whole community scale.

In Glyncorrwg, the coal mining village where I worked from 1961 to 1992, we started in 1968 to screen the whole population for important, treatable health risks, so that current knowledge could be so far as possible fully applied. Because even very high arterial pressures rarely cause symptoms until they have already caused serious organ damage, this important health-related variable needs to be measured in every adult, at intervals of about five years throughout life. This was therefore our first subject for screening, beginning in 1968 and completed by 1970.[74] Of those aged 20–65,[75] we reached 100% of men and 98% of women. This created what was, so far as I know, the first community in the world in which everybody's blood pressure was known and everyone likely (on contemporary evidence) to benefit substantially from treatment was helped to receive it for the rest of their lives.[76] Between 1968 and 1987 we then searched systematically for other common treatable causes of ill health in everyone over 20, mainly using ordinary consultations to collect data beyond that required for the usually minor complaints presented. At review in 1989, of all 1,207 adults in this age group, 44% had chronic chest problems, 36% were current smokers, 19% were obese, 16% needed treatment for high blood pressure, 11% had serious alcohol problems and 3.5% had diabetes, all using defined diagnostic criteria. Most of these problems overlapped with each other.[77] There were not only too many health problems for referral to specialist care to be feasible, the problems were also too complex for specialists to handle. They all needed skilled community generalists; only a few needed hospital-based specialists.

Was all this case-finding[78] and anticipatory care[79] – very hard additional work, none of which was paid for in those days – justified by evidence of eventual health gain? It certainly was.[80] In 1987 we compared death rates under 65 for the five years 1981–86 in Glyncorrwg (which had developed this cumulative proactive programme since 1968) and in the neighbouring, socially similar community of Blaengwynfi[81] (which had received only traditional demand-led care from three successive doctors between 1968 and 1985, all conscientious practitioners of traditional demand-led care). Age-standardised death rates under 65 were 28% lower in Glyncorrwg, the community receiving planned, proactive, anticipatory care, than in the control community receiving only demand-led care. Differences were mainly in deaths in the first year of life and for cardiorespiratory causes of death, the pattern expected when medical interventions are more effective.[82]

Our techniques were based on very high customary use-rates typical of all coal mining communities, with long traditions of free care, heavy burdens of sickness and injury, and frequent dependence on state benefits. They were based also: on very high response rates to our research studies,[83] secured through the trust generated by experience of continuing and emergency care readily provided;[84] on staff embedded in the local community, with all the efficiencies inherent in caring for people already well known; and on well-kept personal medical records, always available, used at every clinical contact and reinforced by frequent informal contacts in non-medical settings. Above all, they rested on a registered, accurately defined population, so that every audit numerator had a population denominator – the absolute precondition for any sort of research relevant to health care policy.[85]

Repealing the Inverse Care Law

The world over, the more any community needs good medical care, the less likely it is to receive it – a banal truism I summarised in 1971 as the Inverse Care Law.[86] High objective scores for social deprivation,[87] low average community incomes per head, high morbidity and premature death rates, and high primary care workload[88] are all consistently associated with high consultation rates (where these are free) but low average consultation time.[89] Poor people get more and earlier illness than rich people, but their communities are least attractive to doctors,[90] and far more potentially clinical time has to be wasted on legitimation of entitlements to the host of miserly benefits required to keep a mass workforce going even when employers don't need it, above all certifications of illness and entitlements to benefit.[91] Repeated experience of mass unemployment, with devastating and lasting consequences for social and biological health, is the most important common factor shared by all these communities.[92]

The Inverse Care Law is an effect of capitalism, which relentlessly subordinates human values to pursuit of profit. It is a human construct, not a law of nature. By taking health care out of the marketplace, it could and should eventually be eliminated. And by forcing already partially socialised health care back to the market, it will be reinforced, a crime for which politicians who have driven this policy, many of them still claiming to be socialists, should be held responsible.

The pre-'reform' NHS provided a framework within which it was possible for GPs, at high personal cost in lower net income, to initiate systematic proactive care as well as good traditional reactive care.[93] We eventually got some evidence that we were succeeding. In 1981–89, ranking all 55 electoral wards in the County of West Glamorgan for deprivation using the Townsend Index, both villages lay in the five most deprived wards. Ranking the same 55 wards for age-standardised mortality under 65, Glyncorrwg lay in third place (alongside the most affluent areas of Swansea). Blaengwynfi ranked 32nd. Good demand-led care in Blaengwynfi had obviously made a difference, but it probably could have been substantially more effective if it had been supplemented by systematic search, recall and planned clinical policies applied to the entire population. This evidence is limited by small numbers and 'natural experiment' design, but on this policy issue, it is still virtually all the evidence there is on this subject, at least for the UK.[94]

Two paths

All governments have now taken the first step towards a rational understanding of health care. They all recognise it as a production system, with measurable inputs, outputs and efficiency, and that it can no longer be a quasi-religious institution exempt from measurement or criticism.[95] But they see nothing beyond that. They assume that the internal economy of the NHS essentially resembles the external economy of commodity production, susceptible to similar measures of input and output, similar fragmentation of work and responsibilities, similar relations between providers and consumers and between management and staff, similar motivations to maximise profit rather than service, similar competition between providers and search for profitable consumers, and consequently similar destabilisation of established customs and loyalties. Led by ideas from the US, the world's most wasteful and socially inefficient medical economy, Thatcher's successors in government, including New Labour, have accepted their view of the nature of progress.[96]

The contract most recently agreed with GPs in 2004 is designed around primary care as a production process, aiming to raise efficiency by an extremely complex and administratively costly and demanding combination of rewards for attaining targets and penalties for failure.[97] This encourages an industrial approach to care processes, maximising GP incomes where all specified boxes can be ticked, but ignoring areas of practice which have as yet no defined boxes. There is good evidence that this policy has indeed resulted in higher output of all the activities which attract these rewards. Inevitably, there is also some evidence of what economists call 'gaming' – perverse provider choices aimed only at maximising income, regardless of their effect on health outcome. When GPs were paid extra money for home visits after 10pm, calls coming in at 9.30pm tended to be kept waiting for an extra 30 minutes. When targets were set for patients to be given appointments within 48 hours of requests to see the doctor, GPs stopped booking appointments a few weeks or months ahead (which are needed for monitoring chronic disorders), and made all their patients apply for appointments within the last 48 hours. Playing the system is an inevitable feature of business planning. It is a mode of thought which erodes professional conscience and trust between providers and patients. Sticks and carrots certainly provoke movement, but in very complex systems requiring frequent judgements between conflicting priorities, it is stupid to apply methods developed for donkeys to intelligent men and women.

Mutually competing Hospital Trusts are now funded in essentially the same way. In extraordinary detail, clinical functions have been divided into component parts which can be costed, and their performance recorded. Production targets are set for these components, and if the boxes can be ticked, the hospital gets the money. A competing provider which can tick more boxes faster and at lower cost will get more money at the expense of its competitors. For a large majority of staff at all levels, the entire approach seems nonsensical. An army of managers, accountants, computer programmers and data-processing staff are applying a commercial theory to clinical production processes, which are entirely different in nature from those of manufacture, commodity service or retail distribution. They have imposed this set of ideas on an entire generation of civil servants, who can now expect to move across the boundary between public service and commerce in either direction, their judgements depending on business ethics.[98]

Way back in 1973, Sir Richard Doll warned that:

> We can estimate the cost of a disability or saving a life, but we cannot express the value of the product in economic terms in such a way that we can compare the prevention of mental deficiency in a child with saving the lives of so many men and women in their 60s. Decisions have to be made subjectively, and in practice are usually the result of a judicious balance of competing pressures. It is a field in which gardening is real and botany is bogus.[99]

This expresses exactly the feeling of most NHS staff today. Of course, the best gardeners learn from botany, and even themselves become working botanists; they combine theory with practice, modifying each from the other as they gain experience. The problem with most of our health economists is that they select for study only the few processes that can somehow be constrained to fit into classical economics as conceived by Adam Smith's successors, who have looked only at commodity production and ignored all other sources of wealth.[100]

Byproducts: social stability and scientific literacy

Health problems are all social as well as personal, because humans are social animals. Health care is conventionally separated from social care, but is in fact a subset of social care quite hard to define except arbitrarily. This conventional separation has in many ways been useful for analysis of problems in isolation, but as soon as we look closely at any particular problem in its real-life context, we have to recognise that these divisions are arbitrary, depending mainly on patterns of intervention.

Just as health and social problems are ultimately so interdependent that neither can be fully understood by itself, so are their solutions. If the NHS has a measurable product, much of this must be a shared social product, as well as a personal gain for individual patients. Because the foremost aim and claim of the NHS is to produce personal health gain, its authority rests on this. All other social products are usually considered as byproducts, if they are considered at all. But again, the distinction is arbitrary, reflecting a society which crowns individual consumers as kings, but deprives them of any power other than selective consumption.

We have already considered the NHS as legitimiser of the state. As well as treating and preventing illness, the pre-'reform' NHS produced social stability and consensus. It helped to limit the socially destabilising effects of market society. It helped to stabilise society sufficiently for wealth to accumulate in an increasingly unequal and therefore precarious distribution.[101] This stability assisted concentration of wealth, but it also helped workers to campaign successfully for substantial legal protection, much of it now swept away. Being itself a successful product of solidarity, the NHS also reinforced solidarity, gave it new social forms, and provided a protected site within which strong public service could grow. To the extent to which the NHS can develop its own distinct internal economy and culture, it can serve the interests both of people who live from what they own (whose interests lie in undisturbed accumulation of apparently self-replicating wealth) and of people who live from what they are required to do (whose interests lie in solidarity, in defending what they have and developing customs and institutions on which a cooperative society might eventually be founded).

The NHS acts also as a mass educator. This is rarely even a conscious activity, let alone a planned output, but every clinician, and everyone with hands-on responsibility for care, knows this is true. Long before explaining things to patients became a formal duty, an increasing proportion of doctors tried to explain to patients what they wanted to do, why interventions were needed and, in simple terms, how interventions were intended to operate and what the consequences were likely to be (including unintended and negative consequences). Where doctors failed to do this, nurses, or even hospital porters, increasingly tried to make up for this deficiency. As interventions became more effective they also became more complex, and patients had to do more than swallow medicine or permit surgeons to cut whatever they liked. Everyone could rely less upon blind obedience and faith, and more upon knowledge and understanding. As interventions became more sophisticated, both staff and patients could see that explanations must follow the same path. Added together bit by bit, these explanations transmit understanding of human biology as an incomparably more complex, more uncertain, more doubtful and therefore more experimental area for activity than engineering or physics. This is a paradigm shift from the first phase of scientistic medical care in the 19th and early 20th centuries, when mechanistic concepts of science provided the dominant model, and the colossal gap between optimal theory and actual practice had to be filled by deception and wishful thinking, tacitly agreed by both sides.

The NHS as a whole became an interface between expert understanding of science and mass understanding of science, mediated by personal experiments in health care. It is a learning interface, based on personal experience on both sides. It is a safe rule that experts who cannot explain their work to lay people in simple terms do not really understand it themselves.

The NHS as an expanding employer

Another byproduct of the NHS is stable, dignified, useful creative work. As machines replace human skills, as subsistence wages in developing economies replace dignified wages in advanced economies, and as casual employment displaces lifelong commitments, work of any kind is in diminishing supply. If we ask how government can justify the huge subsidies from public money which it gives to the weapons industry, media and politicians remind us of the jobs which depend on its continued prosperity. The NHS also creates useful and satisfying work. Unlike the weapons industry, it not only saves lives but is also increasingly labour intensive rather than capital intensive, and its expansion depends largely on developing the skills of its workforce. Through expanding public health care, we could all win and nobody lose.[102]

In 1993 US economist William Baumol predicted huge changes in composition of the US economy in the 50 years 1990–2040.[103] To simplify his argument, he assumed that existing productivity growth rates in each of three sectors, health care, education and manufacture/agriculture, would remain roughly constant. By 2040 total output of the US economy would then increase by about 350% in value. Materially, the nation as a whole would become three and a half times richer.

With the same assumptions, he then considered expected changes in total spending (public and private) on health care, education and manufacture/agriculture, each as percentage shares of their combined total. Because of rapidly rising productivity in manufacturing and agriculture through replacement of human labour by machines, their share of total spending would fall from 81.7% to 36%. In contrast, productivity of labour in education and health would still depend on increasingly sophisticated human skills and interactions with students and patients, acting as co-producers rather than consumers. Productivity in this sector would therefore grow much more slowly. Spending on education would rise from 8.7% of total spending in 1990 to 29% by 2040, and spending on health care would rise from 11.6% to 35%.[104]

While industry and agriculture would become ever less labour intensive, quality health care and education would become ever more labour intensive, both relatively and absolutely. Health and education professionals would become relatively more costly to employ. Assuming this divergence continued at the same rate, by 2040 proportional spending on education and health care would rise more than threefold, while proportional spending on commodity production would be halved.

Over 80% of costs for both education and health care are attributable to wages. A predicted threefold rise in spending therefore implies not far short of a threefold rise in employment in these two fields – close to the three-and-a-half-fold rise anticipated for output of commodities. Baumol concluded that because total output of wealth (as traditionally understood) would rise by three and a half times, there would be plenty of this to fund higher spending on education and health care (and on high culture – orchestras and opera were his own principal interest). It would only depend on social and political choices.[105] The wealth would certainly exist, and 'society' (whoever that was) could choose how to use it.[106]

Baumol's ideas about how political choices are actually made were naïve,[107] but there are other reasons for believing that continued expansion of health care and education as public services will eventually have to be accepted, even by more intelligent rulers on behalf of rich people who rarely lift their heads far enough from the trough to see any further than their personal interest. First, only as public services, wholly separated from pursuit of profit, can health professionals work efficiently to maximise their product as health gain, rather than as a rising torrent of commoditised procedures chasing consumer demand, continually promoted by advertising.[108] The contrast between pre-'reform' NHS administration costs at 6% of total spending, and US administration costs averaging over 20% (and 34% higher in US hospitals run for profit than in those run as a public service)[109] speaks for itself. Other gross inefficiencies flow from fragmentation of care and misdirection of investment. Second, only as public services, separated from pursuit of profit, can the NHS and education provide a stabilising frame for an evolving society, given rising conflicts of interest between people who live from what they own, and people who live from what they do (and conflicts within those who try to live both ways). When either of these public services becomes seen as a business, they lose this stabilising function.[110]

Summary and conclusions

The NHS is a production system with health gain as its main product. Gains in life expectancy are easy to measure but hard to interpret. Gains in happiness and relief of pain have been substantial. They are harder to measure, but that's no excuse for not trying. Meanwhile, age–adjusted mortality rates are a useful proxy for NHS output as a whole.

Assessments of the contribution of care to health gain have swung from naïve optimism, when doctors enjoyed a special relationship with the rulers of society, to equally naïve pessimism, as this relationship moves towards conflict.

Though medical care is of less importance to health than life circumstances, it has been applied very incompletely to whole populations, even in care systems outside the market. Where everyone can be brought within the scope of continuing anticipatory care, large gains in all dimensions of health are possible.

As an independent gift economy, the pre-'reform' NHS had social authority and public trust. As a principal byproduct, it helped to provide a robust social framework both for accumulation of wealth and for development of new social customs and institutions for a future cooperative society, and new patterns of useful employment.

THREE

How does it produce?

As a production system, the NHS as a whole can be regarded as a black box, with inputs into one end, outputs from the other and a mystery in the middle. What happens inside this black box we call process – all the extremely complex chains of decision and intervention that somehow transform inputs into outputs. This is a generally agreed metaphor for all modern industries, in which production processes have become too complex for non-specialists to understand in the ways that earlier and simpler processes, for example production of coal, steel or cars, could be understood in the past. I hope to show that the nature of what goes on in the black box producing health gain and its social byproducts is qualitatively different from what goes on in black boxes producing commodity goods or services. Health gain is always an addition to national wealth, but it need not be a commodity – and has never in fact functioned only as a commodity, in any modern economy.

To analyse the functions of this box for any theory of political economy, old or new, we have to make some simplifying assumptions. Most health economists assume that within the NHS black box a hierarchy of professionals provides a range of services for patients, first creating, then transferring these services as commodities to patients as consumers, but with the price of sale met in full or in part by the state. Health economists recognise that unlike other transactions in the ideal world of classical economics, consumers of health care in all state systems, whether based on taxation or insurance, are so hugely less informed than providers, so shielded from immediate cost penalties and so vulnerable to abuse by providers through sometimes desperate fears, that major modifications of classical theory are necessary and inevitable.[1] However, they still retain classical theory as their core belief. For most health economists, patient-to-professional encounters remain transactions, conveying applied medical science as a commodity from professional producers to patient consumers, with satisfaction of consumer wants as its most visible and measurable product, not health gain. Wants can be defined by one person alone, the archetypal consumer of classical economics. To define needs, on the other hand, requires at least two people, a patient and a professional, working together. The transactional model puts this in question, because it

presumes a conflict of interest between the provider and the consumer
– *caveat emptor*, let the buyer beware.

There is not a single example of any developed economy in which
medical care for everyone is provided through a normal commodity
market, without some component of risk shared by the state. Private
medical trade can exist only as a parasitic adjunct to some sort of
state-aided system. Mass care alone provides enough experience of
uncommon or extreme events to support medical education and
research and maintain expertise in these fields, and a large enough
pool of shared risk to meet the exceptional costs of exceptional cases.
For many centuries, optimal state-of-the-art clinical knowledge has
been derived from care for a small sample of the many poor, reaching
teaching hospitals in large cities. This knowledge could then be applied
to care of rich private patients, which did (and still does) follow
a transactional model, though self-employed doctors have always
concealed this, from themselves if not from their patients, through
codes of honourable behaviour to mitigate the more ruthless pursuit
of profit by corporate providers and insurance companies, permitted
by their more anonymous decisions.[2] In Britain at least, the modern
care system originated from prepaid care for industrial workers, not
from private care for the affluent. Even in the US, the prototype free
medical market,[3] about 60% of all costs of care are met by the state,
albeit transmitted so far as possible through commercial outlets.[4] In
other developed economies, for all but a small fringe market, actual
purchasers are state agencies, insurance companies or other third parties
(or most often combinations of these) buying on behalf of consumer
groups, not individual patients. Though this must change market
behaviour fundamentally, productive contacts between health care
professionals and patients are still seen by most health economists as
essentially provider–consumer transactions, albeit substantially modified.

Empirical study of the actual processes of clinical judgements,
decisions and interventions shows that this classical view, however
modified, is only one way of looking at care processes, and not the
most effective, efficient or enlightening way. There are others which,
if more appropriate to the extremely complex and evolving nature of
relationships between patients and professionals, might offer wider and
more effective opportunities to increase productivity and create new
opportunities for health gain.[5]

The consultation process

In 1960, using contemporary gendered and disease-centred terms, the great paediatrician Sir James Spence defined the consultation as:

> the occasion when, in the intimacy of the consulting room or the sick room, a person who is ill or believes himself to be ill, seeks the advice of a doctor whom he trusts. *This is a consultation and all else in the practice of medicine derives from it.* (My emphasis)[6]

If we broaden this to include all other kinds of personal health problem and all other kinds of health professional, and if decisions taken in such consultations set the course for all consequent processes throughout the health care system, then any economic theory trying to understand the operation of personal care systems as a whole should start from analysis of how players relate to each other at this initial point of production. This is the elementary particle of health care economy, as atoms and molecules are the elementary particles of physics and chemistry. If you get the shape of this basic block wrong, you will meet problems similar to those of a builder trying to make a rectangular structure from elliptical bricks.

Note that though intuitively right for most experienced health professionals, Spence's simplistic view is rarely shared by health economists, journalists or politicians, not for the good reason that it omits all reference to collective public health functions or planning and organisation of care (discussed later on), but because technical interventions are the focal point of their vision, rather than the complex personal (or, for public health, social) interactions that surround these interventions and make them possible. As usual, they ignore the social relations of production.

Most health economists assume that whether writing a prescription, performing a surgical operation or interpreting a diagnostic image, all these interventions are commodities sold as items to patients as consumers, even if the ultimate purchaser is some public agency. Because some clinical interventions resemble other less complex forms of commodity transfer, say cars or mortgage services, these (rather than decisions to initiate them) are their preferred focus for analysis. To this most experienced health professionals would answer that, though clinical procedures need to be performed competently and with thrift, the most fundamental issue is not whether they are done well or at best value for money, but whether they are done at all – whether any particular procedure is in fact the optimal solution for a patient's personal problems, yielding maximal health gain at minimal costs in the patient's time, pain, unhappiness and added risk, as well as in NHS resources. Entry to each level of the care system hierarchy entails at least some creative negotiation, at best a collaboration, between patients and professionals, not merely a consumption. The consultation ends with decisions either to do nothing, or to intervene at primary care level, or to proceed upwards to a higher specialist, sideways to a different part of primary care, or back out of the care system altogether to some other more appropriate social agency, including back to patients' and their families' own resources. The appropriateness of these decisions is critical to solution of patients' problems, and thus to productivity, effectiveness and efficiency of the NHS as a whole.

In defining consultations as the elementary particles from which the health care economy is formed, Spence left unanswered three important questions: how do these episodic consultations relate to each other – as isolated choices or linked into sequential stories? Do health professionals and patients relate to each other as providers and consumers, or in some other way? And finally, where is public health and the planning and organisation of care in all this? Spence's view concerned reactive personal tactics, with little to say about public health and proactive care strategies. Answers to these three questions are linked. How most professionals, most patients and most governments view them is still ambiguous.

Episodic and continuing care

With enough money in their pockets, and for such health problems as seem easily separated from the rest of their lives rather than inseparably bound within them, most people still seem to see themselves as episodic consumers. On the other hand, for health problems which seem inseparable from life problems and which seem still insoluble by body repairs, they still seek continuing care for themselves personally as a lifelong process rather than as a series of disjointed episodes. They also assume that local and national government will try to assure a socially healthy and biologically safe society in which they can live, a continuing and collective experience which is not seen as an occasional consumption. In these two capacities they see themselves not as consumers, but as citizens using shared public agencies.

When people look at the NHS not as spectators but as experienced participants with real problems, they want much more than a consumer role. Complex, continuing problems, including both biological and social factors, present the most difficult challenges to clinical medicine, and account for a high proportion of overall workload and costs. In the US, over 45% of people outside institutional care have one or more chronic health problems, and these chronic problems account for 75% of US health care expenditure. In the late 1980s when these studies were done, most of these people with chronic problems were neither elderly nor disabled.[7] With ageing populations this proportion of people with chronic problems will rise. In 1948, when the NHS was born, it promised care from the cradle to the grave. Though successive governments have never fully accepted this responsibility,[8] and since 1979 have sought actively to reject it, it still endures as a public expectation, and people still get angry when they find it has vanished.

Most acute episodic problems arise from these continuing problems, often because they have either not been treated at all, not been treated effectively, or treatment had not been sustained. Both medical professional and popular cultures prioritise acute care. A study of GPs in Liverpool showed that they rated acute physical problems as appropriate to their responsibilities twice as often as chronic physical problems, and more than three times as often as psychological problems.[9] Chronic problems require continuity – patients' stories need to be already known, not endlessly repeated to successive strangers.[10] Episodic interventions fragment care, tending to keep patients passive and to promote inappropriately heroic roles for professionals, because salvage, whether or not it is successful, always trumps prevention. Acute demands are inescapable prompts to professional action in a freely accessible service, whereas chronic needs can always be postponed. Acute crises have therefore dominated GP medical culture, supplemented by hospital emergency departments for episodic crises beyond GPs' competence or capacity, even though many of these crises need never have occurred, given efficient continuing anticipatory care.

As primary care has become more rationally organised to control risks and prevent a rising proportion of crises, continuing primary care has become an area susceptible to forward planning. Providing that numbers are large (thousands rather than hundreds of people at risk), clinical content of work and case-load are broadly predictable. It can therefore be planned, with opportunities to develop a wider variety of health workers, working at much lower cost than the acute interventions that arise when continuing care has not been given. Failure to develop systematic continuing care, doing a few simple, relatively inexpensive things well for all who need them, has costly consequences. Terminal salvage prompted by crises is dramatic and heroic, but almost prohibitively expensive and much less effective.

Analysis of costs in an intensive care unit in Los Angeles showed that 8% of the patients used half the resources, though over 70% of these high-cost patients died while using them.[11]

Continuity

More rational care implies a shift in both professional and patient behaviour back from crisis interventions and body repairs towards continuing care – more attention to causes, as well as to consequences, greater interest and investment in the uncertain beginnings of disease, where clinical and social care meet the boundaries of public health.[12] All these shifts depend on greater continuity: continuity of care, continuity of experience, continuity of thought and continuity of information across inter-professional boundaries.

Studying how errors occur, a group at the Veterans' Administration Patient Safety Center of Inquiry of the University of Chicago[13] found that in care systems more complex than the elementary doctor–patient particle considered by Spence, there were inevitably many gaps between people, stages and processes. Analysis of clinical errors showed that though there were many gaps, few of these seemed to produce errors. They concluded that safety was increased by understanding and reinforcing the normal ability of all players (including patients) to bridge these gaps and thus maintain continuity. This view contradicts the usual industrial management view that to become more efficient, systems need to reduce their dependence on human judgements and interactions, assumed to be inherently less reliable than machines. To maintain continuity despite necessary division of skills, care systems need to become more human, more flexible and more open to judgement, not more tightly controlled.[14] It also contradicts the nostalgic view that continuity can be assured only by retreating to single-doctor, single-patient relationships, discarding the advantages of teamwork.

Consumer choice?

Think-tanks like the King's Fund, their ears always prudently ('realistically') tuned to state and corporate sponsorship, endorse wider consumer choice as a self-evident path toward more participation by patients in their own care. They underestimate and accept as inevitable any damage to continuity that consumer choice between competing providers must necessarily cause. They fail to recognise the value of mutual support already achieved in a unified national public service, and how this is being undermined by fragmentation of providers encouraged by consumer choice in a competitive market. Rivalry and commercial secrecy deliberately promoted by policies based on competition inevitably destroy cooperation, which has often taken decades to establish. The general public, and to a lesser extent medical and nursing professionals, now face both ways. People want future technology but dread its apparently inevitable consequence – that human contacts will become ever more infrequent, fragmented, tenuous, impersonal and potentially adversarial. They want more body repairs, but tend fatalistically to accept that the price for these must be less personal, less continuing care, because this association has been their common experience.

Spence's elementary particle ignored the public health strategies within which personal care needs to operate to be effective. This indifference is still shared by most patients and most clinicians, but is better understood (and generally deplored) by health economists and policy makers. Historically, public health functions have always been divided both from repair and from care. If we accept that health care systems should produce health gain, some professional and institutional agency must exist to translate this aim into material, measurable terms across the whole population, not just the person sitting in front of you. This agency must set strategies for the system as a whole, with latitude for tactical decisions at points of production. Such a system would include both personal care, in which consultations would operate as elementary particles, and collective or population care. This is difficult, perhaps impossible, to achieve in a system decentralised and fragmented into units competing for consumers. If it can be achieved at all in such circumstances, this will be by tight state regulation, compelling entrepreneurs to address public needs before profitable wants. Such regulation would then be pilloried as a constraint on natural consumer choice and pursuit of profit, and as a burden on business, which is always most profitable when left alone to do as it wants, by the claque to be expected when most sources of information and opinion are not only owned by top business people, but are themselves businesses run for profit. Orthodox health economists and policy developers address these problems as they address all failures of the market to meet social needs, by building parallel regulatory and supplementary structures to perform the functions which markets neglect because they are not profitable. These bolted-on solutions are always liable to attack as parasitic bureaucracy and burdens on the taxpayer.

In fact, given political will and real respect for participative democracy, Spence's perception could easily be expanded to include public health decisions about groups and populations. Public health decisions also should entail consultations, though in a loftier sense than Spence ever intended, in which the same players are collectively rather than individually represented. Most public health doctors have in the past had the same arrogant, paternalistic and condescending attitudes to their public as clinicians had to their patients. Though many were progressive, all were by contemporary social conventions compelled to be despots. To make democracy real, both public health and clinical professionals must find ways to accept their communities and their patients as equals, when it comes to either personal or collective decisions. If they succeed in this, both individual and collective consultations can still form fundamental units in a productive NHS economy.

Accepting that all sustainable change should start from where we are with the people we have (building sound structures upwards rather than dropping lightweight prefabricated modules from the sky), the solution to this hitherto insoluble problem of integrating personal and community care must lie in redefinition of the nature of primary care. This must include collective responsibilities within communities for the many health problems that are soluble only through collective action. We need to reconnect collective public health with personal clinical medicine.

For most people in Britain, personal care in the NHS is still seen intuitively as a collective gift based on shared responsibility. In the pre-'reform' NHS this was already evolving towards a less unequal consultation process, as a natural development led by a less deferential public. Fewer health professionals have been entering practice without undergraduate education in the social nature of their work, and though their social composition has not changed (more than half of all UK doctors have been privately educated) they are generally far more ready to listen to their patients than earlier professional generations.[15] As deference gives way to a long overdue rise in public self-confidence, this could follow two alternative paths. It could be expressed either as consumer demand, or as rising citizen expectations, not just to receive more, but to participate constructively in producing more: by participating in both their own personal care and in the progress of the NHS as a local and national public service. Consumerism was never the only option, though this was assumed by the New Labour government, and accepted by news media and the commentariat.

The patient–professional interface

When sociologists first started studying medical consultations objectively in the 1950s and 1960s, they were impressed by the extraordinarily high sustained rate of major decision making, especially in primary care. By 'major' they meant, for example, decisions that patients' problems were or were not appropriate to the care system, that patients were or were not sick, that symptoms did or did not require further investigation or referral to a specialist, that health problems required treatment or were best left alone, that patients needed referral to this rather than that specialist, or to some activity or agency right outside the care system. Each of these decisions concerned next steps on pathways leading either sideways and away from the care system, further and deeper down into it, or back to continuing care at primary level. Few of these were what most clinicians thought of as big decisions, but they looked big to sociologists, they felt big to patients and had big implications for rational functioning of the NHS and its costs.

These big decisions had to be taken within spans of 5 to 10 minutes, often less.

Needles in haystacks

For clinicians, especially in primary care, the size of many decisions is clear only in retrospect. As a typical example, pneumococcal meningitis is a rare, insidious, frequently lethal disorder, usually in very young children, initially presenting as a slight fever with minimal illness – much like any other minor viral respiratory infection. Early treatment with appropriate antibiotics is life saving, but escalation to irreversible brain damage or death may occur quickly if diagnosis and treatment are delayed by even a few hours.

The problem of handling 10,000 or more minor viral upper respiratory infections in such ways as to prevent one death from late diagnosis of pneumococcal meningitis (occurring at any random point in that sequence of 10,000) depends mainly on how apparently trivial problems are first handled, and what indications worried mothers understand for contacting the NHS again, perhaps only hours or even minutes after their first encounter. How such contingencies can be handled safely over the telephone, by nurse-practitioners who can't even see their patient, no advocate of nurse-led telephone advisory services has yet explained. Nor are out-of-hours agency doctors, or hospital A&E departments, much better. Their staff don't know either the mothers or the children, and at the very early stage in this illness, when decisions can be most effective, they are less well placed than GPs to decide at what point to initiate the investigations needed to confirm or exclude disease through referral. Of course the situation is rare, but similar situations precede most of the unexpected deaths in children which still occur. The care system should be organised to respond to these in ways that are affordable and sustainable, and can be applied to the entire population equally.

Outcomes of care for exceptional problems depend on the nature of care for routine problems (it might be worth repeating that sentence a few times: it deserves to be memorised). Early recognition of life-threatening, rapidly progressive, treatable disease of this kind remains one of the most important processes of primary care, though it has rarely been studied prospectively because of the huge numbers needed to provide even a few such events for study.[16] It depends always on delicately balanced relationships between two groups of players, health professionals and patients, merging evidence from both to synthesise effective decisions that create an eventual health product. In this scenario, there are no consumers, only two different kinds of producer.

I have chosen this example because I have experienced real cases, some with happy outcomes, others ending in tragedy. Broken into successive episodes with successive decision points about what to do next, one of these with a fatal outcome was used for a videotape at Birmingham University Medical School, teaching clinical skills to doctors in primary care training. The 'right' and 'wrong' answers appeared to change at each successive decision point, in ways which at first seemed counter-intuitive to most students. The task at first contact with such a mother and child could not include invasive search for every one of a vast range of possibilities, most of them so unlikely that most doctors would not see more than one or two in a whole working lifetime. Nor should it entail blunderbuss treatment with powerful wide-spectrum antibiotics for every apparently minor infection, just to prevent an occasional major infection, not least because this, more than any other factor, promotes antibiotic-resistant bacteria, endangering many more people than it could possibly protect.[17] Defensive medicine, diversion of effort from solution of patients' real problems to anticipation of doctors' hypothetical problems if faced later by charges of malpractice, erodes trust, incurs prohibitive cost and impedes the clear thinking necessary to recognise exceptional situations before it is too late. At the same time, it is vital that whatever the decision at each point in the story, this must not obstruct or exclude some possible, though unlikely, later development.

Initiative must remain with the mother, because she is the only observer of her child who can be constantly present and is familiar with her child's normal behaviour. She is the expert. This means that at each stage in the story she must feel completely confident that any decision she may make to use her time to renew contact will not be dismissed as a waste of professional time. This was the 'right' answer to questions posed by this videotape early in its course, not instant application of a diagnostic or treatment sledgehammer to every apparent peanut.

However hard this may seem, professional and lay time must in such situations be equated. To assume that doctors' or nurses' time is more valuable than patients' time has dangerous consequences for these infrequent, unpredictable but (on a whole population scale) calculable and foreseeable outcomes. These cause a large and rising proportion of premature deaths as their frequency diminishes, to become concentrated in fewer and more exceptional events. Between this mother and her doctor, evaluations of risk and consequent decisions needed to be shared so fully that responsibility for their eventual results, whether successful or catastrophic, would also be seen and felt to be shared almost equally. This implies a relationship between patients and professionals approaching the relationships within families, not as a virtually unattainable ideal for sentimental reasons, but as a usually achievable aim for practical reasons. 'Our doctor was almost part of the family' is still a familiar phrase, not quite a folk memory. It represents a powerful weapon we should fight to retain or, if already lost, to regain.

Less than ideal experience

Everyday experience for most patients falls far short of that ideal. The following true story comes from Andrew Herxheimer and Ann McPherson's DIPEx archive of patients' accounts of their own experiences of illness:[18]

> OK, last August one Sunday evening I was reaching over on my desk to get a pen and felt a dreadful pain inside my right breast. Prior to that I had had some itching, my nipple was itching very, very intensely and, er, I didn't think about it, itchy nipple to me didn't mean anything suspicious. But when I felt the pain and the lump, er, I immediately was struck with fear and foreboding and didn't know what to do. My family were away visiting the in-laws and I had a dreadful night, but I had an appointment at the doctor's for the next day for something else, something totally

unrelated. When I saw the doctor that day, the next day after finding the lump, er, when we'd finished about the prior consultation I mentioned that I'd found a lump in my breast and I was terribly afraid. He sent me in to see the nurse, the practice nurse, and, er, she basically dismissed it as being hormonal, my age, '80% of breast lumps are nothing, don't worry, go home, keep a diary'.

I went home feeling still very anxious and very worried and, er, kept a diary. That was on the Monday. On the Thursday I hadn't slept for two nights, I felt dreadful and, er, so I phoned the nurse again and told her. And she said 'You need an appointment with me and the doctor so can you come in on Tuesday?' That was eight days after the original appointment, which I agreed to. I went to the surgery that day and sat in the nurse's room for 22 minutes, half naked, feeling absolutely ghastly. She came into the room and said that the doctor was too busy to see me. That was like somebody stabbing a knife in me. Er, she took my blood telling me that this was all hormonal and I had nothing to worry about, go home. I went home, I went outside of the practice and broke my heart in the car. It still hurts to talk about this bit of my treatment because I felt as if I wasn't worthy of even seeing a doctor at that point. To be told that the doctor is too busy to see you when you have an appointment, when you're very worried and you've got a breast that won't even fit in your biggest bra was dreadful.

Anyway I went home and my sister, who was a mammographer of all things, was away on holiday. She came back on the Saturday and I confided in her. It was at this point that my life was turned around. She made me promise her that I would go to the doctor's and demand an examination. That I did on the Tuesday. I had the appointment for the results of my blood test and I walked into the doctor's, put my diary on the table, and said 'I demand an examination'. The doctor said he had examined me and I told him he had not and he said 'OK, let's examine you now, I'll go and get the nurse.' Prior to this the nurse had told me she wasn't qualified to examine breasts, but that appointment she did examine my breast with the doctor there. Again I felt as if I wasn't worthy of the doctor's attention, that the doctor was shunning me again but at least he did the right thing and he sent me straight to hospital.

I sat in a largely medical audience listening to this patient's account of her experience, in a presentation about the DIPEx project. It was initially greeted with incredulity. Most of the audience seemed to think it lay outside normal experience of NHS care, in a sphere of criminal rather than clinical behaviour, like Dr Harold Shipman's deliberate murder of more than 250 of his patients, discovered a couple of years earlier. I'm afraid it had not surprised me. The range of behaviour of doctors and nurses is as wide as that of their patients.

Effective clinicians learn that no observed human behaviour lies outside our normal experience, even including Dr Shipman's. The aim of the DIPEx database is to understand the full range of patients' experience, just as the collected databases used for evidence-based medicine aim to include all clinical research experience. For both a GP and a nurse so obviously to fail even to try to understand their patient's fears, and so recklessly to dismiss the possibility that she was right and they were wrong, was certainly unusual – but cancer of the breast also is unusual, in that a large majority of lumps in the breast are indeed not cancerous, and this was the nurse's justification for dismissing her patient's fears. Even more unusual was my first example, pneumococcal meningitis presenting to me as apparently transient minor illness in early childhood, but professionals have a responsibility never to forget such possibilities.

Shipman's example also is apt. The only rational explanation I have seen for his behaviour was addiction to power – power of life or death over patients he had particularly encouraged to depend on him as their friend (he was much loved by his patients, and encouraged their emotional dependence upon him). Potential origins for such addiction exist for every student of medicine or nursing, because some use of this power is central to their work. Wherever practice becomes *de facto* unaccountable except to personal conscience, conditions exist for addiction to power and escalating abuse. Patient-murderers like Dr Harold Shipman and Nurse Beverley Allitt were extreme examples of dysfunctional professional behaviour, just as child torturers and murderers are extreme examples of dysfunctional parenting, but all these crimes lie within the limits of human behaviour, not outside it. Like Hitler, these criminals are not monsters from some other species, but extreme versions of our potential selves. They look like us, and most of the time, they behave like us. To isolate them as 'pure evil' is to evade our own responsibility always to remember these potential behaviours in ourselves and our own society. As a group, caring professionals have a long way to go before their relationships with patients always reach the quality they would like to receive when they themselves need care.

Viewed not as consumers but as fellow-workers in production of health, patients also have much to learn. When these two groups are encouraged to bring their skills together, both learn from each other to become more tolerant, thoughtful, effective, better informed and therefore more open to doubt. In this as in all social change, speed is less important than direction. The seeds of this change have always been there, in all consultations. We have always had some real, not mythical, examples of close, continuing and productive relationships between caring professionals and their patients, who have shared their evidence and have each respected the expertise of the other. The real problem has been to achieve care systems that promote rather than impede and interrupt sustained growth of these relationships, which develop naturally in contacts between equals.

Material preconditions for optimal decisions

As I write, average face-to-face time available for consultations in NHS general practice has risen slowly from about 2 minutes in the 1950s to about 8 minutes by 2000, and probably around 10 minutes today.[19] Though these averages have always concealed wide ranges depending on the content of each consultation, there is a finite lower limit set by the time needed for a patient to get in and out of the consulting room, and between these to sit down and say what they have come for.[20] Most UK practices now reach averages around 10 minutes, without including a generally new dimension of nurse time, but there are still plenty with booking times of only 5 minutes per patient. The lowest average consultation times have always been in industrial (now mostly post-industrial) practices whose rates of complex morbidity, particularly psychiatric morbidity, are highest and therefore require most time for appropriate decisions.

In the 1990s, of those NHS patients who had received only 5 minutes of consulting time or less, only 30% thought this was insufficient,[21] disturbing evidence of dangerously low expectations. Doctors of the sort who engaged in objective studies of their own work before managed care policies compelled them to record data routinely (from whom almost all published research on generalist practice now derives) are more aware than many patients that every measurable variable relating to quality improves with more time available, and all deteriorate with less,[22] at least within the fairly short consultation times customary in NHS primary care. With times around 30 minutes available in Sweden, Denmark and Finland, differences may be less critical (but in Sweden and Finland at least, more time in each consultation seems to be associated with long delays in access). UK doctors who work faster do less listening, less explaining and transmit less information to their patients. They allow less patient participation,[23] and probably do less critical thinking, though so far as I know we have no evidence on this. Studies of trainee GPs in the late 1970s showed that, unless they had special teaching using audiovisual feedback, with increasing experience they learned to work faster but to communicate less.[24] This association was probably causal: that is, they gained speed by reducing communication to the bare minimum required to devise a diagnostic label. GP and undergraduate training has greatly improved since then in most centres, but under excessive (in most places, usual) workloads this trend soon reappears. Quality of care always depends mainly on time available, which is the real currency of clinical medicine.

Studies of family doctors in North America (again selective for the minority of doctors willing and able to participate in research) show average consultation times over 20 minutes for new patients.[25] Despite their more generous time, research in 1984 showed US physicians gave their patients an average of only 18 seconds to tell their story before interrupting and diverting them to their own preferred topics.[26]

The story in Europe is mostly the same.[27] Having enough time in consultations, and having GPs with time and inclination to listen, explain and encourage discussion of problems (which are patients' highest priorities and usually result in substantial clinic over-runs),[28] conflicts with administrators' higher priorities for starting and finishing times required for managed care targets.[29] Only in Sweden and Finland is there good evidence that decisions in primary care can really have optimal time, averaging around 14 minutes for somatic problems and 30 minutes for psychological problems.[30] Average consultation times of less than 1 minute are usual in public care systems throughout the former colonial world, for those who can afford access to medical care of any kind, now that consultation charges have been restored almost everywhere as a precondition for assistance from the World Bank.

Even within the consultation times now available for grossly under-resourced health workers in many care systems, a start can be made in helping patients to bring their own full potential to making decisions in primary care more accurate and relevant to solution of their problems. Much more can be achieved in a short time if good records are created and maintained, with clear story lines and cumulative (preferably graphic) display of tracking variables such as weight or blood pressure, which patients can see and understand, and if patients see professionals they know in a stable team. This requires continuity of care, not shopping around. When patients begin to participate in decisions, they may gain confidence as citizens to support staff demands that they be paid for the time and diversity of skills necessary for truly shared decisions, making the situation less impossible than it was.

In a beautifully simple research study in former Yugoslavia, Igor Švab showed that letting patients present their own problems without interruption had virtually no effect on consultation length,[31] but yielded gains in goodwill and consultations more relevant to real problems. Contrary to GP and media folklore, most patients do worry about saving their doctors' time, they are not only concerned to get time for themselves. Most patients consciously limit the time they use to make more available for others with more difficult problems.[32] Given the slightest encouragement, most people understand that health care is a shared social asset.

Medically unexplained symptoms

For about 30% of symptoms presented to GPs, and about 40% of symptoms referred to specialists, no evidence of any organic cause can be found. Similar proportions of unexplained illness seem to have prevailed ever since the birth of universal public care systems after the Second World War. They were probably even greater in the less accessible but more fear-ridden and consumer-oriented medical trade preceding them. Because medically unexplained symptoms more often involve fear of disease than disease itself, higher prevalence of organic disease in others prompts higher prevalence of fear of disease, and consequently more medically unexplained symptoms. Organic morbidity is therefore always positively related to functional morbidity, and never displaces it.

Of medical outpatients referred to a London hospital in 1952, 39% showed no evidence of somatic disease. This study was repeated the next year, when that figure barely shifted to 40%; so, at least locally, this seemed to be a virtual constant.[33] Four decades later, studies in the Netherlands showed about half of all patients referred to general medical outpatient clinics had no detectable organic abnormalities.[34] Studies of UK primary care in the 1980s and 1990s showed 20%–25% of adults consulting GPs had no detectable somatic cause for their symptoms.[35] Wherever and whenever we look, we find a lot of it.

Though most of these symptoms are minor, transient and self-limiting, over one third of them persist, causing distress, disability, frequent consultations and ultimately referral to specialists and numerous costly investigations, often followed by cross-referrals between specialists, eventually ending with a psychiatrist.

Many if not most of those initially referred to medical specialists are sent for symptoms suggesting serious but early disease, suspected by patients or primary care staff. When no evidence of disease can be found, this positive outcome is as important as confirmation of disease followed by appropriate treatment. Even so, later progression may reveal that early serious disease was in fact present. There is horrifying evidence of this from practice in the heyday of Cartesian dualism, when hysteria was a common dustbin diagnosis, and few doctors seemed able frankly to admit that they did not know what was wrong with a patient. At London's National Hospital for Nervous Diseases at Queen Square, between 1951 and 1955, Eliot Slater managed to follow up 85 out of 99 patients initially diagnosed as suffering hysterical symptoms, an average 9 years after this diagnosis.[36] Of these 85 presumed hysterics, 12 had died (4 by suicide), 14 had become totally disabled and 16 were partially disabled. Only 43 (50%) were still able to live independently, and only 19 were free from symptoms. By the time of follow-up, only 33 (40%) still lacked any sign of organic disease. Even among these, 10 now showed good evidence of psychotic mental illness.

Trying to answer the question why these referred patients had in effect been dismissed, he found two features they all had in common. First, they had no physical signs of disease: but this had to be true at an early stage of virtually any disease. Second, they all had a multitude of symptoms. Since it was unlikely that all the complaints of patients with many symptoms could be accounted for by any organic condition, it followed that some of them must not be organic; but if some of them were not organic, why not all of them? This convenient and common professional assumption was dangerous. It ignored the effects of disturbances in function of other organs and systems on brain function, and of disturbances in brain function on function of other organs. Fortunately even the National Hospital at Queen Square, a stronghold of professional conservatism, was capable of learning. A somewhat similar study repeated in the late 1990s showed that, of 73 patients with medically unexplained motor symptoms (an important difference), only 3 were found 6 years later to have a previously unrecognised neurological disease.[37] Slater not only destroyed hysteria as an acceptable label, he buried the dualist paradigm that gave it birth, at least among neurologists at Queen Square level. There really has been a steep decline in gross errors of this sort, probably at all levels of care.[38]

Apart from the risks of misdiagnosing serious organic illness as minor disorders of emotion, thought or behaviour, we have consistent evidence that people with all forms of mental illness have much higher mortality from organic disease.[39] The burdens on patients and on society caused by mental illness generally exceed both in volume and distress those caused by somatic illness.[40] A US cohort study of people over 65 showed that depression was associated with a rise in all-causes mortality of about 24% regardless of age, sex, lifestyle or type of physical illness.[41]

Thought is a function of brains, as ticking is a function of clocks. If you smash brains they stop thinking, just as if you smash clocks they stop ticking. People who believe in consciousness without a brain or souls without bodies can still work effectively in health care, but only by separating the credulity needed to sustain their mystical beliefs from the scepticism necessary for safe practice. Without a distinction between ideas and things, between what we wish to exist and what verifiably does exist, no useful understanding of health or illness is possible.

There are few tissues and no organs without some ultimate central connection to the brain, including parts of the brain mainly concerned with conscious thought. Every external input to the brain can therefore potentially modify thought, and every internal thought can potentially modify perceptions, including pain and other common sensations like weakness, fatigue, the sounds of blood flow through the inner ear, or thumps from beating of the heart, and all the other noises and vibrations associated with normal operation of body machinery, which are usually suppressed from consciousness. All thoughts can, in some circumstances, induce change of some kind in all those organs or tissues that have some ultimate central connection to the brain cortex.[42] These peripheral changes may in turn be centrally perceived and reinforce thoughts and fears about their cause, and so on in a rising spiral of fear. All disorders therefore have potential psychosomatic components, organic disease is a common and potent cause of mental and emotional illness, and mental or emotional illness (or robustness) may modify the course of organic disease, though evidence of substantial objective effects is much harder to find than our most enthusiastic psychosomatists sometimes claim.

As there can be no such thing as a conscious patient without an active brain, thought modifies the natural history of every human disorder. This has nothing to do with moral strength or weakness. A patient usually disabled by severe pain may still be able to dance, sing or read a book, and may then suffer less pain, or even none at all, while doing so. This is not evidence that the pain or the disorder causing it is not real, it simply demonstrates that pain is a subjective sensation, whose perception changes in different states of mind.

Symptoms that commonly turn out to represent no recognisable underlying disease include chest, back or abdominal pain, tiredness, dizziness, numbness, headache, shortness of breath and sleep difficulties.[43] These presenting symptoms together account for roughly half of all first episodes of illness met in primary care. When followed up a year later only 10%–15% are found to have been associated with detectable organic disease.[44]

Do consultations for medically unexplained symptoms represent over-use?

The high proportion of consultations for symptoms which prove in retrospect to have no organic medical explanation provide the main material evidence for myths of NHS over-use or abuse, particularly at primary care level.

In industrial and post-industrial areas this myth gets some support from local knowledge (real or imagined) of the extent to which consultations are inflated by claims for benefit. These once formed a high proportion of GP workload in industrial areas, though much less in white-collar residential areas. Administrative reforms over the past 20 years have greatly reduced this function for GPs, but it remains a powerful folk memory, reinforced by the mistaken but common belief that costs of social insurance benefits come from the same purse as funding for the NHS.

The myth that consultations for retrospectively diagnosed 'non-illness' represent over-use or abuse is refuted by evidence, but this has not deterred advocates of NHS 'reform' from using it as a weapon in argument. Bosanquet and Pollard have long been vigorous advocates of NHS 'reform' towards a commercial model. They know how difficult it is to redefine care as a commodity once people have become accustomed to it as a civic right in an NHS gift economy. They correctly perceived that public perception of NHS over-use was their best weapon for their attack on social solidarity. In a well-conducted survey of public opinion in the 1990s, they confirmed the grip of this myth:

> almost two-thirds say that people visit their GP when there is no real need, simply because the service is free at point of use ... it is the public's readiness to concede over-use ... that points the way forward [to reform]....With 64% saying that there is over-use, there is a strong moral as well as practical case for a charge ...[45]

As a well-informed academic who had studied primary care and GP behaviour for many years, Bosanquet surely knew of a classical research paper by Hannay and Maddox, who compared the numbers of people in Manchester who consulted their GP for minor symptoms (as judged by themselves), compared with the numbers over the same two weeks who decided not to consult their GPs despite having symptoms that were painful or they thought might be serious.[46] There were more than twice as many in the second group as there were in the first. Moreover, there is no way that any care system can function without the number of people consulting about worries greatly exceeding the number whose worries eventually prove justified. Though two-thirds of people may believe that other people over-use their doctors because consultations are free, how many of them believe this of themselves?

The assumption of over-use is irresponsible and dangerous. For example, rectal bleeding is an important signal of possible bowel cancer. Early surgery may be life saving, but the disease is still commonly recognised too late. About 20% of adults have some rectal bleeding each year, but less than 1% of them consult a GP, and the proportion referred to a hospital specialist for further investigation is 10 times less even than this.[47] For this example alone, and there are many others, there is overwhelming evidence that patients use the NHS too little rather than too much.

A case for systematic over-use can be made against proactive care, screening apparently healthy people for possible pre-symptomatic disease, where this is not supported by consistent research evidence of probable and substantial net benefit. Where screening is driven only by concern for public health, and where it is limited by competition for scarce staff time in primary care units responsible for the full range of primary care in whole, socially inclusive populations, we can be reasonably sure that proactive care will be undertaken only where there is good evidence of substantial net benefit. In their book *Ready for Treatment*, Bosanquet and Pollard's openly declared strategy in 1997 for eliminating what they saw as a nonsensical gift economy in the NHS was not to deny its attractiveness in a world more generous as it got richer, but to deny its viability in a world that was bound to get meaner, whether we liked it or not. It was a powerful strategy, which has penetrated almost all media for public discussion over the entire period of New Labour government. They correctly perceived that the most potent weapon for replacing public service by commerce was the intense pessimism of both public and professional opinion, the disbelief of most people in their own power to change society, and their readiness to mistrust their fellow citizens.[48]

The real risks of over-use begin when we go down precisely that care-as-commodity path which Bosanquet and Pollard and other 'modernisers' want us to pursue. For example, screening for prostate cancer by measuring Prostate-Specific Antigen (PSA) still lacks convincing evidence that it improves outcomes, or consensus endorsement by international medical science.[49] Despite this, by 2003 PSA screening in the US and Australia was too big and too profitable to accept any limiting evidence without a struggle. Autopsy studies of representative samples of men over 50 show that about 30% harbour cancer cells in their prostate glands, but only 8%–10% develop clinical cancer during their remaining lifetimes. It is therefore not surprising if some microscopic evidence of cancer is found when six or more biopsy samples are taken.[50] Over 80% of clinical prostate cancers in men under 60 occur at PSA concentrations below the conventional screening threshold at 4ng/ml.[51] Even with this threshold there is gross over-diagnosis and over-treatment, if the aim is to achieve not normal microscopic appearances, but longer and healthier lives. Attempts by expert professional groups to draw public attention to this evidence in Australia and the US have led to concerted personal attacks in the media, largely through patients' groups funded and used by the professionals and companies engaged in the private screening trade and consequently inflated surgery.[52] As profit enters motivation, thrift, caution and scepticism depart. The limits of marketed interventions are set not by evidence, but by what the market will stand: in this case, by the readiness of frightened people to spend money on their own false reassurance, and media editors to promote circulation at the expense of truth.[53]

What evidence is there that user charges, known to health economists as co-payments, have the selective effects on consultation rates required to restrain over-use, even if that were a real problem?[54] Obviously user charges discourage use, but economists have good evidence that consulting behaviour has little elasticity. Poor people will give higher spending priority to consulting a doctor than to food, if they believe medical advice is needed.[55] The effect of user charges is simply to reduce all consultations across the board, regardless of the nature of the problems that prompt them. The effect is selective only for those with lowest incomes, least able to afford them, but most likely to be sick.[56] In the early years of the African AIDS pandemic, user charges were imposed at state-funded Sexually Transmitted Disease clinics in Kenya on advice from the World Bank and as a precondition for international aid. Consultation rates fell by 60%.[57] Public care systems have collapsed throughout Africa: no money, no treatment.[58]

It looks as though user charges are advocated not to promote more rational behaviour, but to shift public thought and behaviour 'corrupted' by experience of a free public service back to a 'normal' commercial pattern. Co-charges are always a tax on illness, weighing more heavily on the poor than on the rich.

Emotional illness

At any one time, about 20% of people are in sustained emotional distress.[59] About one third of these consult their GP about this,[60] and in about 66%–75% of these the nature of the problem is recognised.[61] Many people also fear organic illness, particularly when a friend or relative has recently suffered some unexpected and catastrophic event. Emotions, particularly fear, create their own symptoms: rapid and audible heartbeat (palpitations), rapid breathing, difficulty in breathing or swallowing, and perception of internal processes that are normally excluded from consciousness.[62]

The content of primary care is ultimately defined by patients, not doctors. The most powerful predictor of a successful outcome of consultation is agreement between doctor and patient on a list of main problems.[63] A Canadian study in the early 1980s showed that both parties agreed the same agenda for 76% of organic problems, but for only 6% of psychosocial problems.[64] It is not patients' fault that only a minority have any of the important but infrequent diseases which used to dominate the curriculum in teaching hospitals and questions in examinations, and still dominate thought in many hospitals. If patients accept the costs in time and lost independence entailed in seeing a doctor, their problems should be taken seriously, even if time is short. The possibility of serious early disease is never absent. It should not be dismissed solely on the grounds that it is statistically improbable. However, misdiagnosis of emotional illness as organic disease can be just as destructive as vice versa. Either way, experienced and effective clinicians give priority to positive evidence of problems (mental as well as physical) which patients probably do have, rather than negative evidence purporting to exclude problems they probably don't have. Mental and emotional illness deserves positive diagnosis in its own right, mainly from patients' own stories and opinions as initially presented, before they are modified to suit a professional audience. Its diagnosis should not appear to be a punishment for not having detectable physical disease.

Who decides what qualifies as illness, and why?

The scope of medical diagnosis is defined socially, not biologically. All life is by definition biological, so which aspects of life are regarded as within the scope of health care depends on conventions, which in turn depend on whether a problem seems more likely to be soluble by medical care or by some other route. This judgement must eventually depend on agreement between patient and professional. As care comes to depend less on symptoms, and diagnosis becomes more an anticipation of impending risks, the initiator of this process may increasingly be a proactive professional.

Problems that can be solved quickly and completely by medical treatment, like meningitis or acute intestinal obstruction, are obviously a very important medical responsibility, but cure of this kind is an extremely small fraction of NHS work. Particularly in mental and behavioural health, the border between what is and is not medical is much less obvious than it may seem within contemporary conventions. Judgements do have to be made. From time to time the idea is resurrected that all mental illness lies only in the eyes of beholders, and is defined only by transgression of ruling social conventions. That idea may be reinforced by experience of treatment, which has often been, and sometimes still is, worse than experience of disease. Once a disease label has been applied, often on weak evidence, it may be hard to remove.[65] However, none of this proves that mental illness is not real (for both patients and their families)[66] or potentially fatal.[67] Mind is a function of a material organ, the brain. Why should the brain, alone among body organs, be immune from disease?

For example, as well as systematic studies of how thought and behaviour in schizophrenia differs from normal in a wide range of cultures,[68] and impressive evidence that it depends little if at all on environmental experience,[69] we now have a huge accumulation of evidence about ways in which the biochemistry of thought in schizophrenia differs consistently from the biochemistry of thought within its very wide normal range. Continued search for better ways to modify this abnormal chemistry is rational and probably, though not certainly, appropriate to the problem. We have good evidence that established treatments are effective,[70] and more so when applied early, in the first presenting episode of the disease.[71] Treatments should include psychosocial interventions,[72] which are very labour intensive, as well as medications, which are very much less so, a difference which often leads to virtually exclusive reliance on medication.

We need to remember that harmful side effects even of current treatment may be substantial and often irreversible, and to bear in mind at least 200 years of history in which a long list of behavioural, physical and chemical interventions have been imposed on people with schizophrenia. Many of these interventions have entailed violence to patients, applied with a ruthless arrogance which is in retrospect breathtaking.[73] How can we be sure that our present interventions are any better founded or less cocksure than those of the past? Only by *not* being sure: by awareness of our own fallibility, even though we know far more now than we did then. We need to approach management of mental and emotional illness with extreme caution and sensitivity, and recognise that in this field, more than any other, every intervention is experimental, and none can ever have a completely predictable result – but also to remember that patients and their caring families need and want effective treatment, not philosophy.[74]

Mental illness in childhood

These judgements are hard enough in adults, but in children they become almost impossible. Starting in the US, professional perception of childhood mental illness justifying medication began to rise slowly in the 1970s, and steeply after 1980. The proportion of children who are unhappy most of the time, and the proportion whose behaviour at home or at school disrupts family life or teaching, are probably also rising. Probably every generation tends to think the next is going to the dogs, but even allowing for this, something very ugly seems to be happening to many of our children, as the full force of consumer society gets applied to ever younger age groups, and parenting becomes further marginalised by the demands of two-income families and the demise of a single wage sufficient to provide for a family.

As in adult psychoses, measurable biochemical and even biophysical differences can be detected between the brains of affected children and 'normal' children. This is hardly surprising. Since brain behaviour operates biochemically, so that anger or despair are each accompanied by measurable biochemical shifts, different behaviours will inevitably be associated with at least transient biochemical differences. However, if some biochemical intervention can be found which improves behaviour more or less consistently, this creates an opportunity for diagnosis and medication. Doctors who want to help children and their parents may feel justified in exploring that opportunity, and companies in search of new markets will be only too eager to assist them.

This evades another much more important question: why are these children unhappy, or why is their behaviour impossible for parents or teachers to cope with? If we knew the answers to those questions, we might start to address causes rather than modify effects by starting children on medication while their brains are still growing and their development is still most easily modified (for good or ill).[75] But perhaps that question is too big, would take too long to answer, or the answer might lie beyond the power of doctors, parents or teachers to apply? The prudent, middle-of-the-road course is just to carry on prescribing whatever pharmaceutical companies have developed to replace their old products, as each in turn becomes discredited. So the long list of medically approved abuse continues through its depressing cycle of alternating credulity and disillusion.[76]

The perceived incidence of childhood depression, attention-deficit hyperactivity disorder (ADHD) and autism have all risen steeply over the past two or three decades.[77] In Britain the incidence of first diagnosis of ADHD seems to have peaked in 1996, and changed little between 1996 and 2001, suggesting that whatever it is,[78] it seems now to have stabilised at a prevalence of about 5.3 per thousand boys aged 5–14, compared with between 40 and 260 per thousand in different surveys in the US.[79] ADHD behaviour usually improves when these children are given methylphenidate (Ritalin), a drug closely related to amphetamine.[80] For a stimulant drug to help over-active children seems paradoxical, but empirically it seems to be so, with benefit sufficiently obvious to impress even sceptical parents and clinicians. Diagnosis and treatment in Britain have lagged far behind the US, leading some doctors and many parents and media commentators to claim that the NHS and our schools are neglecting a large remediable problem.[81] In the US, on the other hand, the new fashion prompted enough concern among educators that behavioural disorders were being over-diagnosed and over-treated for the Federal Drugs Administration (FDA) to commission an inquiry by the United Nations Narcotics Control Board. Researchers at the University of California reported that in 1994 50% of children diagnosed as needing methylphenidate treatment for ADHD by 380 paediatricians had not received any psychological or educational testing, but were diagnosed and treated without any formal assessment. Between 10% and 12% of all boys aged 6–14 were using the drug.[82] Most seriously of all, this study confirmed others which have shown that methylphenidate also improved concentration in 'normal' children not diagnosed with ADHD. This brings into question whether ADHD can usefully be regarded as a disease, rather than an extreme normal behaviour.[83]

British child psychiatrists and psychologists seem still to be divided on this issue, between unrepentant advocates for more active diagnosis and treatment, and sceptics calling for caution.[84] A Working Party of the British Psychological Society has warned against the rush to label naughty, inattentive children as needing treatment for a disease.[85] However, most special-needs teachers know children receiving methylphenidate from their GPs, despite never having had any skilled formal assessment. This was bound to occur after so much public discussion in news media, with distraught parents pleading for prescriptions directly to their family doctors, often after a diagnosis made by parents themselves after trying out the 'miracle tablets' recommended by their neighbours.

These parents and neighbours may also be familiar with amphetamine, popularly known as 'speed'. This was originally used to keep the Second World War commandos and bomber pilots awake and concentrating long after their bodies told them to sleep, and later by all-night dancers and people needing to lose weight, reduced appetite being a major side effect. When I came to Glyncorrwg in 1961 I found addiction to and dependence on amphetamine (readily available from an alcohol-dependent local pharmacist) was a major local problem. At that time the pharmaceutical companies denied any risk of addiction or dependence with amphetamine, and most expert psychiatrists agreed with them. By the mid-1960s addiction to amphetamine and dexamphetamine was recognised everywhere as a major problem, and by the 1970s most countries had legislation to limit its use. Why should methylphenidate, its close chemical relative and with a similar stimulant action, prove to be any different? As with earlier experience with amphetamine, manufacturers now deny any risk of dependence or addiction, but there is already plenty of anecdotal evidence that this is a growing problem among teenagers prescribed this drug, and this has been accepted by the FDA as a real risk.

In reaching these extremely complex judgements, children, parents, family doctors and child psychologists and psychiatrists can be sure of simple and unequivocal advice from at least one source which entertains no doubts whatever. In 2001, these became the first prescribed drugs to be advertised directly to the US public, over the heads of their doctors, to create consumer pressure for diagnosis and treatment, and consequently more prescriptions and sales.[86] In 2003 the companies launched a sales offensive on UK and other European countries to promote prescription of methylphenidate and dexamphetamine for ADHD. Per capita sales in the UK were still 10 times less than in the US, and 20 times less than in France and Italy, but UK prescription rates were rising and sales were improving. Though both drugs had been listed by the FDA as having addictive potential, prescribing in the US still rose more than sevenfold between 1992 and 2000, so that between 4 and 5 million US children out of a total child population of 80 million under 18 were estimated to be taking stimulant drugs, a legal market worth about US$1bn annually.[87] Something ugly is happening in all market-driven societies, which their leaders seem unable to admit even to themselves.[88]

Pressures on consultation time lead to hasty, impulsive clinical decisions using inadequate evidence, either from what patients say and think, or from considered professional thought in peer-reviewed journals. Pressures from pharmaceutical companies, and any other agency whose profits depend on clinical decisions, offer simplified and attractive but biased choices which distort those decisions. Consultations are a delicate construct, which should be treated with more care, respect and protection from commercial pressures than they now have.

Stories

On average, about 85% of the evidence used to reach any definitive medical diagnosis comes entirely from what patients say – from their own stories. Physical examination adds about 7% to this, and investigations like X-rays, blood tests and so on add another 7%.[89] Accurate diagnosis therefore depends overwhelmingly on careful, thoughtful, unhurried talking by patients and listening by professionals to patients' stories, and then careful interpretation of that evidence. Optimal quality of diagnosis requires inputs from patients for interpretation of their stories. One study in primary care found roughly one third of the ideas offered by patients about the causes of their problems, when they were invited to do so, proved useful for forming a diagnosis.[90] Every experienced clinician knows all this, but still we hear suggestions that if all this talking, listening and interpretation might somehow be replaced by technology, care could be made more cost-effective (and profitable to those providing the technology).[91]

Diagnostic weapons cannot be aimed accurately and economically without a diagnostic hypothesis, which can be established only by talking and listening, and often some waiting-and-seeing.[92] This must include the 50% of usually minor symptoms which eventually turn out to be self-limiting disorders of small consequence. In otherwise healthy people, policies of delayed labelling, waiting-and-seeing for two weeks or so, rather than rushing straight to complex investigations or referral, are safe, effective and still acceptable to most UK patients. Advancing consumerism makes such cautious and tentative approaches increasingly difficult, by exaggerating expectations and by promoting litigious recrimination.[93] Providing patients get intelligible and truthful explanations of what's happening, a balanced assessment of risks, and assurance that their carers will always be open to new evidence and revised opinions, few have persistent symptoms they cannot tolerate for two weeks.

Somatised mental illness

Minor and usually transient symptoms caused by emotional states, particularly by fear or minor depression, generally respond well to a combination of attentive listening (with particular attention to patients' own ideas about possible causes), careful examination and possibly some simple investigations, and explanation in simple terms, together with a positive invitation to return for review if the symptoms or worries persist.[94] This is a field in which inappropriate investigations and treatment are not just wasteful, but destructive. In the words of Jerome Frank:

> With many patients the placebo may be as effective as psychotherapy because the placebo condition contains the necessary, and possibly the sufficient, ingredient for much of the beneficial effect of all forms of psychotherapy. This is a helping person who listens to the patient's complaint and offers a procedure to relieve them, thereby inspiring the patient's hopes and combating demoralisation.[95]

A minority, around 5% of patients consulting in primary care, have a major problem of somatised mental illness.[96] Some of these originate from patients presenting initially with minor symptoms, whose anxieties have been reinforced by early resort to defensive measures designed to exclude problems they probably don't have in their bodies, with little or no effort to find what they probably do have in their minds. Patients with major somatised disorder tend to get disposed of by hasty and excessive disease labelling, investigation, referral, cross-referral and inappropriate surgery.[97] They become 'thick file' patients, dreaded by doctors and frequently off-loaded to a series of specialists (ending with a psychiatrist), incurring mounting costs and misery as they go.

Somatisation disorder is therefore a big problem, with big effects on NHS costs, effectiveness, efficiency, and morale of staff and patients. It seems to be much more common in people who have suffered physical or sexual abuse in childhood, the results of which in adult life seem to be identical. Surveys in the UK, the US, Germany, Switzerland and Australia all show around 20% of women and 8% of men admitting to experience of sexual abuse as children.[98] Among patients who consult their doctors often, around 25% admit to experience of either sexual abuse or serious domestic violence in childhood.[99] Looking at it the other way round, about one third of people who experienced such abuse have a reported psychological problem, compared with about half as many among people who deny such experience.[100] As for domestic violence between adults, that social iceberg only began to be revealed in the 1980s, but has always generated huge fears, mostly undeclared.[101] Most people are surprisingly tough, but as Katon, Kleinman and Rosen said, if the only way you can draw attention to sadness or fear is to have a headache or palpitation, that is how you learn to complain.[102]

All this is confusing, as complex and difficult as most other aspects of human biology. We are a complicated species. But our greatest problems arise not from the always doubtful, uncertain and ambiguous nature of human health and behaviour, but from cocksure refusal to admit this, and faith that putting human problems into a dehumanised black box with medication as its sole machinery can produce an efficient and useful output.[103] If doctors or patients can find any reason, however implausible, for a mechanistic explanation of symptoms or a somatic label, most will seize this with relief, rather than enter the bog of their innermost fears and anxieties, which they may share as much as the patient. If any trace of even the most doubtful evidence of somatic disease can be found, preferably with some apparently simple surgical solution, both doctor and patient can return to short consultations about body engineering and repairs, and keep away from the dangerous ground where causes so often lie. On the other hand, to have any hope of rational care with measurable health outcome, we must pay the price in more staff, longer consultation times and wider, more sceptical and more compassionate imagination:[104] a black box designed from experience of handling human problems, not from managing assembly belts.

Discretional surgery

So far, we have considered only the black box of primary care, and ignored hospital inpatient and outpatient care (secondary care). And rightly so, because about 90%–95% of first consultations end at this point, and decisions at this level largely determine not only whether people are referred to hospital-based specialists, but who they will see and what will be done when they get there.[105]

The simplest and most familiar examples of specialist care, which have almost monopolised media attention to the NHS since it began to be pushed back into the marketplace, come from planned, discretional surgery (also called interval or elective surgery): coronary bypass grafts and stents, hip replacements, cholecystectomies, hysterectomies and so on. Surgeons necessarily work in a culture of clear decision and vigorous interventions of an engineering kind. However, rational surgical practice is as complex and replete with difficult choices as rational medical practice. It requires equally sceptical shared decisions, unbiased either by management pressures or by economic rewards or penalties.

Common surgical procedures in this discretional category include tonsillectomy and adenoidectomy for recurrent sore throats, grommets for middle ear disorders, hysterectomy for excessive menstrual bleeding, cholecystectomy for gallstones and unexplained abdominal pain, hip and knee joint replacements, and the different operations now available for grafting or stenting diseased coronary arteries. All these have great latitude for decision even within evidence-based consensus guidelines.[106] As surgical procedures are applied to people of ever-increasing age, decisions to operate entail increasingly complex judgements balancing inevitably transient health gains against immediate losses. Inevitably, because their problems tend to be even more complex and interdependent, decisions in older people are about twice as liable to error.[107] Patients and their families need to participate in these decisions, confident that professional judgements are unbiased either by economic incentives or clinical pride.[108]

For example, for hysterectomy alone, there are huge differences between countries, even between those with advanced economies, supposed to share a common evidence base. US and Australian rates are twice as high as British rates. These in turn are half as high as Norwegian rates, despite similar prevalence of rational indications for hysterectomy in all four.[109] It has been truly said that to study the indications for hysterectomy is to study the interface between medicine and society.[110] Hysterectomy removes more than a uterus. For some women it assures a welcome end to reproduction, for others this finality seems a disaster. For some it justifies withdrawal from an unhappy sexual role, for others it threatens a happy sex life.[111] Surgery may have placebo effects at least as great as those of medical treatment.[112]

Evidence-based decisions, checklists and guidelines

Evidence-based medicine (EBM) is a concept introduced in the 1980s, with the Canadian David Sackett the most influential of its many parents. He defined it as 'the conscientious, explicit, and judicious use of current best evidence in making decisions about the care of individual patients'.[113] This is a platitude with which few doctors could ever have dared to disagree for the past several hundred years, but behind it lay three new developments which gave it new force:

(1) After the Second World War clinical research shifted from intensive before-and-after studies of handfuls of interesting cases in a few teaching hospitals, to randomised controlled trials with first hundreds, then thousands and eventually hundreds of thousands or even millions of patients, either networked in many hospital clinics, or in people sampled from many communities.[114] The content of medical journals shifted from anecdotal accounts of interesting cases and intuitive reasoning about their significance, to reports of randomised controlled trials with reasoning based on formal logic and statistical analysis.[115]

(2) Beginning with mechanised information technology (IT) in the 1950s and electronic IT in the 1960s, data could be accumulated, stored and selectively accessed, at first centrally, later peripherally at points of clinical production, at vastly higher speed and lower cost in office labour than in the days of case-notes, marginal perforated cards or Hollerith machines. By 1995 almost 90% of UK practices used computers, and 55% used them to access clinical data or other information during consultations.[116] Medical brains could therefore be used less for remarkable feats of memory, releasing them for better-informed and more sceptical thought.

(3) By the 1990s worldwide evidence from human experimentation in trials and meta-analyses of trials became available in concise summary form to every clinician with access to IT. This is now centrally reviewed and edited by the International Cochrane Collaboration (ICC), and available everywhere through the internet.

Worldwide health care reforms are intended to rationalise care by applying this evidence systematically, gradually replacing use of procedures still unsupported by controlled evidence that they are effective. Selected and condensed into clinical checklists[117] and guidelines,[118] systems of managed care try to make routine practice more consistent with evidence from clinical trials.[119]

What at last made systematic application of evidence feasible 'at the bedside' was IT, and through this a central store of cumulative knowledge, summarised by the ICC. The ICC was founded by Iain Chalmers, one of Archie Cochrane's apprentices, who had already pioneered evidence-based obstetric practice, delighting most midwives but infuriating many obstetricians. The ICC brought together a global network of expert committees able to produce meta-analyses merging data from numerous small trials to reach consensus conclusions, and from these to develop guidelines for everyday practice. All this cost money, readily forthcoming from governments convinced that if medical care could be made rational it would also be more cost-effective and easier to manage.

Guidelines are certainly necessary and useful. A study of 24 East London practices in 1994, all of which had already established disease registers (and were therefore above contemporary average quality), showed that only about one third of all diabetics had ever had their weight recorded, and less than a quarter had smoking status recorded.[120] Just over one third of all asthmatics had ever had any aspect of lung function recorded, and less than 20% had smoking status recorded. Of course these tasks needed urgently to be done, rational care was not possible without them, but consequent staff workload had either been ignored or grossly underestimated by NHS authorities.

For staff in the front line, all this encouraged extremely sceptical if not cynical attitudes to guidelines. Because their earnings are increasingly tied to evidence that guidelines have been followed and targets have been met, this rejection may be superficially concealed, but for most medical and nursing staff it remains a chilling and obvious truth. EBM and its guidelines may make their work visibly more difficult, without making it obviously more effective.

Guidelines have some great advantages. They provide evidence-based expert consensus views on optimal solutions for clinical problems thought to be commonly encountered in practice. Decision trees can be designed for continuing management of common health problems, so that these optimal solutions can be applied by health care workers with much less training and experience. Thus, albeit in somewhat rigid form, continuing health problems can be followed up on a mass scale at low cost but to a higher standard of quality than the erratic performance of the past, even in the best practices. Their systematic use in the NHS, strongly reinforced since 2004 by the Quality and Outcomes Framework (QOF), which rewards GPs for applying guidelines to detection and follow-up of several of the most important chronic impairments and health risks, has led to rapid gains in all measures of process in primary care – so rapid, in fact, that in the first year or two GPs' incomes greatly exceeded expectation, and nearly bankrupted the NHS.[121]

However, guidelines also entail serious risks. First, and above all, they encourage thoughtless ritual and discourage clinical imagination. Nobody seems to have noticed that guidelines centrally devised by experts were a main feature of the Soviet national health service, helping the state to control pandemic typhus, syphilis, and other serious infectious diseases in a remarkably short time in the 1920s and early 1930s, with a rapidly recruited and hastily trained workforce, led by a few fully trained and experienced doctors. They could never have achieved this without some simplified system of this kind. However, when I looked back from what still survived from the ruins of this system in Kazakhstan in 1995, it was obvious that these guidelines had soon become tramlines, stifling critical thought, innovation and imagination, and encouraging legalistic and authoritarian management.[122] It was better than nothing, the alternative available then and now for most poor people in most poor countries, but that is not the situation in developed economies.

This complex problem will never have a simple answer, even if we move to a more rational system of primary care that encourages the new sorts of generalist we need. There is a necessary and inevitable tension between respect for organised past experience, and imaginative judgements within immediately present experience. To develop an effective care system that does not freeze into ritual, this lesson has to be learned repeatedly at every level of education, both by staff and by the public.

Second, if pharmaceutical companies, or any other sectional interest, can influence the content of nationally adopted guidelines, this may have economic implications too large for professional integrity to resist. Researchers in Toronto who studied 200 authors of 44 clinical guidelines used in North America found that 87% of expert advisers had undisclosed financial links to pharmaceutical companies.[123] We all hope that equivalent British agencies like the National Institute for Clinical Excellence (NICE) will be able to resist corruption of this kind. So deeply is NICE detested by some pharmaceutical companies that the vice-president of the Center for Medicine in the Public Interest, a pressure group in the US protecting them from government regulation, has likened it to a terrorist organisation, and denounced its decisions as morally indefensible. NICE acts not itself as an assessor of cost-effectiveness, but as a commissioner for such research, which is actually carried out by seven different UK university centres.[124] However, even

NICE has had to be warned by WHO about the company connections of some of its advisers.[125] WHO itself is extremely circumspect when it criticises powerful commercial interests, and even more so the states which support them and can threaten the funding of WHO. The ICC probably will stay independent of commercial pressures if this is possible, but it will be a fight. It devoted a world conference with around 1,000 delegates to this subject in 2004, but increasing commercial penetration of university departments, encouraged by government, makes independence for all agencies increasingly difficult.

Evidence from patients

These problems will be much easier to solve when we all accept that EBM as generally understood still lacks a necessary dimension, namely evidence from patients.[126] Substantial progress is probably impossible without this. We have already seen that at least 85% of personal diagnosis derives from listening to patients' own stories, and that, outside hospitals, patients or their informal carers become 100% responsible for actually carrying out whatever treatment has been agreed. Failure by patients to perform either of these tasks impedes production of health gain just as much as failure by professionals. Patients are just as able to benefit from guidelines, and they are equally confused by guidelines devised by experts ignorant or careless of the real world in which they must operate.[127] Cumulative research evidence about patients' experience of illness and treatment is as necessary and feasible as cumulative research evidence about medical or nursing experience.

Thanks mainly to Andrew Herxheimer and Ann McPherson, this evidence is becoming available through the International DIPEx Library and website, now rechristened www.healthtalkonline,[128] from which we have already seen an example. This excellently designed, user-friendly website provides essential learning material for all health professionals. It is now beginning to be used for undergraduate and postgraduate medical education. DIPEx provides a potential foundation for Chief Medical Officer Liam Donaldson's programme to facilitate development of Expert Patient networks throughout the UK, giving further education to volunteers with experience of particular chronic disorders to assist in their own care.[129] Seven years after inception of this programme, it still omits development of any of these expert patients as teachers to help other patients with similar problems, though that is surely the logical next step.[130]

As yet, few doctors seem ready to welcome patients positively as co-producers, rather than embarrassingly well-informed potential critics. In

1999, only 21% of doctors in a random sample welcomed the Expert Patients idea. Fifty-eight per cent predicted it would increase GP workload, and 42% thought it would increase NHS costs. Only 12% thought it would improve doctor–patient relationships.[131] Another poll in 2003 found that 76% of pharmacists, 63% of doctors and 48% of nurses thought better-informed patients would take up more of their time, be more demanding and be harder to deal with.[132] Objective studies of patients receiving more education about how to manage their disease show exactly the opposite: after patients had received more information, consultation rates fell by 42%.[133] The professional response has been not more vigorous promotion of Expert Patients, using this evidence, but capitulation to these intuitive fears. A *BMJ* editorial on the subject welcomed suggestions that the Expert Patients Programme be renamed as the Involved Patients Programme, or Autonomous Patients, or Resourceful Patients[134] – anything, apparently, so long as health professionals would not have to accept that patients do indeed have intelligence, information and expertise, which might assist care rather than impede it, if they were encouraged and expected to take a more active role.

Used as a foundation for development of Expert Patients as an extension of teams both in primary and hospital care, and combined with evidence from controlled trials through the ICC, DIPEx could provide an expanding patients' international database to complement the Cochrane Library, which now also accepts inputs from patients. From these two sources truly evidence-based practice could be developed at all levels, from international and national policies to the most peripheral primary care units developing their own guidelines. Whether this possibility is ever actually realised will depend on whether professionals have enough maturity, self-knowledge and political realism to welcome more informed and assertive patients as their allies, or, as the evidence cited in the last paragraph suggests, they continue to see intelligent patients as just another problem. Perhaps some would prefer to be veterinary surgeons rather than doctors. In England, at least, they can expect no leadership from government, but as their fears are refuted by experience, and hopefully with some professional leadership, perceptions may change. Progress will depend also on whether enough patients retain their dignity as citizens, and refuse demotion to consumer status. For both groups, this is a political and social challenge rather than a technical problem.

Managed care: who for?

Accessible databases of professional plus patients' evidence are preconditions for optimally effective EBM, but they do not of themselves ensure that decisions in practice will use this evidence.[135] Respect for evidence from patients, including collective local experience of care, requires escape from a deeply rooted traditional culture of medical dominance, appointed rather than elected local managers, and public deference. At best this has been expressed through paternalism, and at worst it is becoming subordinated to corporate trade. Both oligarchies have systematically ignored, minimised or embezzled the always necessary but customarily invisible contribution of patients' evidence to diagnosis and treatment.

As always, progress may take either one of two opposed directions. Patients' evidence may be used to encourage more discriminating choices by individual consumers in markets of competing providers – the path now favoured equally by leaders of New Labour, Conservatives and Liberal Democrats, and by many patients' problem-specific pressure groups which, however loyal they may try to be to the NHS, find themselves allied with commercial providers, prepared to fund any lobbying group that may promote their sales. This eventually self-financing trade would be peripheral to core services still provided by the state as an ultimate human right for the indigent, preserving token loyalty to the NHS as conceived in 1948. New developments would occur at the innovatory commercial periphery, not at the stripped-down NHS core. The system might thus eventually become a self-financing commodity market, its proportion of all health care determined by what the market could bear and voters would tolerate. In this scenario providers and consumers would confront each other as in any other transaction – *caveat emptor*, let the buyer beware. This process would proceed at the same pace as gentrification of the population as a whole, limited only by the rate of expansion of the real economy.[136] People still unable to pay for necessary care would still get it, in suitably spartan form, from what would remain of the NHS, but as more wealth spilled from the tables of the rich, everyone could hope eventually to be included. State care could then wither away, taxes could fall, consumers would be kings, and doctors would finally be put in their place – regulated by government, managed by their corporate employers and restrained by their own need to charm customers and avoid litigation. Suitably regulated to restrain outright fraud, this consumerist scenario is the solution towards which global capitalism has been moving since the 1980s.[137]

Regardless of the declared intentions of policy makers, in this consumerist scenario, evidence from providers and consumers would remain divided, because they would serve opposed interests. Each might learn from the other, but only as all providers and consumers must try to understand what their opponents are up to.

The alternative is that patients and professionals combine their two sets of evidence to form something new, a human biology including the full range of human experience and behaviour, its cultural and behavioural foundations as well as its material basis in anatomy, physiology and pathology. In this way medical practice could begin not just to use science, but itself become part of science, unique among sciences in that both its subjects and its objects would be ourselves. Having made huge gains in effectiveness through respect for scientific thinking, health professionals continually seek new ways to bring their practice closer to scientific methods, recognising the essentially experimental (because not fully predictable) character of all interventions in health care. This has brought some of our most conservative professionals to recognise that without developing patients as equal partners, health care cannot advance beyond episodic repairs for advanced pathology. Effective action to promote and preserve health depends on often very simple tasks undertaken jointly with all of the people, not just the minority already in obvious breakdown. In this practical and material fashion, most health professionals are already immersed in a *de facto* alliance with their patients and the populations they serve. However uncertainly, their feet are already set on a path toward participative democracy in a broad social alliance.

Citizens or consumers?

With socially informed imagination, virtually all consultations provide opportunities to develop new relationships between professionals and patients, in either of these two opposed directions. At first, their divergence may not be obvious, but if we look at populations as a whole, it quickly becomes so. As consumers, an already confident and well-informed minority of usually affluent and conventionally educated patients will become ever more confident and better informed as it picks its way through an NHS of diminishing scope, and avails itself of a widening variety of commercial alternatives. This issue has been powerfully raised by development of very expensive new treatments for lethal or very disabling diseases, most notably some cancers. This list will inevitably increase as new treatments are marketed, at prices set (like all others) not by cost of production (including research), but by what an often irrationally fearful market will stand, because often they deal with matters of life or death, where even marginal gains may command high prices. Because in the NHS the purchaser is the state, this becomes a political as well as an economic issue. It is compounded by our need to retain the NHS as a unified service. If some treatments become so expensive that the NHS cannot pay for them, and if individual patients are allowed somehow to find the extra money themselves, then the many advocates of consumerism and a return to commercial care will have the next step they need in their war of attrition. On a token scale, for some innovations (real or imagined) in cancer chemotherapy, this process has already begun.

In any publicly funded service, there must be a limit to what the nation is able to spend to extend a single human life, often by small margins. This may be less than a billionaire consumer might wish to spend on himself, and will certainly be less than a pharmaceutical company would like to receive. In 1999, NICE set this ceiling at £30,000 (€38,000, $54,000) per Quality-Adjusted Life Year gained.[138] This ceiling was arbitrary. It has been unchanged since it was first set more than a decade ago. Inflation at roughly 3% a year has steadily drawn it down. So there is a strong case for change, perhaps an index-linked formula. However, the principle that the NHS must have some way to limit what it spends on one patient is the real issue, not the level at which this limit is set.

British news media have no doubt who to blame for this dilemma. In suitably vulgarised language, the *News of the World* christened the director of NICE: 'Dr Death ... a bean counter in a posh suit with the power to tell people to eff off and die'. The *Daily Mail*, *Daily Express* and *Daily Telegraph* headlined a Conservative Party claim that NICE spent more on spin than on assessing drugs. NICE's published accounts showed that in fact it spent less than 1% of its budget on its press office.[139] The real target of the Conservative press is not Dr Death (later re-invented by Sarah Palin in the US) but the NHS gift economy. For the past three decades we have seen a procession of tragic victims of rare but lethal diseases, most of them young and beautiful, their personal cases espoused by newspapers willing to spend millions of pounds on supporting their personal case against NICE, in certain knowledge that their added sales will more than compensate for whatever they spend.

This development poses two fundamental questions, neither of which seems to have been addressed by any of these newspapers, nor by the broadcast commentariat who follow their agenda.[140] What is the value of a life – not just this particular life, but any human life? And what sets the price of new treatments – do any new treatments really need to cost more than £30,000 per year of life saved?

Why not negotiate a lower price, putting the pressure on pharmaceutical companies, rather than the NHS? The NHS is still virtually a sole purchaser, with immense power as a negotiator, if government allows this power to be used.[141] Pharmaceutical companies supplying the NHS already have a guaranteed 20% or so return on investment across the board, for all of their drugs (guaranteed by government). Why should new drugs attract more than this? If the scientists who develop new treatments are motivated only by super-profits, they deserve to be sacked, but is this in fact the case? I have never met such a scientist, and doubt if any exist. On the other hand, there is clearly no limit to the greed of company executives or shareholders. A regulator trying to set a decency limit to executive earnings would have an even harder task than the director of NICE.

For patients to develop their full potential as co-producers of health, trusting relationships have to be rebuilt on a new basis, not on faith or deference but on evidence. In a public service where all risks are pooled, and everyone depends on everyone else, patients have to become mature citizens, not just consumers. The old trust in professionals rested on myths of omniscience, supported by both professionals and patients so as to preserve hope. Doctors in competitive trade could not afford to admit either that science had as yet few useful answers, or that even if answers existed, they did not know what they were. Doctors in competitive trade could never afford to say 'I don't know, but let's find out', and then reach for a book or search a website, in full view of their patients. They could not afford to reveal in practice that biological science rests on doubt, not engineering certainty, and that doctors' heads are not books. When their useful knowledge was small, the profession behaved as though it knew everything and patients knew nothing. Both parties colluded in this deception, because placebo effects were virtually the only weapons they had, and placebo effects depended on faith. This seemed a fragile asset best left undisturbed. Though now severed at its roots, much of this culture of mutual self-deception still persists, a withered plant which needs actively to be cleared away, by patients together with professionals.

Medical and nursing records[142]

Clinical records provide most of the evidence we have from which to measure the quality of decisions which initiate processes within the black box. They provide the verifiable continuity between clinical episodes, between different professionals in a single unit.[143] They provide data for the links between units in the generalist–specialist referral hierarchy, between the NHS and other social agencies, and between the NHS as a whole and the population it serves.[144] Many errors and inefficiencies arise at these linkage points, rather than in performance of the clinical tasks they connect.

By most professionals even today, records are tolerated rather than loved. They provide verifiable evidence about decisions often so blurred by doubt and uncertainty that some errors are inevitable. For many NHS staff, some evidence actually used to make important decisions seems safer in their heads than when written or entered into a computer. They see records as evidence that may be used by administrators to apply either punishments or rewards, rather than as their own indispensable aids to effective, self-critical work as independent creative workers, from which they can see the consequences of their decisions and learn.

For primary care of industrial workers and their families, medical records scarcely existed before the NHS. Nominally created by the 1911 Insurance Act, records usually contained only lists of medicines prescribed and certificates of incapacity issued, with at most a cursory diagnostic label.[145] They rarely contained any of the evidence on which such diagnoses were supposed to be based. Though most GPs knew their patients fairly well, they carried their life and health stories in their heads, inevitably with gross simplification and stereotyping – caricatures of real lives.[146] In almost all cases, the only elements in these records containing any useful evidence were hospital letters from specialists, usually stuffed into the record envelope without regard to date order, and rarely, if ever, consulted. These letters could be really useful, because most consultants wrote them primarily as succinct case-summaries for their own use, with information to GPs as a byproduct. Somewhere in the patient's record, it was important for hospital staff to have a summary making some sense of what seemed to be going on. If this could be found at all, it was in these letters.

When evaluating different international care systems, quality of primary care records is a good indicator of maturity in the system as a whole. Slowly and erratically, GP records worth reading began to appear in a few UK practices in the 1960s, became commonplace in the 1970s, and were almost universal by the 1980s. Today over 95% of all NHS GPs use electronic computer-held records for at least some aspects of patient care, and since 2004 GPs' contracts have become virtually unworkable without them.

Plans are now in hand for all UK patients to have direct access to their own online primary care records.[147] There is evidence of substantial popular demand for a patient's right to enter their own data in them.[148] A small but growing proportion of practices with fully computer-held records have direct computer links to local hospital diagnostic and outpatient departments, so that results of laboratory tests, X–rays and other direct-access diagnostic data go straight to the GP.

The rate-limiting factor for development of a single unified NHS record, usable at any level, is the still generally primitive and un-coordinated state of hospital records compared with GP records. A much lower proportion of hospital data is computer-held, and a single NHS record usable throughout all levels of the service remains a promise possibly 10 years ahead if we are lucky, though we are still paying for similar promises made periodically at colossal cost since the 1970s and still unfulfilled.[149]

Several explanations have been offered for the backwardness of UK hospital IT compared with IT in primary care. Patients referred to specialists tend to present more difficult clinical puzzles, poorly suited to the still primitive capacities of computer programmes depending on essentially obsolete systems of disease labelling.[150] A more fundamental problem is that in order to develop a viable system, programmers must understand the processes their programmes will serve, in biological, social and economic terms. These purposes are probably better agreed and more clearly defined in primary generalist care than in hospital specialist care. Primary medical care is not divided between rival specialty fiefdoms, and largely thanks to the Royal College of General Practitioners (RCGP), it has developed a unified postgraduate teaching programme with a coherent, unified philosophy over the past 50 years. This still cannot be said of the specialists who together comprise hospital medical staff, or of their various Royal Colleges, who all had to agree on a common language. Before they managed to do so, development of IT in hospitals had been seized by the new breed of administrators and managers drawn from industry and retired senior military officers. Their main aims have naturally been to keep their hospitals solvent against competitors in the NHS quasi-market, to satisfy higher management and government demands to control waiting times, bed occupancy and staff deployment, and squeeze ever more process from fewer skilled staff, not to help clinicians to work more effectively.[151] Some of these process measures are important, but they should follow from clinical process, not lead it.

In line with government policies to encourage competition and consumer choice in the NHS, a 'Choose & Book' function was included in the new IT system (National Programme for Information Technology: NPfIT) launched for NHS England in 2005. This was supposed to be available throughout England by the end of that year. In theory, all patients would, at the point of referral by their GP, be given options of time, place and date. The referral could either be booked there and then, or the patient would be given a reference number and phone numbers to confirm an appointment later. GPs were promised this would take them 20–30 seconds, but at a demonstration session in summer 2004 three experienced GP trainers struggled with it for half an hour.[152] The new system was not integrated with any existing GP systems, though these were already sophisticated enough to be able to communicate with each other. In 2007, a report by the House of Commons Committee for Public Accounts found that the new NHS electronic record programme was running two years late, and suppliers were struggling to deliver. After four years of the programme, costs estimated initially at £6bn were now expected to reach £12bn, and benefits were still unclear.[153] Though the English NHS IT agency, Connecting for Health, had forecast in January 2005 that 151 acute hospital Trusts would have installed administrative parts of the new systems by April 2007, by February 2007 only 18 had actually been deployed. Today, five years later, the system 'Choose & Book' is still not fully operational.

'Choose & Book' was only one part of a general system intended eventually to replace all GP and hospital records with a single computer-held record that could be used at any level in the NHS, but because it was essential to New Labour's vision of patients shopping around throughout the UK for hospital specialists with the lowest waiting lists and operative mortality rates as shown by league tables, it was the dominant part. Software programming for the system as a whole was put in the hands of the privatised former UK telephone provider, British Telecom, which had bought into IDX, a computer program lifted directly from the existing systems of US hospital administrators. It seems scarcely credible, but this system was developed without regard to any of the existing IT systems already in use by the NHS, or any of the systems used by virtually all primary care teams for many years, enough to have accumulated a great deal of experience of their possibilities, limitations and pitfalls. The plan seemed to be that if and when this program was completed, this product of theory without practice would then displace the IT systems already functioning in primary care.[154]

Both hospital-based specialists and politicians still seem to assume that all worthwhile innovation has to come from hospital systems, preferably in the US, even though government policies encouraging consumerism were first presented as 'a general practice-led NHS', and later as 'a consumer-led NHS'. To anyone familiar with how referral pathways upward and discharge pathways downward actually operate, it was obvious that the way to avoid another immensely costly IT disaster would have been to build on what already existed in primary care, extend it upwards to hospital specialist care, and from this to create a truly integrated system. This would not have needed to include trading functions which nobody except the private sector lobby ever asked for. Though there are still several different competing primary care IT systems, all of these are already able to exchange data between them, and there is already a single system used by almost half of all practices.

By 2008, the new integrated NHS IT system was five years overdue, one of its principal contractor companies had backed out, and optimistic informed observers doubted if it could be in place before 2015.[155] Informed pessimists are now predicting that the entire project may soon have to be abandoned, at a cost of at least £12.5bn, but estimated by some well-informed observers to be closer to £30bn.[156]

Use of computers: who for?

Devolved governments in Wales and Scotland, which have stayed at arm's length from the English IT project, have quietly taken the lead and developed rational programmes, starting from where they were, with the people they had, and within a framework of thought that reflects how the NHS actually operates, rather than how it might operate as a Japanese total quality control factory. Wales already has a unified system working in NHS hospitals, linked to primary care centres in each catchment, functioning well and at a small fraction of the cost of the programme in England. It had the advantage that this was designed from the beginning to serve cooperative clinical needs rather than competitive commercial requirements.

Local, regional and national planning all need intelligence systems to make evidence-based rather than intuitive or passive decisions. At all these levels, gathering this evidence formerly entailed drudgeries so laborious at primary care level that no such evidence was gathered at all, except in a very few practices committed to research, almost entirely at their own expense. Even in hospitals, only the barest outline of their clinical work was visible. Computers now perform in milliseconds work which once required many years of bureaucratic labour. They make locally, nationally and internationally coordinated networks for upward, sideways and downward communication easy, where they were formerly hard even to imagine. At every level of public service, wherever the NHS still serves defined populations rather than shopping-around customers, we now have the means to develop services intelligently, with judgements informed by sound data, routinely collected by staff directly engaged in patient care as a byproduct of their everyday clinical work – because once clinical records are computer-held in a shared pattern, routinely recorded data can be used for any purpose within the system.

Paradoxically, some of the major advantages of computers lie in their inhumanity. Soon after they were introduced, imaginative pioneers discovered their value for gathering human evidence without making human judgements, so that patients could open up their real lives without the embarrassment of a human listener. After an initial computer-led search for concealed problems like alcohol dependence or abusive relationships, evidence so gained could provide a basis for subsequent more realistic human assessment, jointly with health professionals, to reach sounder judgements.[157] The ruthless logic of IT and its capacity to present data in graphic statistical form can reveal truth and make deception obvious even to unskilled lay readers, providing it has been designed to do so.

However, with these powerful virtues come dangerous new sources of error. Most obviously, doctors who spend more time interacting with their computers than listening to their patients, or who place computer screens so that patients can only guess what is going on, may dehumanise consultations and confine them to even narrower and less imaginative agendas than before.[158] This issue is now generally tackled well in undergraduate teaching. Clear ground rules have emerged which could humanise their use in consultations.[159] Use of checklists as a framework both for care and for rewards and penalties required by management is a growing industrialising trend. This is closely bound up with IT, threatening yet again to replace imaginative judgement by ritual.

To write a useful computer programme dealing with human decisions, it is essential to start from a valid model of how these are actually reached in best practice. Fundamental philosophical problems about the nature of clinical information are rarely addressed. Examples cited in this and earlier chapters show that present diagnostic practice is often closer to chaos than clarity, but at least chaos can provide flexibility, choice and a human face. Once locked into the logic of a computer programme, such qualities may disappear. Computers conscript users to theoretical models on which their programmes have been based. This presents exciting opportunities for rationally planned development, but also dangerous possibilities for perpetuation of fundamental error, built into the foundations of entire health care systems and dictating the way people think and work.

Clearly we need one single national, and eventually international, IT language and format in which the evidence used by applied medical science can be expressed. This single language must necessarily incorporate assumptions about the nature of the evidence it describes. In its widest sense, human biology must include sociology, because we are social animals. The evidence used by medical science is not a growing and potentially limitless pile of independent facts, but the story of an extraordinarily complex species, told by itself to itself for its own use, to make its own future more human than its past. It is conceivable, though probably unlikely, that our foreseeable future might still be constrained by the requirements of commodity trade, but medical science cannot in any circumstances accept that its universal language should incorporate this assumption and deny alternatives. If we did, we would close the door to real competition between the recent and hopefully ephemeral philosophy of care as a business transaction, and our ancient but evolving philosophy of care as an expression of social solidarity.

Confidentiality

All four nations in Britain are now trying to develop regionally networked records interchangeable at all levels of the NHS. Obviously these systems must be accessible to all staff using data from them and adding data to them, but with electronic records duplication is easy. Less obviously, their inputs and outputs should be accessible to patients. Present policy in Wales is committed to records designed around patients' life stories, and therefore readable, understandable and potentially open to factual correction by them and their families. These records will include some data that are not readily intelligible to patients, or even to non-specialised staff, but these will be peripheral to the life stories at their core. Consequences will be dramatic for present assumptions about confidentiality and ethics.

These assumptions are often remote from real experience of necessary choices between evils rather than between good and bad, of damage limitation rather than cure. All that is true is not always immediately acceptable. Since the invasion of the NHS by commercial providers, confidentiality has entered new dimensions, as yet virtually ignored in public discussion. In primary care, the NHS already holds computer lists of people itemised by their health problems, often inseparable from social problems, together with their names, addresses, telephone numbers and e-mail addresses. To invite commercial providers to share these with non-profit public services in a single universal NHS electronic record, constrained only by promises to ignore their huge potential for targeting accurately defined consumer groups, is clearly impossible. A company specialising in continuing care of diabetes, for example, will naturally expect to have access to lists of people with that problem. From there it is a small and logical step to identify subsets with kidney failure, retinal damage, or erectile failure. Where do we draw the line between informing potential consumers, and promoting a competing company or its products? Confidentiality would then be defended only by business ethics – in other words, not defended at all.

Apart from these threats to confidentiality from commerce, serious personal problems will arise from a more open and honest approach to recorded stories: for example, past histories of interrupted pregnancies, domestic violence, sexually transmitted disease or suspected but unconfirmed major disease. All these need to be recorded. They will present major problems for sharing information within families, though such sharing will probably be inevitable.[160] These problems could be overcome, provided that innovative culture is allowed to follow innovative practice, each learning from the other as they have in the past. The most important point is that patients should begin to hold records themselves, and gain access to their information in some stepwise fashion that recognises and respects such initial difficulties in moving towards a more open, tolerant and trusting society. People will need time to learn. There have been some excellent examples from UK radio and television broadcasts on how to do this, most notably for teenagers.

Only such records can provide material evidence that patients' participation in care has moved from rhetoric to reality. Fortunately these systems will take some years to evolve, giving us time to ensure that they are flexible, adapted to learning as we go. Provided that the NHS remains accessible to all citizens, that new electronic record systems are made accessible to direct patient inputs, and that fragmentation of NHS care does not continue to the point where defined catchment populations no longer exist and audits of total performance against population denominators become impossible, these records will provide opportunities to merge data in many different ways, longitudinally in time and laterally in populations. Such systems would provide powerful new tools for improving individual patient care, for monitoring performance of the system as a whole, for developing large-scale observational research and even some kinds of experimental research, for redefining both professional and public attitudes to science, and for raising professional–patient relationships to a qualitatively higher social level.

Black boxes: dehumanising or humane?

This chapter has provided a few examples of what happens at some important points of decision within the NHS black box. They were chosen to illustrate ways in which they differ fundamentally from what happens at typical points of production in the black boxes of commodity industrial production, which are designed reduce personal human decisions as far as possible.

What about our NHS black box? This also uses machines, but it is difficult to find any that replace rather than augment and extend human labour and human decision. Even information technology, which has raised productivity in its own field by orders of magnitude, has not displaced any labour I can think of. What it has really done is to create new and extremely useful tasks that were previously unthinkable. Electrocardiograph (ECG)[161] machines now analyse their own results, and do so more accurately and reliably than most non-specialist doctors were previously able to do. No doctors have become unemployed as a result, they just have more time for other tasks requiring more sensitivity and imagination. The same applies to surgical interventions, which, since the advent of flexible endoscopy, closed-circuit television and minimally invasive procedures, are coming to depend more and more on advanced technologies.[162] Far from displacing human labour, this surgery requires an ever-growing number of staff with extremely specialised skills, working to much higher standards of accuracy.

For the sorts of shared decision exemplified in this chapter, IT can also make a huge new contribution; indeed, without it, shared production of health gain would probably be impossible, but it does nothing to reduce the human workforce required. On the contrary, to use IT intelligently and humanely we need many more people, with much higher skills, particularly the human skills of caring and communication.

Our NHS black box is qualitatively different from, and in important ways diametrically opposed to, the black box of commodity production of objects for the market. It has to deal with hugely complex biological and sociological uncertainties wholly unlike the world of engineering. Even in fields that seem most mechanical and suited to commodity trade, for example hip replacement, apparently apt engineering metaphors are illusory. Demand for hip replacement cannot be estimated only from objective evidence from X-rays or scans. A large population study in Sweden found that fewer than half of elderly patients with substantial X-ray evidence of joint damage had any complaints,[163] yet other studies have shown people with severe pain despite normal X-ray appearances. To target joint replacement accurately requires a wide range of carefully evaluated evidence from patients, including subjective assessments of pain, disability, co-existing illness, and social functioning, as well as assessment of joint rotation and X-rays.[164] These criteria can be quantified and standardised, but always depend on careful, shared assessments of patients' personal evidence as well as evidence from machines. When such criteria are applied to whole populations they reveal total needs for replacement about 6% greater than NHS supply, an important difference, but not an infinite gap. With political will, it could easily be closed.[165] Those who deny this seem driven by their need to find impossibilities to justify their 'reforms'.[166]

Post-modernists may discount the relevance of black box commodity production based on the Henry Ford, conveyor-belt model to sophisticated contemporary industrial production in which virtually anything, including ideas, information and all services, can become products. For those who still have jobs in commodity manufacture or marketed services, 'post-Fordist' black boxes differ from their predecessors only by dehumanising commodity production even faster than before, transferring more tasks from people to machines, and finding labour in cheaper and poorer parts of the world. Management policies derived from industrial production, however indirectly and however modified to recognise at least some of the real clinical world, succeed mainly in demoralising staff and stifling all except the most profitable initiatives. The internal processes of our NHS black box depend on becoming more human, more labour intensive, more imaginative, more trusting, with closer and more sustained relationships between staff and patients, disentangled from pursuit of profit, so that mutual trust can grow through sustained contacts and knowledge can accumulate in a secure workforce. To develop this new model of shared creative production we have to do much more than reject the industrial model, but until this first step is taken, we cannot even begin.

Summary and conclusions

The NHS care system operates in ways entirely different from commodity-producing industries. Progress in health care depends on developing professionals as sceptical co-producers of health gain rather than salesmen of process, and developing patients as sceptical co-producers rather than consumers searching for bargains and shorter queues. Productivity in health care depends on complex decisions about complex problems, involving innumerable unstable and unpredictable variables. These decisions require increasingly labour-intensive production methods, with ever deeper, more trusting and continuing relationships between professionals and patients. Though machines may be increasingly useful, they need to be subordinated to human decisions. These decisions need to be based on evidence, freed so far as possible from bias, from either rewards, penalties, or personal vanities. They require an increasingly skilled, thoughtful, labour-intensive service.

By contrast, industrial production of commodities depends on a diminishing number of human decisions, with increasingly exact duplication of standardised mechanical actions, eventually eliminating human decisions almost completely. It starts by reducing workers to machines, and ends by virtually eliminating them from production, other than at a design stage.

When applied to health care systems, management policies derived from industrial commodity production, and incentive systems of reward and punishment based on that model, are demoralising to staff and patients. They are therefore likely to reduce productivity more than they can promote it. Health care requires an entirely different body of economic theory, only the outlines of which are beginning to become clear, to which health economists have as yet contributed little. Progress and productivity in this field depend on new social relationships between public, patients and health professionals, based on levels of trust unattainable within commercial transactions. Beginnings of these already exist in the NHS, but will develop optimally only within a gift economy and culture, separated entirely from the economy and culture of commerce.

FOUR

Generalists and specialists

Internationally, most people expect successful doctors to be specialists. If you have to admit to being just a GP, they think you must either have fallen off the bottom rung of the ladder of ambition, or never even reached it.

I was a Glyncorrwgologist, the only one in the world. I knew more, did more, and certainly wrote and spoke more about the health problems of Glyncorrwg, than any other doctor. So I became the world expert, a specialist in at least the initial recognition, and often the terminal management, of the entire potential range of health problems in that unique community. I was a broadly informed person able to reassemble into a comprehensible story what an ever-increasing variety of disease-specific specialists had divided. What higher ambition could any doctor have?

Assumptions that community-based generalists are less trained, less skilled, less knowledgeable or less useful than hospital-based specialists rest on apparently logical foundations. If GPs really were generalists, so the conventional argument goes, they would have to know everything. But nobody can know everything. So generalists are bound to fail, and might as well stop trying.[1]

In fact, the existence of effective generalists is a precondition for the existence of effective specialists. And paradoxically, to be effective, GPs have themselves to become specialists, but of a different kind – specialists in their own locality and population, specialists in general responsibility for initial, continuing and terminal care strategies over lifetimes, and for the huge, still under-explored territory between the outer limits of health and fully formed end-stage disease.

To get full value from expert specialists who know more and more about less and less, we need expert generalists who can still see the whole picture, from a standpoint closer to patients, but very much better informed than patients are about what is either possible or probable. Our need for such generalists increases, as specialised divisions of practice multiply. The functions of these generalists must be redefined, from the GPs of the past, who had to cope somehow with whatever chance threw at them, to the resident human biologists of the future.

To get from where we are to where we need to go, British doctors need to understand where British GPs came from – and the same goes for the very different professional histories of other countries.

Origins of the generalist–specialist division

Clinical specialisation began at both ends of the medical hierarchy, the top and the bottom. At the top were teaching hospitals, dominated by the personal doctors of the rich. They gained their knowledge and skills from experience with the small fraction of sick poor people admitted to teaching hospitals. Treatment at home (providing you had a good home, not a hovel) was safer, because hospitals were nests of lethal infection. Physicians and surgeons for the rich controlled formal medical education, and thus defined their profession as a whole. Until the last half of the 19th century, these top doctors were generalists, divided only into surgeons, whose work entailed invasion of the body, and physicians, who kept at stethoscope's length from it. Both were familiar with a wide range of illness, but apart from a very few surgical procedures, were almost powerless to change its course.[2]

Just above the bottom were GPs, general-purpose doctors who could turn their hands to any task presented to them (including a good deal of rough and ready emergency surgery) by people who couldn't afford a physician or surgeon with hospital appointments and membership of a Royal College. GPs far outnumbered physicians and surgeons, but had little professional influence until Lloyd George's Insurance Act of 1911 guaranteed at least subsistence earnings, just before the outbreak of the First World War.

At the bottom, numerous, uncounted and strictly excluded from the medical profession, were several sorts of people with specialised skills but no formal medical education. Their skills were developed from concentrated experience of particular problems, preceded by apprenticeship to someone with the accumulated experience of previous generations, often within occupational dynasties: itinerant tooth-pullers for dental abscesses, couchers for cataracts, bone-setters for fractures and dislocations,[3] abortionists for women who couldn't afford to have a baby, midwives for those coming to birth, sick–nurses for those approaching death, and general medicosurgical handymen, who seemed to emerge in every industrial community, to deal with whatever qualified practitioners did not do.[4] All these unqualified specialists the physicians and surgeons despised, persecuted and, so far as possible, excluded from the scope of medicine as an academic discipline.[5] Arguing from nothing but their own power and authority, any of their own professionals who sought to limit their practice in similar ways were condemned for unethical conduct, essentially because they might compete successfully for fees, and fees were thin on the ground in a narrow and fiercely defended market.

Starting around the middle of the 19th century, new instruments began to make the insides of the human body accessible for prospective diagnosis during life, approaching the standard of retrospective diagnosis already possible after death.[6] These instruments required much practice to acquire and maintain the skills necessary for their safe and effective use. The only way to get this experience was to specialise. For the rest of the 19th century, generalist physicians and surgeons fought a slowly losing battle against competition from these new, medically qualified specialists – eye specialists, ear, nose and throat specialists, skin specialists, eventually venereologists and specialists in tuberculosis – an ologist for every ology. In every case, doctors who did something all the time, and saw plenty of unusual cases, did it better and less dangerously than doctors who did it only some of the time, and saw such cases rarely.

By the end of the century, it was clear that the specialists were going to win this battle for trade. For big things, rich people were not going to bother with generalists, even if they held a teaching hospital appointment. They would go straight to whoever had the best reputation for competence in what seemed to be their own problem. They sought clinical skills derived from concentrated hospital experience with poor people, but they didn't yet want hospital admission for themselves. Hospitals were still dangerous places, designed for poor people with no alternative. As far as the rich were concerned, the functions of hospitals were to offer palliation to a token number of sick poor inpatients as a gesture towards social stability, and, more importantly, to provide experience for medical students and doctors, who could then apply that experience to rich people in their own homes.

Even for major surgery, people who could afford it were generally treated at home until after the First World War, when this balance began to reverse. By the end of the Second World War, the reversal was largely complete. Anyone who could afford it expected virtually all major illness to be at least initially treated in hospital.

Towards the end of the 19th century advances in medical science began to be visibly effective. GPs without hospital appointments saw many of their more affluent patients lost to hospital outpatient departments, where they could be attended by medical students or junior staff without fees, providing they could slip past the lady almoners who were supposed to exclude anyone able to pay.[7] During the first decade of the 20th century this increasingly bitter trade dispute came to a head. Paradoxically, it was resolved not by professionals, but by Lloyd George's Insurance Act of 1911. This gave GPs a basic income from the state for legitimising benefits and meeting local expectations for elementary care, for working men registered with them. Together with whatever private fees they might attract, this was sufficient for them to live in the manner customary for the middle class, without trying too hard to imitate specialists.[8] Hospital specialists, at least in the larger cities, could rely on sufficient private referrals from these GPs to pay for their tailors and chauffeurs and other requirements of consultant status.

The specialists and the GPs reached an understanding, framed as a code of professional ethics, enforceable not in law but by professional custom and the power of ostracism. Until the 1970s, the main concern of medical ethics was not competence, but etiquette: gentlemanly terms of trade and competition. In this new concordat, GPs would not attempt to treat illness beyond their own skills, but would refer problems beyond their competence to specialists with a hospital appointment, with a referral letter as their ticket of entry. Specialists would see patients only if they were referred by a GP, with a letter to prove it. In the words of the superb historian of this process, Rosemary Stevens, 'The consultants got the hospitals, and the GPs got the patients'.[9]

In theory, and usually in practice, when UK specialists had dealt with a problem, they would return the patient to the GP, with a letter explaining whatever else needed to be done for continuing care. Hence the term 'consultant'. Specialists had transient responsibility for an episode of illness, but otherwise only an advisory role. GPs 'owned' their patients, and their patients in aggregate formed the goodwill of their practice. This, along with their premises (often part of their own homes), formed their principal capital, which could be bought or sold in the professional marketplace, until the buying and selling of goodwill was made illegal in 1948.

Arrangements of more or less this sort eventually developed in all industrialised economies, but this happened much sooner and more completely in Britain than anywhere else. Even today, patients in France can refer themselves directly to the specialist of their choice, without consulting anyone in primary care to decide whether referral is appropriate.[10] In every country, rich doctors had rich patients, poor doctors had poor patients, but only in Britain did industrial manufacture employ an absolute majority of workers. Support for fee-earning medical trade by a small-town and rural middle class, the preferred clientele for liberal professionals, was correspondingly weak. This is one reason why Britain was the first capitalist country to develop a comprehensive NHS for its whole population. A wide network of community generalists had developed to select problems appropriate for referral to specialists, allowing these specialists really to specialise. This, the selective gatekeeper function of primary care, was the main secret of its affordable cost.

A consequence of this division was that UK GPs were separated from the hospitals, which increasingly monopolised all technical innovation, as well as teaching and research. To survive in their small corner shops, GPs had to spend as little as possible on staff, equipment or premises, so participation in teaching or research was almost out of the question. If they set aside any time for postgraduate learning, this was only to escape from general practice and try to reach some bottom rung of the specialist ladder. In the industrial areas where most people lived, GPs more or less reluctantly yielded all but the simplest tasks to specialists in hospital, because demand for these simplest clinical tasks was more than enough to take up all their available time, and the Insurance Act paid for it.

Particularly in industrial areas, GPs therefore remained a permanently inferior category, the poor bloody infantry of the medical army. They had much shorter training, lower incomes and lower social standing than consultants, and the useful skills they still had commanded little professional respect.[11] When I was working in NHS primary care, GPs were contracted to provide 'the services normally provided by a general practitioner' (to quote the words of our contract).[12] In other words, GPs were required to do what other GPs did, a resounding tautology which satisfied all governments from 1912 to 1990. Generalism was not developed as a necessary concept. Generalists were not recognised to have an important clinical role until 1966, when GPs seemed about to disappear, but that's another story, told later in this chapter.

Reification of disease

So far, specialisation has been considered in its professional rather than biological implications. Let us now consider it as a way to categorise illness.

Most people tend to think of diagnostic labels as derived from some pathological reality, readily separable from health. This must always be a falsification, though often a useful one. A disease exists always and only in an affected human being.[13] The malarial parasite in a mosquito only becomes malaria when the mosquito sucks blood from a human victim, and spits some malaria parasites back into its victim as it does so.

Even then, malaria does not develop as a disease unless these parasites overcome the varying but often successful resistance put up by their victim's immune system. All disease labels, without exception, represent disordered states of health in real people. No disease can be understood as a thing in itself. The process of thinking it so, of conceiving of diseases as enemies independent of their human vehicles, is reification of disease – turning a process into a thing.

Reification of disease has a long history, and a powerful grip on our language and imaginations.[14] Clinicians as scientists have looked for questions with potential answers, what Peter Medawar called 'the art of the soluble'. Clinicians as entrepreneurs, on the other hand, had to find consumers with wants. As professionals they were compelled to accept both scientific and entrepreneurial functions to at least some extent, so doctors have always had to make a living by addressing real problems as patients perceive them, leaving them little time or incentive to philosophise.

When they could do little about illness, other than state its nature and predict its likely course, their diagnostic labels were built around these descriptive and prophetic functions. As they acquired greater power to modify the course of illness, they devised new labels centred on different treatments. Not only different diseases, but different subsets of disease, and then subsets of subsets of disease, were found to respond better to an ever-increasing variety of interventions.

Searching the border between their expanding knowledge and their consequently expanding volume of perceived ignorance ('What we know we don't know', as Donald Rumsfeld would say), to have any hope of success scientists have had to divide this actually continuous boundary into manageable sections. They have simplified, and therefore to some extent falsified, the realities they study, in order to make a start, doing what they can, one bit at a time. In practice this reductionist approach has proved effective for beginning to solve many health problems. It provided the foundation for specialism.

An important consequence is that once any new field has been well developed, new advances tend to occur along its outer boundaries with other specialties, rather than at its core.[15] This potentially re-integrates fields that were formerly separate, in an endless cycle of initially useful but eventually counterproductive divisions, eventually succeeded by rediscovered unities. These may in turn prove more useful until they also have to be reconfigured in new ways, with greater explanatory and predictive power – always the tests of usefulness and provisional truth, closer to reality.

Multiple labels, and cascades of misfortune

By the 1960s, few people in developed economies were dying young from infectious diseases. As major causes of premature death, infections were disappearing, to be replaced by injuries, auto-immune diseases, cancers and degenerative conditions of the brain and circulation (AIDS had not yet arrived, and tuberculosis had not yet been reborn). None of these causes resembled invasions by parasites like malaria or diphtheria, though this was still the way most people thought about them. They were more like internal mutiny or decay.[16] With an appropriate weapon aimed accurately by a correct diagnosis, doctors could kill pneumonia or meningitis with a quick burst of fire over a few days, with little risk of injuring their patients. They had much less need to know them personally, than when their main weapon was the placebo effect. Internal mutinies and decays, on the other hand, were inseparable from the lives they impaired or shortened. To prevent, recognise or delay them required lifelong supervision and follow-up,[17] and intelligent participation by patients themselves – in some ways, a reversion to the more personal knowledge required before the development of impersonal medical science.[18]

From middle age onwards, most diseases now no longer appear singly. Perception of more than one disease label (co-morbidity) has become the rule rather than the exception.[19] This multiplicity increases with age,[20] and also with descending social class.[21] This is partly because misfortune is fertile: the more problems you have, the more you are likely to get. Life for many people becomes just one damned thing after another, a cascade of cumulative misfortunes, social as well as medical. Each downward step falls harder, further and faster, adding more problems to those already there, finally galloping down to an abyss from which there is no escape. There is no mystery about social class differences in morbidity or mortality, which increase at every stage of human development throughout life.[22] Every experienced worker in primary medical or social care knows families so beset with multiple and multiplying problems that hope shrinks down to survival from one day to the next, plus whatever comfort people may find in mystical beliefs.

This cascading process is enormously significant for the economy of health care. Early interventions, requiring little technical skill but much time and thoughtful social experience and judgement by a few locally known primary care staff, can be far more cost-effective than late crisis interventions using high technology, large teams and refined expertise.[23] Yet over and over again, resource-starved acute services provided by end-stage specialists are compelled to steal from the anticipatory care budgets of primary generalists, so as to sustain crisis care and thus hopefully avert public scandals, pillorying by journalists and the ire of politicians losing votes at the next election. No one with their feet on the ground can justify withholding care in a crisis because anticipatory care for those not yet in crisis would be more cost-effective. Consequently, crisis care is our everyday reality in most generalist public services, in social services even more than in the NHS. When services are grossly underfunded overall, as they were in the UK for at least the last three decades of the 20th century, anticipatory care of people not yet seriously ill is forced into grossly unequal competition with heroic end-stage salvage by specialists. In such conditions, which are likely soon to recur as the British economy slides closer to bankruptcy, generalists and anticipatory care will always lose, until they get protection from planned investment in primary care with clear clinical strategies, in an NHS using its own intelligence rather than abdicating responsibility to contractors competing for consumers in a state-subsidised market.

Specialist probabilities, generalist possibilities

Reified disease becomes a counterproductive concept whenever we look back from end-stage diseases to their origins. This is where primary generalists may find their best opportunities to reverse, delay or arrest progression to gross disease requiring specialist care. Late or necropsy diagnosis, from which our entire classification of disease and system of clinical thought was developed in the 19th and early 20th centuries, concerns converging probabilities in people sick enough to enter teaching hospitals, established as museums of gross, end-stage pathology, now dominated by specialists.[24] Early diagnosis, on the other hand, the chief concern of all health professionals in primary care, concerns diverging possibilities in people not yet ill. Generalists hope to keep most of their patients out of hospitals, and possibly free from sickness of any kind. Generalists need a different system of thought, including management of end-stage disease because this will never disappear, but far wider in scope to include the first origins of disease, often much earlier in life, when the future, positive or negative, is far less predictable. Generalists deal mainly with divergent possibilities, specialists deal mainly with convergent probabilities.

Data produced by specialists are often misunderstood by everyone else – generalists, media and the public – because they fail to take this difference into account. It is a fact, known everywhere since the 1950s, that smokers have a roughly 20-fold greater risk of getting lung cancer than non-smokers. But it is also a fact that of all smokers averaging one pack a day, only about one in eight ever actually gets lung cancer (though a much higher proportion get coronary heart disease and/or chronic obstructive lung disease, often ending in deaths more unpleasant than those caused by cancer). So for each lesson from personal experience that smoking kills in this dramatic way, there are another seven lessons from personal experience that it does not. Similar figures exist for virtually all known truly causal risks for specific disease.[25]

If you cross even a fairly busy road blindfold, you probably still have a greater than 50% chance of reaching the other side unharmed. Nobody concludes from this common-sense observation that this is a safe way to cross the road, because we are all familiar with the many different variables involved in the probability of a collision. Unfortunately we have not yet learned how to think about or to present wider aspects of human biology in similar terms. A major reason for this is the way we have become accustomed to discuss diseases as if they were things rather than processes – reification. People are generally aware of what is likely to happen around them, at home and at work – and of what is unlikely to happen. Overstatement of risks or benefits, above all by expressing them as percentage rate increases or rate reductions (relative risks) rather than as changes in absolute risk,[26] simply confuses people and promotes sceptical views of scientific evidence.[27] It also invites reversion to fatalism, superstition and denial, particularly in poorer populations with heavier and more complex burdens of ill health.[28]

For either the general public, or for generalists providing primary care in the community, clear thinking usually requires much broader categories than those used by specialists to manage specific diseases. If we tackle the earliest processes likely to lead to later disease, moving closer to initiating causes, instead of dividing health problems into ever smaller fragments for ever narrower specialties, we may be able to synthesise and unify solutions more comprehensible to patients and ourselves, with less duplication of staff, using simpler resources.

Though seven out of every eight smokers may escape lung cancer, they are very unlikely to be otherwise healthy. On average, lifelong smokers die about 10 years sooner than lifelong non-smokers, from a wide variety of terminal diseases. At any stage, stopping smoking is associated with longer average remaining lifespan than not stopping. Broadly speaking, the same applies to other unhealthy behaviours. Sustained intakes of energy from food larger than outputs of energy through physical activity cause obesity. This is causally associated with earlier average age of death, at least up to late middle age.[29] Together with smoking, obesity has become the most visible outward indicator of social class.[30]

Central obesity,[31] high blood pressure, type 2 diabetes, high blood cholesterol, and early disease of coronary and other major arteries, can all be gathered into a single category of insulin resistance (the metabolic syndrome).[32] Until they have already caused the major organ damage which their treatments are supposed to prevent, all of these so-called diseases are defined by points on a continuous distribution in any large population. What determines where these borders between health and disease lie? In theory, they should mark the point at which we have good evidence from clinical trials on appropriate populations that expected health gains from medical intervention substantially exceed health impairments caused by those interventions.[33] In practice, such evidence often does not exist, mainly because few large trials include patients similar to those most often seen in primary care. Participants in trials tend to be much younger, with less complicated health and social problems. For these conditions, the points of transition from health to disease are in practice set by expert consensus, dominated by specialists, and by powerful though usually indirect pressures from pharmaceutical companies to include ever higher proportions of people without symptoms, identified by some sort of screening.

The necessity of generalists

In 1966 there was a crisis of recruitment into British general practice. The work of GPs, particularly in industrial areas, was seen as 'perfunctory work by perfunctory men'.[34] They specialised if they could find a post, and if not, they emigrated, mainly to Canada, Australia and New Zealand. GPs were disappearing even faster in the US, because specialists' earnings were (and still are) very much higher than generalists' earnings.[35] NHS administrators looking across the Atlantic realised that the collapse of general practice in the US was creating a professional system which even the US couldn't afford – a system where every doctor would soon either actually be a specialist, or pretend to be one.[36] All but the least serious diseases would be dealt with in hospitals by specialists, and nobody would be left to deal with the 90% of problems which did not need that level of care.

The result was a turning point for British general practice: the GP Charter.[37] Its most important features were: a rapid rise in GP incomes, approaching equivalence to the lower rungs of the specialist ladder; state funding for GPs' buildings, and majority funding for their office and nursing staff; and state funding for their postgraduate training.

Organisation of this last was effectively handed to the newly founded Royal College of General Practitioners, giving it assured funding for its development, and an important reason for its continued existence and significance. This led in turn to eventual creation of departments of primary care in all British medical schools, and a much less hierarchical relationship between generalists and specialists.[38] The 1966 Charter succeeded in stemming what had been a catastrophic out-migration of British graduates to the US, Canada, Australia and New Zealand. It raised the status of general practice to create for the first time a large cohort of GPs for whom this career was a positive choice, rather than a last resort after failing to specialise.

Primary care as a medical specialty, emphasising continued development of generalist skills, originated in Great Britain. Progress was soon much faster in the Netherlands and Scandinavia, where government funding was eventually more generous and political support was more consistent, but the British NHS was where it began.

From this new origin, British general practice developed rapidly for the next two decades, though more slowly in industrial (and in later years post-industrial) areas, than in affluent areas, because very high workloads made progress more difficult; because industrial employment and unemployment generated high bureaucratic workloads almost unknown in affluent suburbs and market towns; and because independent contractor status left investment in the hands of GPs, with powerful incentives to invest in more staff and better buildings where property values were rising, but perverse incentives to invest as little as possible in poorer areas, where property values, populations, and therefore practice earnings were all falling.[39]

For the most part, this development looked in an entirely new direction, away from the technical skills and biochemical knowledge developing in hospitals, towards interpersonal and social skills required to select accurately problems appropriate for care in the community, or for referral for care by specialists based in hospitals. Even today, these interpersonal skills command far less respect than technical skills, but without them, technical skills cannot be applied appropriately.

Productivity in primary care

By the 1980s, government was again turning its attention to generalist care in communities, as a more affordable alternative to specialist care in hospitals.[40] Our experience in Glyncorrwg, already referred to in the last chapter, apparently provided part of the outline model for what eventually became the GP contract in 2004.[41] A speech in

1989 by Conservative Secretary of State for Health Kenneth Clarke signalled an entirely new agenda for primary care, followed by every government since.[42]

Before Clarke, no minister for health (including Aneurin Bevan) had ever taken the clinical product of primary care seriously. Governments had been concerned almost exclusively with satisfying users, rather than verifiably improving either their health, the health of their communities, or even the efficiency of GPs as gatekeepers to hospital-based specialists. The task of GPs had been to take responsibility for whatever was either as yet untreatable by hospital-based specialists, or could be considered too trivial to merit their attention. In this view, hospital specialists provided the engine for the NHS, primary care provided the clutch, and patients in populations provided the extremely variable road surface. GPs connected hospital specialists to popular needs, while defending them from the full impact of undifferentiated, unprioritised public wants, in a service where the specialist engine was always overworked and underfunded.[43]

Unlike hospitals in the US or most other West European countries, NHS hospitals could concentrate on work appropriate to them, because access to specialists in the NHS was obtainable only through referral from GPs. Accident and emergency (A&E) departments[44] provided an alternative direct pathway, but until recently this was generally regarded as a serious weakness in the primary care system which ought to be remedied, rather than as an inevitable feature of hospital care requiring additional specialist staff and hospital resources, and finally a plurality of access scattered around any supermarket willing to act as a contracted provider. Apart from socially marginalised groups, such as homeless people and prisoners, almost everyone in the pre-'reform' UK NHS had free access to a GP functioning as a personal doctor,[45] acting also as gatekeeper. Gatekeeping GPs were supposed to act both in the interests of government concerned to contain costs of hospital care, and in the interests of patients concerned to avoid iatrogenic risks disproportionate to probable benefits.[46]

More than any other single factor, this gatekeeper function made the NHS more cost-effective than any other Western care system, as in most other Northern and West European systems patients had direct access either to specialists,[47] or at least to 'specialoids'.[48] However, governments concentrated their attention on what they wanted to see – that primary care was much cheaper than hospital care. They saw also that primary care was often slipshod, poorly organised, understaffed and badly equipped – a primitive cottage industry. As GPs were independent contractors, this could plausibly be attributed to professional greed rather than government parsimony. Once the usefulness of GPs was recognised, the remedy seemed obvious – primary care needed an order-of-magnitude larger investment, to raise its work to standards comparable with hospitals. GPs acting only as signposts and selectors for referral of about 5–10% of their consultations to hospital-based specialists were cheap for the other 90% or so of consultations which GPs dealt with themselves. However, accurate choices for referral depended on generalist skills of high quality and sophistication, and on sufficient consultation time to exert those skills. All these requirements raised the real costs of primary care. Patients' acceptance of gatekeeping depended on confidence that primary care was appropriate and effective for the responsibilities it retained, and that the gate was opened or closed in their, the patients', interest, not just to save money for government in an always underfunded service. Investment in primary care would have to rise if its clinical functions were to become effective enough to justify and sustain this trust.[49]

This unwelcome conclusion seems to have been about as far as UK central government was willing to go, keeping within the bounds of conventional opinion about primary care. The quality of undergraduate and in-service postgraduate training and teaching for GPs has been generally excellent for the past two decades, and is set to improve even more over the next few years, with a very impressive programme of compulsory postgraduate training, eventually over five years. It is even now much better organised (for its own purposes) than equivalent training and education for specialists. In 1948, the obvious way to increase investment in primary care and develop it in new directions would have been to organise it in the same way as hospitals – to nationalise whatever provision already existed, and make GPs salaried professional employees on terms similar to those agreed with specialists in the nationalised hospitals. At some time in the future this must return to the political agenda.

Meanwhile, government must somehow contain costs by raising the efficiency of specialist care, and by using skills which most community generalists now possess. Above all, we need more selective and accurate referral, but both New Labour and Conservative policies fragment the gatekeeping function on which this depends.[50] Doctors and nurses graduating today have far greater skills than their predecessors, when GPs were just regarded as a clutch for the hospital specialist engine. A large part of hospital outpatient care is done by junior medical staff in training, so with suitable buildings, and nursing and office teams, they should be able to do it later in primary care.

Slimming down the outpatient department

In 1979, John Fry compared the health care systems in Britain, the US and the USSR. He suggested that the NHS occupied an intermediate position between almost completely unsocialised, marketed care in the US, propped up by a multitude of ad hoc state agencies and charities on the one hand, and the rigid system of specialoid care in Soviet polyclinics on the other.[51] In particular, he noted how Soviet polyclinics apparently eliminated the need for hospital outpatient departments, whose continued expansion in the British NHS seemed both unaffordable and unstoppable. A large part of the medical work of NHS outpatient departments was being done by young doctors in training, roughly half of whom would end up working as GPs, but evidence showed that they then seemed to lose this competence, with frightening consequences for the safety of patients.[52] If some way could be found to develop primary care so that GPs could continue to perform relatively simple clinical functions they had learned while training in hospitals, huge reductions in cost might be possible, and GPs pining for more concentrated clinical experience of the familiar kind might find greater satisfaction in their work. Everyone would win, nobody would lose.

There was no danger then that anyone elsewhere in Europe would rush to replace GPs with polyclinics. The USSR was no longer a convincing model for anyone. However, in 2008 these were proposed by Lord Darzi, an eminent rectal surgeon and oncologist chosen by the New Labour government to reorganise primary care in England (of which he had no personal experience) and integrate it with specialist care.[53] Contracts to plan, manage and recruit staff for these polyclinics were opened to corporate bidders of any kind, either commercial or consortia of professionals, funded more generously than traditional providers. They were apparently intended to provide a 24-hours-a-day service, but for at least some of this time they relied entirely on a staff mix of specialist medical skills, with no GPs at all. In one leap, consumers were invited to bypass primary care and take themselves to the specialist of their choice.

Whether this scenario will ever be implemented outside London now seems doubtful. Operating costs would be high and profit margins low, at least for the first couple of years, while some semblance of public service would have to be maintained. As the global economy slides into recession, private sector investors are becoming more sceptical about likely profits from health care, particularly from really sick people, and several corporate providers have already withdrawn from this market.[54] Even if these plans continue, they seem to rest on a strategy completely contrary to all research evidence and experience from primary care. They repeat the strategic error of post-war Swedish governments, ignoring the need for generalists at the periphery of the NHS, at the interface between health and illness, to discriminate efficiently between people who need referral and those for whom this would probably be counterproductive. Within conventional thinking, primary generalists seem to face mounting difficulties, not only because of pressures to privatise public services,[55] but because the value of generalist skills is still so poorly understood, even by otherwise well-informed people. Just because polyclinics should not be parachuted onto existing primary care services does not mean it would be wrong to plan a general shift of outpatient care away from hospitals, back to primary care. It has long been obvious that much of what medical students and junior staff learn in hospitals is lost and wasted after they leave to work as primary generalists in the community. Strong departments of primary care, which now exist at all UK medical and nursing schools, are producing staff who should be able to adapt hospital outpatient follow-up techniques to work in community centres, with many advantages over hospitals, provided they do not imagine they have nothing to learn from experienced staff already working in primary care and the body of research they have already produced, and provided that staff numbers are appropriately increased. For people well enough to lead more or less normal lives, hospitals have never been the right places for continuing care. Serving families in small, relatively stable communities, the knowledge which staff can gain and friendships they can build from a wide variety of sources can be cumulative. This would make it much easier to develop patients as colleagues, co-producers of their own and each other's health, with minimal drop-out, error, waste and bureaucracy. Some committed GPs in poor urban areas, even with annual patient turnovers well over 30%, are in fact managing to follow patients with common chronic health problems at least as successfully as outpatient clinics did in the past, and probably more so. Despite sustained encouragement of consumer choice by government and media through league tables and divisive competition, most people remain as stubbornly attached to their local doctors and local nurses as they are to their local hospitals, so the opportunity still exists.

Moving some of the simpler work of specialists into primary care is a sensible step, which everyone should welcome so long as it is properly funded (an essential proviso which is by no means guaranteed). Work might then be done to at least the same standard as it was in hospital outpatient clinics, and probably better, because drop-out could be much reduced. By itself, however, this does nothing to develop generalist skills and attitudes.

Is your generalist really necessary?

Dr Geoffrey Marsh, a pioneer of teamwork in primary care in the 1970s, believed that future GPs should delegate most if not all first contacts with patients to practice nurses or nurse-practitioners, and that this could release doctors to deal with more concentrated clinical problems, more appropriate to their costly skills.[56] This was and still is a plausible argument, and all the more attractive when health workers of all kinds usually gain higher incomes and status from more specialised functions and technical management of well-defined disease, depending less upon interpersonal skills. It appeals particularly to managers accustomed to industrial divisions of labour, where gains in efficiency often seem to depend on standardised tasks, with minimal human judgement.[57] Within this paradigm, primary care is not the foundation of the NHS as a whole, but its outermost boundary, the border between health and sickness. Decisions at this point plausibly seem less important, requiring less education, less thought and less precision than they do at points more central to the system. The idea is exemplified by the role of the triage nurse in A&E departments, whose task is to sort patients at entry into broad categories of need, before they see any doctor at all. This role has recently appeared in some large group practices, which implicitly accept the same philosophy.[58]

This case is rarely stated in such stark terms. Rhetorically, GPs are often flattered, and flatter themselves, as the cream of their profession. They are said to provide a warm familiarity with clinically unimportant details of everyday life, often lacking in specialists. This reassuring image underlies the term 'family doctor', supporting cosy memories of past social stability. When it comes to real priorities for investment in staff and development, this nostalgic sentimentality soon evaporates, and primary care is returned to where it belongs, at the back of the queue for material resources. As everyone knows, the cosy image does not, and never did, represent the real experience of most ordinary patients, or the GPs who served them.[59]

About one quarter of all NHS doctors work in primary care as GPs. In 2007 they employed about one twentieth of the entire nursing workforce as practice nurses, in an average ratio of about one practice nurse to two GPs. About four times as many nurses, including home nurses, midwives, health visitors and several kinds of specialised public health nurses, work in the community outside hospitals. Most of them work in patients' homes. Initially they were employed by local government, then, since 1974, by NHS authorities.[60] Like GPs, community nurses have always formed a stable workforce, with the cumulative knowledge, friendships and efficiencies of long local experience. Urban practices are often very dispersed, with different families in the same street registered with different GPs, so it would have been more logical to attach GPs to community nurses, than the other way round. Though many think it is now too late to change, urban practices are now tending to become more concentrated, with more of them applying rational zoning policies for recruitment, so we may get back to locality, even in cities.[61]

As we have seen, throughout the UK, central and regional government policies aim to shift as much work as they can away from hospital outpatient departments, into primary care. This implies that the community and practice nursing workforce must expand faster than the acute hospital nursing workforce. In England at least (I have no figures for other UK regions) this does seem to have been achieved. Between 1996 and 2006, whole time equivalent (WTE) practice nurses increased by 48% and community nurses by 38%, whereas hospital nurses increased by only 29%.[62] Over the same period, the number of WTE GPs rose by only 2%. New GP contracts include powerful economic incentives (through QOF) for GPs to produce evidence that they are identifying patients who need continuing care for chronic health impairments and risks, and that they are treating them, monitoring their progress and reaching target levels of control. The only way this evidence can be produced is to delegate an increasing proportion of this work to non-medical staff, initially to practice nurses, now increasingly to health care assistants, usually with at least some training, but no specified qualification, and sometimes simply two or three school-leaving grades.[63] Quality control in this field seems to be approaching a dangerous state.

Delegation of tasks to less-qualified staff absolutely requires guidelines. Guidelines for continuing care of single diseases in patients believed to have no other health problems are probably valid for the small minority of patients in this simple condition, but after middle age, most are not. Adding together all the guidelines for patients with multiple problems, assuming that each diagnosis and each treatment is independent of the others, cannot be right – but in practice, that is what we are doing. Even annual reviews of care may be delegated by some less conscientious GPs to less-qualified or even unqualified staff, because the role and training of health care assistants are still not defined. Added risks incurred by delegated work following guidelines may be small, but so are the health gains to be expected from each treatment, if we look at the scientific evidence rather than the advertising or the opinions of eminent clinicians getting thousands of dollars for lectures that just happen to endorse the medications sold by their corporate sponsors. No doctor is compelled to listen to pharmaceutical salespersons, but about 80% still choose to do so, and thus receive their postgraduate education from systematically biased sources.[64]

How sure can we really be that probable gains exceed possible losses? The benefit of the doubt is seldom so obvious as first appears. At best, it depends on interaction between professional information and judgement, and patients' circumstances and priorities, synthesised to an agreed conclusion. At worst (and more often), it depends also on whether the money spent by pharmaceutical companies on all forms of promotion (greater than what they spend on research) succeeds in its purpose.[65] As this spending still continues, evidently it does; companies do not deliberately waste their money.

Obviously this extremely complex role cannot be played by practice nurses or health care assistants operating only as cogs within a guidelined and tick-boxed machine. When most routine contacts with patients are with narrowly trained staff, constrained to think and work within guidelines designed for the smooth highway of trials in hospital clinics rather than the rutted and potholed alleys of care in the community, the product may be more process but less outcome. These very complex decisions need far more professional thought than they have had in the past, more and better evidence, and more participation by patients in decision making. This particularly concerns priorities, above all in the very young and the very old. People approaching the end of their lives know very well they have to die. They are entitled to choose their own priorities more than most are now able to do. Precisely because they have less education, practice nurses and health care assistants often seem more friendly and accessible than doctors, but if they are encouraged only to perform tasks rather than think about them and question them, they cannot even begin to learn how to help patients to become critical participants in decisions about their own care.

Primary care needs to operate within a new paradigm, almost entirely different from the industrial commodity production or provision of standardised services from which conventional views of medical economics are ultimately derived. Of course primary care needs to be planned and managed, with rational resource allocation geared to national wealth and consensus priorities, but its efficiency depends mainly on imaginative use of all human interactions by a growing and ever more labour-intensive and more educated workforce, not on replication of standardised procedures by a shrinking workforce with narrower skills, in an ever more capital-intensive industry.

Trust

Public opinion surveys have repeatedly confirmed that people trust doctors and nurses more than any other occupational group. In spite of generally unforgiving media comment on medical errors over the past three decades, 91% of the British public still trust doctors to tell them the truth, compared with 88% for teachers, 77% for university professors, 76% for judges, 20% for politicians and 16% for journalists (these figures preceded recent political scandals).[66]

To maintain trust in their effectiveness as well as their truthfulness, advancing knowledge needs to be applied as well in primary care, as specialists apply it in hospitals. For both to reach comparable standards, this will require more material resources and staff in-service development, and larger and more diverse teams, implying a substantial shift in the balance between investment in primary care and hospital care. If public investment on the scale required continues to be routed through GPs' pockets as independent contractors, running small businesses where profits depend on how much of this money they keep for themselves and their families and how much they spend on care for their patients, it may be used less efficiently than it is now used in hospitals. Without bringing GPs into a single framework of salaried service employing all NHS staff, this development will probably not occur.

However, even if primary care were organised consistently as an area public service rather than a local business, and GPs were salaried like hospital specialists and doctors in training, there would still be a problem. Heroic salvage of late disease always trumps mundane anticipatory care, a robust tendency clearly visible in commissioning by Primary Care Trusts (PCTs) in England and Local Health Boards in Wales. Determined leadership will be needed from the top, to make space for workers in primary care to measure the quality of their work in their own terms, rather than the ways specialist care is measured in hospitals.

Good primary care is not a cheaper alternative to specialist care, either in hospital departments or in outreach polyclinics. We need to look more imaginatively for successful models of care in the community – not GP corner shops, not corporate supermarkets, not specialoid modifications of specialist outpatient departments, but units organised to take full advantage of the trusting relationships possible for local primary care teams known personally to their communities, by making personal responsibility and continuity of care central to every strategy.

Forgotten models for primary care

Before the advent of penicillin and streptomycin, syphilis and tuberculosis were major causes of incapacitating illness and premature death, with a huge impact on society. GPs working as shopkeepers were unable to develop the teamwork needed to address these problems effectively. Measures were therefore taken in every advanced economy to create networked clinics specialising in their early detection and control – chest clinics and venereal disease clinics. Throughout the UK, every local government authority had responsibility for establishing and maintaining these clinics, through their public health departments, led until 1974 by Medical Officers of Health.[67] Treatments for tuberculosis were almost completely ineffective before streptomycin, but transmission at work and within families could be controlled by educating patients in safe disposal of sputum, and by isolating them in sanatoria, often for several years until their deaths, so this strategy did help to control spread of the disease. Treatments for syphilis with injections of arsenic derivatives were effective, but very unpleasant and potentially dangerous, requiring skilled medical supervision. Even after antibiotics made treatment of these diseases more effective in the 1950s, treatments needed close supervision to be effective and prevent emergence of resistant disease. At every point, staff at both these clinics had to bear in mind not only treatment, but from where the disease had come, and where next it might go. They had to think about the social conditions in which tuberculosis and sexually transmitted disease thrived, they had to educate patients about the nature of their infection and how they could prevent transmission to their partners, families and friends, and they had to persuade patients to accept treatment not just in their own interest, but the interest of their partners, their children, and of society as a whole. They could never rely only on what patients wanted, they had to consider what they, and everyone else they were in contact with, needed, while still maintaining goodwill sufficient to keep patients coming to the clinic. All this work had to be done within bounds of confidentiality, set more by experience than by managers or expert committees. To work effectively, staff needed profound and subtle understanding of the communities they served. They had to discard judgemental and punitive attitudes, and concentrate on damage limitation rather than scolding or preaching.[68]

All these qualities closely resemble those we need now for effective primary care for the full range of health problems, not just these infectious diseases. We need to remember that many disorders, other than those caused by bacteria or viruses, are infectious. Behaviours are infectious: eating dangerously, drinking dangerously, drugging dangerously, domestic violence, neglect or abuse of children – existence of any of these in one person has damaging effects on others, and promotes similar behaviour.

One important feature of these clinics seems to me particularly important for development of effective anticipatory care today. At the end of every clinic session, members of the staff team considered the no-shows – the patients who had failed to attend – and what should be done about them. We could not allow patients with tuberculosis or syphilis to drift out of view, without finding their reasons for non-attendance, and if possible, winning them back. This could not be done with a heavy hand. Laws did exist, which might have been used to compel attendance, but I never saw them applied. If they had been used, I suspect they would have been counterproductive. Every non-attender was followed up, by a telephone call or a home visit, usually by a specialist community nurse.[69]

Imaginative and responsible work of this sort, adapted to what individual patients and particular communities want and can cope with, is the direct opposite of the narrow, task-oriented work allocated to GPs by current guidelines, and largely delegated by them to their practice nurses and care assistants. By apologists for the provider–consumer model of care, it will be dismissed as paternalistic. People who use that term need to think more about what it actually means. Most fathers are not bullying patriarchs. Primary care teams should aim at relationships with their patients that do indeed resemble those in stable and affectionate families and friendship networks – fraternal care. So-called paternalism may be a step toward this higher state. As a first step on the way, 'maternalistic' might describe better what is immediately feasible in most circumstances. Patients who want only an impersonal relationship with a completely detached expert on everything must somehow be fitted into our pattern of care, but such expectations are primitive, and we should aim higher than this. A good team learns to adapt its work to all sorts of people, but it also needs to know where it is going – toward expanding citizenship, not consumerism.

Teaching and research in primary care

The huge advances made by specialists in both curative medicine and public health medicine cannot be applied effectively or efficiently without an equal development of generalists in primary care, with two principal tasks: to bring together the amazing products of specialised analysis into clinical syntheses appropriate to the usually unique requirements of real people leading independent lives; and to apply the general measures devised by public health from evidence from large, anonymous populations, to small, local populations with names, personal stories and local community histories.

These generalists will have huge responsibilities. We cannot go on pretending that a patient in her 60s with diabetes, high blood pressure, nicotine dependence, chronic obstructive lung disease, a periodically depressed husband, one grandchild with Down's syndrome and another who evades school and is in trouble with the police can be helped just by adding together seven different guidelines and following all of them, for so long as she will tolerate such interference. Complex problems of this sort, which account for most of the work of primary care (and will account for much of the work of hospital care if primary care fails), have to depend on clinical and social judgements.[70]

Even with small list sizes, personal doctors and continuity, care of this sort will need team care, with more staff and a wider variety of skills. All the health workers concerned in such complex cases need to exert judgement, because real patients do not restrict their participation in care to consultations with doctors – on the contrary, they often find it easier to start with staff less distant from themselves in education and culture, and more easily approachable. In any case, nobody working in primary health care should be made to work, or even allowed to work, without thinking about what they are doing or why they are doing it. This means that the whole team needs to meet regularly to discuss outstanding problems, and agree on responsibilities for their solution. It means that everyone in the team needs to participate in some sort of learning and teaching. Learning and teaching should begin from personal, local experience, because this is most efficient and effective. That means they need also to participate in data collection, to provide evidence of where the unit has come from, where it now stands, and where it is going, in relation to its denominator population. This is continuing audit, the most elementary form of research, an essential function for every unit of the NHS: to be able to describe the population it serves, and the service it provides, in terms comparable with other units serving other populations.

Every primary care unit needs to teach, every primary care unit needs to research, because teaching and research keep staff awake, inquisitive and self-critical and minimise the dangers they present to patients, and maximise their output of health gain. These should not be optional or exceptional functions. They are just as essential to efficiency as the provisional strategies suggested by guidelines. The teaching need not be formal, nor part of a centrally planned structure like the GP registrar scheme. It may simply consist of organising practice so as to encourage education of patients in the nature of their disorders, and clinical education of practice staff, so that everyone shares in the continuous expansion of applied medical science. The research need not aim at publication, or even application outside the practice. Research simply means trying to discover anything that is not yet known, but seems likely to be useful. Nobody will know much about the problems or opportunities of your local population until you organise to find this out, and nobody will know what your unit actually does until you audit its work. Collecting data required by government to justify practice income, of which QOF data are an obvious example, is research for a different purpose, with different sources of error. Data of that kind may end by concealing more than they reveal.

Until practice of this sort becomes commonplace, it will be hard to get far beyond this tentative outline. As Barbara Starfield has argued, even in the new age of applied genetics, cell biochemistry, organ replacement and nanotechnology, either primary care will become one of the largest, most important and influential areas for research, or most of the potential benefits of these other advances will not reach most of the people who need them.[71]

A new kind of doctor

To insist that GPs, hitherto the lowest form of medical life, should all immediately accept far wider responsibilities than specialists, hitherto the highest exponents of applied medical science, is not realistic. We must start from where we are, with the people we have. They are in any case already far in advance of those who know everything about medical science but nothing about the circumstances in which their colleagues have to apply it.[72]

Way back in 1995, when the world seemed simpler than today, it was already estimated that a general physician would need to digest 19 articles a day, 365 days a year, just in order to keep up to date with the whole field of internal medicine, never mind surgery, gynaecology, child health, geriatric medicine, psychiatry or public health. Obviously, even the specialists weren't really doing this. Even enthusiastic clinical teachers were claiming only to spend about two hours a week reading professional journals or books.[73] If specialists already find it impossible to know all they should, and generalists need to know even more than specialists, then progress must have ended long ago.

The reality is that those estimates were wrong, because most of the assumptions on which they were based had never been thought through. Relatively little of the professional literature is designed to be useful for making either clinical or organisational decisions. What there is has never been concentrated in the journals or books easily available to doctors or nurses directly responsible for patient care, nor has much of it been written in ways that connect easily with common experience. People read and do what they find useful. Very little of what gets published in medical journals seems useful to clinical generalists, so many of them stop looking at them.

New entrants to primary care now leaving UK medical schools generally have extremely high standards of education, high expectations and a generally better experience of clinical decisions in primary care than their colleagues in hospital care, because GPs involved in undergraduate teaching have adapted their ordinary service work to accommodate student experience much better than have the managers of large teaching hospitals. These undergraduates and new entrants should be the main targets for the much higher expectations and more imaginative performance we shall have to demand from primary generalists in the future.

General causes are at least as important as special effects

Next to smoking, obesity is the most serious recognised health problem facing advanced industrial and post-industrial societies (though bigger still, demoralisation is not yet a recognised problem). Dr Colin Guthrie, a Glasgow GP who has tried harder and more imaginatively than most to control it, reached the sensible conclusion that prevention of obesity was not a medical problem. As he pointed out, an extra 3 miles of walking every day could eventually enable 4kg of weight loss, reducing personal risk of developing diabetes by 58%. But 60% of the green space used for London housing in the past 10 years had come from the sale of playing fields.[74] His conclusion was that prevention of obesity and type 2 diabetes was an environmental problem, not a medical problem; patients understood this, doctors did not.[75] Or perhaps neither group would ever really understand it until they got together to demand and help to build a more rationally ordered society.

Doctors, community nurses and counsellors in primary care may all be of some use at the edges, but the central problem is the gigantic shift in society from domestic and industrial economies based on physical labour, where people moved about on their feet and worked with their backs, arms and legs, to a society where physical labour is increasingly replaced by machines, and people use only their fingertips. This need not be the final state of human society. We still have choices, and community-based generalists are exceptionally well placed to force this onto local and national political agendas, once they accept that their job includes this wider responsibility.

Social problems require social solutions. Medical professionalism (and all the other health care professions that follow its model) and patient consumerism have both been almost always oriented to personal rather than collective choices, actions and solutions – because nothing else has seemed possible. Was it inevitable that as men and women stopped having to work like cart horses, they would have to spend their lives standing beside machines, seated in front of computer screens, or in cars? Labour-saving machines should have released time for people to live, but in fact they were used to shrink the workforce, reduce labour costs and augment profits, because all the decisions remain with employers of labour, and they must above all make profits. Healthy life includes using all of one's body and all of one's mind at full stretch, but these ends have never been pursued either by employers, or by governments that serve them. In practice, profit comes not from expanding lives, but from shrinking them down to ever narrower tasks. Post-war plans to provide safe access to work by bicycle were abandoned as soon as most people had cars, forgetting that in many poor areas at least one third of all families still do not own one. Between 1974 and 1994 cycling to and from work fell from 25% of human traffic to 1%.[76] Local initiatives to promote safe urban cycling, like the good beginnings made by Ken Livingstone as Mayor of London, were never generalised as UK policy. Sport in schools was actually downgraded after 1979, and schools, local government and the NHS were encouraged to sell off public open spaces and playing fields to developers.[77] Sports and fitness facilities have expanded, but almost entirely as for-profit clubs without free public access. Even publicly owned swimming pools charge for entry, except in Wales, where they are now free for all children and pensioners.[78]

Time spent in supporting and leading local initiatives to make it easier for people to do things actively instead of just watching them on television could be far more effective in promoting health than our largely futile attempts at individual control of obesity. Even when people accept that body weight must ultimately depend on the balance between energy consumption and energy expenditure, they usually start by concentrating mostly on energy input – the nature and volume of food consumed – simply because this has been what most doctors talked about, was easiest to research,[79] seemed most susceptible to personal control and seemed least dependent on a way of life most people felt powerless to change. If you look for them, you find many examples of patients who are actually well ahead of professional practice, who have developed their own programmes for active exercise. The problem is to make these numerous personal advances into a general demand for more physically active lives, at home and at work.

Why cannot community generalists help to generate and lead local demand for change? Primary care staff have lists of names, addresses, telephone numbers and e-mail addresses, they know which of their patients are actual or potential movers and shakers, they can organise election of representative committees to agree on projects with potentially mass support. So rapid mobilisation of civic action should be possible. With little evident difference today between any of the major political parties once they get into power, old political loyalties have lost most of their meaning. It should therefore be easier to mobilise inclusive social alliances for civic objectives, while still respecting traditions of professional neutrality.[80]

People get the public facilities they are willing to fight for, and keep fighting to retain. In this necessary and continuous community struggle, primary care staff should be leaders, not spectators. Doctors and nurses serving local communities already have immense public authority and respect. If they use these imaginatively to promote collective health measures, elected politicians will listen to them, if only for their own re-election.[81]

Summary and conclusions

Since the early 19th century, medical specialisation has been driven by two forces: by science, through analysis of physiological and pathological processes, with consequent division and subdivision of these into apparently separate parts; and by a more general culture which tends to compartmentalise civic responsibility, leaving major societal decisions to operation of the market. Continuous human stories are thus divided into episodic parts, with isolated problems, classified into specialised groups. They may then be handled with apparently greater efficiency, and much of this has been real.

Generalists have always existed, but until the 1960s – in many places, much later – they were a residual category. The number of generalists was a measure of backwardness, and the number of specialists was a measure of progress. As the complexity of problems of real patients in the real world comes to be recognised, we need to develop generalists with wider and deeper skills to coordinate the inevitably increasing number and diversity of specialists.

The main reason why from 1948 to 1979 the NHS was more cost-effective than any other socially inclusive health care system was its (inadvertent) retention of community generalists as gatekeepers to specialist care, and as familiar and trusted guardians and interpreters of patients' life stories, who could hold the specialised fragments of care together as a comprehensible whole. Continued advance of effective specialist care depends on parallel advance in this integrating and synthetic function of generalists. In the presently dominant culture of NHS management in England, developed from business experience and following an industrial model, this is not recognised. This is leading to demoralisation of staff and confusion of patients. If commercial and scientific cultures could again be separated, and public service be restored as an independent developing gift economy, the integrating and synthetic function of generalists could develop faster and more cost-effectively than ever before. This will not happen unless health care professionals accept much wider social and political responsibilities, as leading citizens in the communities they serve.

FIVE

Ownership

Production systems may be owned by health professional entrepreneurs (singly or collectively), by senior managers and shareholders, by cooperative collectives or by the state (with varying degrees of public accountability or participation). All except a few idiosyncratic single-handed practitioners now have office staff, nursing staff, and land, buildings, equipment and so on – a team essential to effective work. For each of these players, ownership is always a centrally important question. For each of them, ownership is differently conceived and defined.

Because patients are increasingly compelled to accept roles either as consumers (for whom the ownership of a providing agency is a matter of indifference: what matters is the commodity they provide), or as co-producers of health gain (for whom ownership must be important, because this determines the motivation of their professional partners in the production process), so the ideas of patients about ownership of the service, and of its subordinate parts, have become as important as those of all other players.

Ownership relates not only to the buildings, equipment and other requirements for effective work in health care, but to the work itself. Adam Smith recognised that people work more productively for their own gain than to help others. This was his justification for the profit motive, which in itself he did not admire, referring to it as 'self-love'. This explained the higher productivity of capitalism than the feudal agriculture it replaced as foundation and legal framework for commodity production. It also explained the higher productivity of serfdom than slavery. However onerous their tithes, taxes and tribute to landowners, sharecroppers worked more productively than slaves because they could, to at least some extent, work for themselves. With transition from craft skills to machine minding, we see both a huge rise in productivity from human labour plus the labour of machines, and declining craft skills and a fall in their value, as their productivity compared with machines declines. In industrialised labour, people themselves become tools, to be hired or discarded as market requirements and the progress of machinery dictate. Ownership of one's own work in imagination is as important as, and potentially distinct from, ownership of the material requirements for participation in work.

Origins of property in health care

Together with specific treatments made possible by knowledge gained almost entirely in the past 150 years, recovery from illness requires the same factors as those required to maintain normal health. These have been known for thousands of years: clean air, food, water, shelter, sewage disposal and security. Social conditions providing access to these for everyone should therefore be the primary aim of any rational global economy. Their active provision for sick people should be the first step for any care system.[1] For an overwhelming majority of people in the eras preceding industrial capitalism, the tasks required for care of people too sick to care for themselves were initially done by families, almost entirely by mothers, daughters and grandmothers, outside any marketplace. Where support from extended families or neighbours failed, a main task of all the main world religions was to provide it in similar terms. Almost all of this was nursing. Whereas if nobody nursed seriously ill people they died, hardly anyone died for lack of a doctor, and many might have had a better chance of survival without one. This religious tradition of care persisted in Catholic Europe even to our own day. In England, it was virtually destroyed in the 16th century when Henry VIII dissolved the monasteries – our first nationwide step towards organisation of capitalist society.

The first person in Britain to think quantitatively about the nation's health as a whole and in economic terms was Sir William Petty in 1690, the pioneer of public health in England, and intellectually a product of the English Revolution of 1643.[2] Most originally, he regarded the whole population as a measurable economic asset for the nation, rather than mostly a liability. Shift from the common, unspecialised labour of subsistence agriculture to the divided, specialised labour of industrial capitalism was at the expense of domestic labour, including the tasks of caring. This made it harder either for well people to maintain their health, or for sick people to restore it, without aid from their employers, from their own mutual aid organisations or from the state. Such aid began here and there from the late 18th century onwards, becoming more widespread through the 19th century as industry advanced. Mostly it supplemented or supported nursing aid still provided by families, chiefly through cash benefits, so that families with a sick breadwinner could survive until he recovered. Medical care was added more to control distribution of these benefits and provide emergency care for accidents than for any effect it might have on the course of illness.

To make a living within the huge majority of the population who could not afford the fees of physicians or surgeons, doctors as individual entrepreneurs had to find ways to introduce clinical medicine and surgery into this informal support system. Much later, professional nursing faced the same task – not to invent a new social structure of its own, but to find ways to enter an old one that had grown through a combination of state authority and local custom. Because clinical interventions produced little or no net health gain until the early 20th century, doctors were a relatively weak social force – much less powerful than many medical historians have until recently seemed to believe. The framework for care within which modern British medicine had to grow in practice was led chiefly, though not entirely, by a compromise between state interests, employers' interests and the expectations and demands of industrial workers. The leadership role of doctors as individual entrepreneurs serving patients who could pay for state-of-the-art care was small, much less than in continental Europe.

Origins of property in institutional care

For the first half of the 19th century, state interests centred on social engineering, made necessary by the privatisation of virtually all common land, the subordination of domestic agriculture to manufacturing industry, and the concentration of population in industrial cities. The instrument for this was the workhouse, invented by the Poor Law Amendment Act of 1844, and largely designed and driven through by Edwin Chadwick. He is remembered today as the founder of UK public health, but in the 1840s he was reputedly the most hated man in England.[3] Workhouses warehoused indiscriminately the indigent sick, disabled, senile or insane, together with anyone fit enough to work but unable to find employment. They were deliberately designed and operated to resemble prisons, and with men parted from women and children from fathers, and all set to hard, repetitive handwork, stone breaking or on treadmills. As successive Enclosure Acts drove peasants from the common land, they were forced either to find employment in a continually diminishing agricultural workforce, to move to factory towns, or to enter the workhouse. The workhouse provided elementary nursing, midwifery and medical care for the indigent of its neighbourhood, though often on little more than a token scale, but its main function was to drive redundant labour out of the countryside, into industrial slums.

Huge hospitals for the insane, built in the late 19th century, generally followed a similar cultural pattern, with warehousing and social isolation as dominant functions. Most of the hospitals inherited by the NHS had been built and continued to function as workhouses or giant insane asylums right up to its origin in July 1948. Workhouse attitudes persisted for at least a decade after this. Converting county hospitals and asylums from custodial to caring and curative functions required leadership and pioneering of an exceptional order, patchy and often late in coming.

These state-owned and state-serving institutions provided important employment opportunities for all health workers, for which there was fierce competition. Promoting their professional and social status, first doctors and then nurses did all they could to separate their ideas of professionalism from this squalid reality. What the state institutional care provided by the Poor Law Boards of Guardians (who employed doctors to provide at least nominal attention for the indigent sick),[4] the workers' mutual aid societies (Clubs), and even the local enforcement of sanitary laws through Medical Officers of Health all had in common was that they applied to all, or nearly all, of the common people. They were entirely separated from the care of the gentry. In particular, they applied to people, or to functions necessary for society, that were unwanted by private medical trade. Doctors needed as many rich patients as they could attract, because the number of poorer patients they could afford to help depended on subsidies from the rich, paying fees according to the estimated value of their homes. Thus, care for the poor remained on a token scale until employers found it impossible to maintain or develop a stable industrial workforce without it.

The ideological base for medical trade (rather than health care for the people) was developed in large teaching hospitals, first in London, Glasgow, Edinburgh, Dublin and eventually in other big industrial cities. These were funded first by the aristocracy, then by industrialists, not for their own care (hospitals were too dangerous) but for the care of their servants and employees. They also served as many of the urban poor as could reach them, and dared to enter, as they had room for, and who had acute diseases or injuries then thought to be susceptible to treatment – chronic illness was excluded. The most important price paid for entry (apart from high risk of cross-infection) was that patients would be taught upon and experimented upon. Teaching hospitals were museums of disease, where students could become familiar with living disease and its mortal remains.

What did the rich and powerful sponsors of teaching hospitals get out of their investment? A recognised personal contribution to civilisation and social stability, important for their position in society; honourable disposal of their sick servants; and connections with doctors who had hopefully become less ignorant as a result of practising and experimenting on hospital patients, and whose skills might prove useful for the care of their own families, in their own homes.

What did the doctors get out of it? In direct payment, nothing at all. They were 'honorary consultants', not paid for attendance. Hospital sponsors had to pay only for building, heating, nursing, cleaning and minor administrative staff, and for cooks and food, not for doctors. These unpaid 'honoraries' had got themselves a good deal. They became rulers of their profession, responsible for teaching and, through their Royal Colleges, for defining the form and content of professionalism. Their reputations among rich people were founded on their experience with poor people. Their private patients were found in the social networks surrounding hospital sponsors, or were referred to them by their former pupils, practising as GPs in the suburbs or countryside. Who owned the teaching hospitals? Nominally, ownership was held by rich benefactors and the cumulative trust funds perpetuating their names; in practice, by the senior consultant surgeons and physicians, eventually joined by nursing matrons. However, virtually none of these professionals would ever disagree with their noble patrons. Together they owned not just the teaching hospitals, but almost the entire medical ideology. The only exception was that slender but potent continuing thread of rational innovation represented by experiment and research, long despised as inimical to the culture of gentlemen. In England, more than any other developed economy (and unlike Scotland), full-time science was kept away from power for as long as possible – effectively, until the late 1950s. The definition of medical professionalism still used today was developed towards the end of the 19th century, long before medical science began to dominate practice, and still carries abundant traces of its origins.

All over the UK, wherever sponsors could be found, small hospitals in market towns developed their own relatively feeble imitations of teaching hospitals. Local GPs with enough training or influence to get appointments to their staff got roughly the same terms as the consultants in teaching hospitals. They got fees from the few patients who could afford to pay, and filled the rest of their beds from patients treated almost for free. If there weren't enough fees or donations, no hospital was built. Together with the teaching hospitals, all these together were known as Voluntary Hospitals, a treasured *de facto* possession of the secure and established medical profession in each locality.

Starting in the 1930s, a third category of hospitals emerged, based neither on the Poor Law nor on voluntary funding. These were County Hospitals, administered through local government county councils, funded in part by the state. Where county councils had the political will, they developed their own hospitals, employing their own salaried staff. Many of these were excellent for their time, sometimes more impressive than most teaching hospitals, because they accepted patients with chronic as well as acute diseases.[5]

Subordination of public health to clinical medicine

For doctors as professionals, personal clinical care has always appeared to be the core of medicine, because this was the way most of them earned a living. Interventions to preserve health, or at least to sustain hope or predict the future course of illness, could always be sold to those rich or desperate enough to pay their fees. The top doctors were not those who served the nation as organisers of public health like Chadwick, Sir John Simon, or William Farr, but personal doctors to the Royal Family, the Court, the aristocracy, and eventually captains of industry. In any rational picture of medicine as socially applied human biology, public health, the health of whole nations, was surely a larger category than personal clinical medicine or surgery, and should have set the aims of all clinical specialties, but in every fully developed industrial economy, and (though to a now slowly diminishing extent) in every medical school, these rankings were exactly reversed. Public health is a subordinate partner to clinical medicine, which still finds it hard to accept that public health should define the scope and aims of its practice. Only the state can own public health, but clinicians can credibly claim ownership of the skills of clinical medicine. This became their most fiercely defended possession.

Despite this, health workers of all kinds have always felt more comfortable if they could serve all of the people according to their needs (as perceived by professionals), rather than some of the people according to their wants and wealth. The first thing students learn in medical school is that all human bodies follow a common design, and fail in similar ways. Unity of humankind has always been built into the foundations of their training, however much professional culture may at times have ignored this in practice. Throughout history, medical care (real or illusory) could never be fully subordinated to the marketplace.

Doctors are therefore open to a dual sense of ownership. They are open to the idea of state ownership of hospitals and clinics and state employment of their staff, if this seems to be the only way they can do their work, but ownership and control of their work itself they will not yield willingly. They want to remain responsible for what they themselves do, for their own clinical decisions. This is true of all health workers, of whatever grade or skill. Though doctors as an organised profession have almost always opposed the first steps toward state funding and therefore control of health care, once they have positive experience of such funding, most of them seem to become its defenders. Very few doctors now working in the NHS want to return to any kind of private or corporate market (though some of these few have loud voices). As an organised profession, they are now defending the NHS as a public service more vigorously than any of the other health service unions. They have also shown more courage than governments in promoting initially unpopular public health causes.[6] This suggests that if governments do not hand them over to employment by for-profit contractors, a large majority of caring professionals working in hospitals or other large institutions could prefer ownership as personal responsibility to ownership as personal property, if this were ever again a political option.

Origins of property in primary health care

Hospital-based specialists had to recognise two fundamental truths long ago, which only began to be generally accepted by British GPs in the 1970s, and are still not fully accepted, even today. First, doctors could no longer work effectively alone. Other medical colleagues were necessary, if only to relieve them of 24-hours-a-day, 365-days-a-year personal responsibility for their patients, tying them to their neighbourhood, and their wives (there were few women doctors) to the telephone. First nurses and office staff, then a host of other assistant primary care staff have become recognised as necessary to provide effective care. As in hospitals, now in primary care, more and more tasks needed teamwork to make them feasible or effective. Even the smallest of these units needed skilled organisation and administration, requiring administrative skills for which doctors have not been trained, and in which most have little interest.

Good general practice needs more than a good memory, a stethoscope in your pocket and a smart car. However, the illusion of being your own boss, paid by society but accountable to nobody, is still often more powerful than reason. Governments were in no hurry to disturb the wonderful formula discovered by Lloyd George in 1912, which made GPs responsible for their own clinical squalor by making them independent contractors for public service. In material terms, the idea of GPs' personal ownership of primary care has therefore persisted, centuries after specialists accepted public ownership of hospitals.

Just as Britain became fully industrialised earlier than any other country, it was also the first country where almost the whole population had access to some sort of care from a qualified doctor.[7] A minority of successful GPs could live entirely from fees from patients who could afford to pay, possibly reaching about one third of the population by the 1880s. Doctors in middle-class areas scaled their fees roughly in proportion to their estimates of the value of their patients' homes. There was no fixed tariff; prices were scaled to what doctors believed patients could pay – not from charity, but from realism. The richest areas were therefore most attractive to medical trade, generally getting doctors able to spend longer as unpaid junior staff in hospitals to get wider clinical experience and therefore greater competence, with pressure of work low enough to permit its application. Richer patients paying larger fees allowed doctors to give patients as much time as full application of contemporary medical knowledge required. These areas provided opportunities to develop state-of-the-art personal clinical medicine and surgery.[8] To doctors they therefore appeared the natural growing points for any eventual public service (the eternal argument for 'levelling up, not levelling down'). Their patients were a treasured and saleable asset. When a GP principal retired, he sold the goodwill of his practice, that is, the loyalty to him of his patients. Patients' loyalty was a saleable property.[9]

This carriage trade never provided the model for publicly funded care in Britain, or anywhere else in Western or Northern Europe. The origins of NHS primary care lie in prepaid systems developed for the care of industrial workers, not in genteel fee-earning practice in market towns or white-collar suburbs. Because Britain was fully industrialised by the end of the 19th century, we developed a universal model of primary care from these prepaid systems, with unlimited free care at a fixed annual payment per capita – capitation. This was initially paid by workers through their own organisations. Later it was taken over and funded by the state.[10]

Primary care without fees

Wherever income from rich patients was insufficient to maintain a medical family, doctors looked for other work, either for the state, through extremely ill-paid salaried service for the Poor Law Boards of Guardians, or for groups of industrial workers able to organise subscription schemes for prepaid care, generally known as clubs.[11] To distinguish them from trade unions (which were by the Combination Acts of 1799 and 1800 made illegal until 1825) they were called friendly societies. These were compelled to register with the state after 1793, so their subsequent progress can be measured. By 1891, almost half the adult male UK population, and a majority of employed industrial workers, were members of such societies.[12]

Some societies became huge national institutions. By 1855 the Odd Fellows had 200,000 members and the Ancient Order of Foresters 100,000. By 1872 both of these had more than doubled. Despite their size, these were still largely organised and controlled by their members through local lodges, where everybody knew everyone else and could watch how their pennies were spent. The lodges provided burial expenses, subsistence during unemployment, illness or injury, and a usually narrow range of prepaid medical and nursing care, often for dependents as well as subscribers. Costs were low because almost all administration was by elected committees of volunteers, and all profits were accumulated as reserves for future benefits. They paid doctors marginally better than the Poor Law.

Miners' medical aid schemes

Mining villages, often in previously remote areas, had to make their own social institutions for themselves, drawing from egalitarian social theory implicit in dissenting interpretations of the Christian Bible. These originated from the Puritan movements of the English Revolution of 1643 and subsequent Civil War, from ideas about temperance born from bitter family experience of alcohol dependence, and finally (from about 1898), from socialist ideas.[13] These three sets of ideas were often fused. Marxism had little impact until around 1910, but then rapidly became a powerful force in the South Wales coalfield, in simplified form. Valleys socialism had strong elements of syndicalism, derived from the fact that engagements between lodges of the South Wales Miners' Federation and boardrooms of the Coal Mining Employers' Federation were the battlefields from which all the most important social and political decisions in South Wales derived. These often led government policy. Local government was incomparably stronger than it is today. Every local council election was a struggle between miners and coal owners for supremacy.

The miners' medical aid schemes were the most advanced of the Club systems. They employed doctors either on contract or on salary to provide unlimited free care for registered patients, paying the going rate for labour in a then over-manned and extremely competitive professional market, in which medical poverty was still a reality. Whereas schemes in England and Scotland depended on fixed rates of subscription, all the miners' medical aid schemes in Wales eventually adopted poundage schemes (usually around 3 or 4 pence for each £1 earned), in which subscriptions proportional to earnings were deducted from wages at the colliery office. In effect, this was a local income tax.[14]

Employers generally favoured these schemes as a stabilising factor in their often stormy relations with their workforce, and as a means of attracting doctors to the often remote communities in which they needed doctors for their own families.[15] The poundage system became a critically important feature, creating possibilities for development of comprehensive services impossible elsewhere.

In all these schemes the doctors' duties included adjudication of fitness for work and entitlement to benefit, exclusion from benefit for illness attributed to 'immoral behaviour' (mainly alcohol and venereal disease), treatment of industrial injuries, and provision of medicines and diagnostic labels for all illness presented to them, with unlimited free access. Major injuries and surgical emergencies like fractures or strangulated hernias were managed by GPs, all of whom were expected to have elementary surgical skills as soon as they qualified.[16]

The friendly societies and miners' medical aid societies were strongholds of probity, sobriety, dissenting religion, and a balance between servility and solidarity which depended on the conflicting local influences of religion, self-help and militant traditions descended from the Chartists of the 1840s, according to the relative strength of these traditions in different communities. Socialist and Marxist ideas, even in the vulgarised forms then available, had little impact in Wales until the Cambrian Combine colliery dispute in 1910, after which they grew rapidly.[17] On the other hand, less radical advocates for self-help turned readily to local employers and gentry for whatever they might give, either as cash or influence, and in most areas such opportunism remained dominant, except in times of crisis. In most of the earlier schemes, employers hired and fired the doctors, expecting and often getting loyal support from them in their many disputes with their workmen. After the Workmen's Compensation Act of 1897 made employers liable for some of the more flagrant consequences of industrial injury, employers' influence over doctors became a major issue. Eventually most schemes were brought under full workers' control to prevent this. The status and accountability of doctors were not generally regarded by employers as a fundamentally important issue. Where workmen were militant enough to press their case, employers gave way and operated poundage schemes through their pay-offices, even if this upset the organised medical profession, and loosened their influence on doctors' 'expert' evidence in court for compensation disputes.[18]

As miners' doctors had to deal with frequent fractures and other injuries, they encouraged their various sponsors – mainly local government and the aid societies, but also local employers and charitable donors – to build small cottage hospitals, usually with only 10 to 15 beds, with a small theatre in which to operate. Moral ownership of these hospitals, and control over access to them for surgical practice, were frequently contended. Local bigwigs were often more generous with their names than their money. The coal-mining valleys of South Wales and the slate-mining valleys of North Wales soon filled with cottage hospitals, variously built and maintained by rates from local government and by local public subscription. Their public face and administration were often virtually monopolised by gentry whose cash contributions might be much less than the funds raised collectively by mining communities and through subscriptions from poundage.[19]

Unsupported by the state until 1911, the friendly societies excluded the very poor, but in all areas of heavy industry they included most employed workers. In Welsh coal-mining communities the medical aid societies included all miners' dependants, and by annual or weekly personal subscription, all council workers, small business people, shopkeepers, teachers and other small occupations surrounding the coal industry – in effect, the whole community.[20]

The most comprehensive miners' medical aid schemes developed in the South Wales coalfield, because of its unique character concentrating whole valley communities around production of coal, iron, steel or tinplate.[21] The small valley towns became culturally self-sufficient, with their own highly developed representative and participative democracy.[22] The poundage system provided funding and administration not just sufficient to maintain primary health care, but allowing some investment in staff and buildings. The communities did their best to provide for all their own social needs out of their own human resources. The doctors they employed had common interests with the communities they served to establish better facilities for care, chiefly through building small cottage hospitals as surgical units and for isolation of infectious fevers.[23] The doctors also had property interests of their own, wherein lay seeds of conflict. Development, control, staffing and ownership of these GP hospitals soon became central to contention between three well-defined local forces: doctors, miners and gentry.

Miners' schemes as models for free care

Though most South Wales doctors saw their ownership and control of local hospitals as inseparable from ownership and control of the leading edge of their work, there were important exceptions. Social service ultimately implies social funding, social funding implies social accountability, and this in turn implies either social regulation or social ownership. If you really serve the people, you must also be answerable to the people, which means salaried service (so that value added by doctors' work can be used to expand the range of health care, beyond the scope of GPs), not entrepreneurial ownership (whereby GPs could mainly expand their own work and incomes, with lower priority for investment in care and, particularly, in additional skilled staff). Though almost forgotten today, there were powerful advocates for salaried medical service in the valleys within the profession, most notably Dr Henry Norton Davies in Rhondda. He believed that poundage, efficiently administered, could support better-than-average salaries for doctors. They would then not need further income from private practice, and could concentrate on work according to patients' needs. He believed salaried service, funded by poundage, could expand health care to include a range of medical and surgical specialties far more imaginative than contemporary general practice – the beginnings of a modern integrated referral system.

Several of the miners' aid schemes demonstrated this. In Tredegar, by the 1920s the medical aid society included 95% of the town's population and employed five GPs, a specialist surgeon, two pharmacists, a physiotherapist, a dentist and one domiciliary nurse, as well as providing free rail transport for access to larger hospitals in Newport. In Rhymney, Dr Redwood was employed by the miners' aid scheme at an annual salary of £700, together with a free house, a dispenser, a cottage hospital and nurses – a better living than most of his 'independent' local colleagues.[24]

These examples show that salaried service, with locally representative lay control, was a viable option, and could be more innovative both socially and clinically than medical shop keeping.[25] The miners' medical aid schemes survived even through the period of mass unemployment which devastated the South Wales coalfield from 1926 to 1941, by reducing subscriptions for the unemployed to 3 pence a week, by employing unemployed men as collectors, and by reducing the cost of its contracted doctors, because, through the poundage system, their earnings fell at the same rate as those of their subscribing patients. The salaried doctors escaped this penalty. With imaginative leadership from a state serving all of the people, salaried service could have lifted all British medical practice to become a source of national pride, rather than the squalid disgrace it actually was in most UK industrial areas when the NHS began,[26] and mostly so remained until the 1980s.[27] By then well over 80% of investment in buildings, equipment and non-medical staff was being met by the state. With rare exceptions, GPs in industrial areas invested huge amounts of their work, but as little as possible of their money, in even the minimum of staff, equipment and buildings expected of any other business.[28]

Regardless of evidence, most GPs held stubbornly to what seemed to them self-evident. They thought it was their job to know what was best for their patients, and this included definition of professional tasks, the scope of services, the nature of staff, planning and ownership of land, buildings and equipment, and how access to these might be divided between patients prepaid by insurance or medical aid schemes, and more profitable private patients. In this they were powerfully supported by the British Medical Association (BMA), whose central principle was total rejection of any kind of lay control. All regulation of doctors must be by other doctors, and even then applied with extreme delicacy.

The central issue of dispute between the miners and the doctors lay in control of poundage funds.[29] The miners presented their case frankly, but the BMA claimed higher motives, warning that the locally elected committees of the miners' medical schemes would try to control the doctors' clinical decisions. As public funding inevitably meant public accountability in some form, this became an argument against any kind of state funding for health care. Though from time to time the BMA made progressive proposals in theory, every attempt to make direct state investment in staff, equipment or buildings for primary care was resisted by the BMA until 1966. It was then conceded only because most NHS general practice in industrial areas had become so squalid that it faced collapse of recruitment.[30]

As most documentation about the many disputes between miners' medical aid schemes and their doctors comes from the *BMJ*, we have little evidence about how the miners presented their own case. However, I have never been able to find any example, either written or anecdotal, where miners, or any other group of workers, actually challenged the opinions of doctors in their own field of clinical expertise. On the contrary, miners seem generally to have taken an even more deferential view than was justified by the real state of contemporary medical knowledge. Such was the authority of doctors that it was probably prudent not to challenge their opinions head on, even if their claims to expertise were obviously being used to disguise economic self-interest.[31] Though letters to the *BMJ* at critical times often show miners' doctors more sympathetic to their patients than to employers or coal owners, these sympathisers were not linked with the minority of radical top doctors advocating a state service. There was then no political party interested in making such connections.

To coal-mining employers, their relations with organised workers were more important than their relations with unorganised doctors, easily replaced from an over-filled profession. They therefore generally agreed to cooperate with the medical aid schemes, even though the men now controlled them. This powerfully reinforced emerging trade union and socialist political culture. Recognising that optimal work from doctors required their undivided attention, in 1905 the Ebbw Vale Workmen's Medical Aid Society instructed its salaried doctors to cease private practice in the area. Supported by the BMA, which they had now joined, the doctors ignored this instruction. The *BMJ* refused to advertise any salaried post, and the BMA threatened to expel any doctor who accepted a salary from any miners' aid society on terms it had not approved. The BMA maintained the incomes of doctors sacked by the society, and in these ways turned the tables. The society retreated to a 10% limit on private practice, but the BMA was now on the offensive, fearing extension of salaried schemes first to the whole Welsh coalfield, then to the rest of industrial Britain.

The BMA demanded that virtually all poundage be paid directly to the contracted doctors, thus eliminating the main advantage of salaried service by putting investment back into the hands of the doctors. The society retaliated by recruiting non-members of the BMA to replace its existing medical workforce. This raised new issues of principle. What was the difference between the solidarity of self-employed GP entrepreneurs, and the solidarity of employed industrial workers? That there was indeed a real difference is not in doubt, but it was a question more complex than has generally been recognised.

From 1905 to 1913 the doctors and the aid societies fought for the loyalties of mining communities in Ebbw Vale, pulled one way by collective ties to their union and the other way by personal ties to their doctors – both substantial forces, because these doctors lived within the communities they served, and often played major roles at critically important moments in their patients' lives. The doctors continued to practise in the area and publicly appealed to their patients to claim repayment of poundage so they could give this to their own doctor. This succeeded in detaching about 10% of the Ebbw Vale society's members. Closely followed by the *BMJ* and by all the other miners' schemes, the dispute grumbled on without a clear victory for either side until 1913, when Lloyd George's National Insurance Act took the ground from beneath their feet.[32] With similar smaller disputes erupting elsewhere in many parts of the coalfield, it became a major item for public discussion in South Wales, then the most dynamic part of the still globally dominant British economy, and Lloyd George's own political base. In designing his Act, he must certainly have had its resolution in mind.

In historical retrospect, the most important issue of this dispute was whether investment in health care for the people would be socially controlled, serving social aims, with doctors' incomes a subordinate charge on this social fund, or be privately controlled by doctors as their own personal incomes, with any further investment coming from their own pockets. All experience confirms that however it may have been obtained in the first place, once money enters the pockets of professionals, spending for any social purpose has to compete with personal acquisition of carriages, cars, holidays and privileged education for their children, leaving little or nothing for the public interest. Capitation-paid independent contractor status proved to be an effective way of limiting the costs of primary care while leaving responsibility for consequently squalid services with doctors rather than government. Again, the underlying issue concerned personal ownership – of personal property, or personal responsibility.

Opportunity lost: Lloyd George's insurance

In Wales in the 1870s, 60% of all land was owned by about 570 people, nobility and gentry. Landed aristocrats were still fattening from royalties on coal found by chance beneath their estates, to whose production they had contributed not a penny, nor a drop of sweat or blood. Popular hostility to this injustice provided foundations for a Liberal ascendancy throughout Wales as complete as the Labour ascendancy which began to replace it in the 1920s, and finished it off by 1935.[33]

An alliance of miners, steelworkers, industrial employers, tenant farmers and slate quarrymen confronted socially conspicuous but otherwise idle landed aristocracy. They were led by David Lloyd George, a small-town lawyer, in the last battle of a revolution started in 1643. After the election of 1906 a newly transformed industrial and imperial Conservative Party began to supersede the dominance of landed nobility, drawing big industrialists away from the Liberal Party as its working-class voters shifted toward the Labour Party, which had appeared in 1903. Since the socialist revival of the 1880s, socialist ideas had first begun to compete successfully with Liberalism, from Fabians close to the top of society, to militant trade unionists close to the bottom.[34] Recognising that the social foundations of Liberal ascendancy were crumbling, Lloyd George embarked on social reforms that gave Liberal government a few more years of power before its permanent eclipse, provided his Labour successors with their eventual agenda for the rest of the 20th century, and finished landed aristocracy as an independent political force. As Chancellor of the Exchequer he attacked the aristocratic landowners' economic power through inheritance taxes in 1909, and their political power in the House of Lords through the Parliament Act in 1911. Finally, he set foundations for state pensions, unemployment and health insurance through his National Insurance Act of 1911, all these providing a new basis for popular consent to rule by the few, with minimal disturbance to industrial power and property.

For an answer to nascent socialism, Lloyd George turned to Germany. Bismarck had simultaneously made the Social-Democratic Party illegal and stolen its most popular social policies for mutual aid on lines similar to the UK friendly societies and miners' medical schemes, but sponsored by the state.[35] Lloyd George intended a similar system for the UK, chiefly to support wage earners during short periods of injury or acute illness, and provide retirement pensions for the usually brief lives of men following retirement at 65.[36] Ever since 1840, the Poor Law had been punitive in intention, deliberately stripping its supplicants of their homes and possessions as a precondition for minimal relief, designed to drive rural labour into the mines, mills and factories.[37] Knowing from his own experience as a small-town lawyer that illness in a wage earner was a major cause of irreversible pauperism for entire families, he designed his Insurance Act mainly to prevent this, by assuring a subsistence income of 10 shillings (£0.50) a week for wage earners during periods of incapacity up to three months, falling to 5 shillings (£0.25) a week for 13 weeks thereafter. Beyond this period, they fell again into pauperism and the grip of the Poor Law. These benefits would be paid for by compulsory weekly contributions, 4 pence from workers, 3 pence from their employers, and 2 pence from the state (promoted to voters as 'ninepence for fourpence').[38] Though elementary medical care was included in the Act, the main function of its doctors was, even more than in the miners' medical schemes, to justify selection for benefit by certifying incapacity for work. Again this became the central feature of medical work in primary care, around which anything and everything else had to be built.

Though Lloyd George took his strategy from Bismarck's Germany, the social customs needed to root it in British soil had already been developed by organised industrial workers, above all by the coal miners. He simply nationalised the social machinery already in existence, and extended it to virtually all other workers on a weekly wage. This solved some problems, but created others. It largely eliminated nascent trade union control either of benefit systems or of local investment in medical care, and put an end to all experiments in local participative democracy that might otherwise have limited the authority either of doctors or of the state. On the other hand, it also destroyed the local social control which had previously limited abuse of benefits. State insurance came to resemble state taxation – too large, too remote and too unshared a property to retain the respect once given to locally owned and organised mutual aid. Those playing the system had little respect from their communities, but were no longer regarded as thieves from their own kind. Ownership and responsibility had passed to the state.

For the next 36 years, GPs serving industrialised populations gave such care as they could find time for through Lloyd George insurance, which outside mining areas covered only employed workers, not their families, nor the growing middle class of lower management, professionals and small businessmen. They took such private practice as they could get, which in industrial areas was small. Affluent areas attracted many more doctors, with much less necessary work to do. Primary care evolved, if at all, as a poor imitation of professional specialism in hospitals.

When the NHS arrived in 1948, even this illusion of progress disappeared. After a long delay, caused essentially by the BMA's refusal to accept responsibility for leading primary care on any terms other than total personal ownership of this part of public service as their own property, general practice in the mid-1960s faced imminent extinction. It was rescued by the state, rightly afraid that without its foundation in primary care, NHS hospital care would become unaffordable. These two fears of collapse led both parties to the negotiating table, resulting in the first major investment the state ever made in British general practice, the GP Charter of 1966, already described in Chapter Four. By the 1970s, it can truly be said that in this domain, Britain led the world (though not for long).

Evidently it was not necessary to own a public service personally in order to work well within it. From the late 1960s onwards, a large and increasing proportion of GPs worked more imaginatively as contractors for a state franchise than they had as struggling entrepreneurs. Perhaps they would have worked better still if they could have been relieved entirely of running a business, and been allowed to concentrate on the work they had chosen, and been educated to do – as salaried doctors in Tredegar and Rhymney were already able to do in 1912. Development of these within-community skills has created a huge new sense of social responsibility and self-respect for GPs, distinct from ownership as personal property. However, to move voluntarily from self-employment to rule by an employer requires confidence in that employer. How can employees have confidence in the NHS, if its senior management is in the hands of people who no longer believe in its continued existence as a unified service, operating within a public service culture entirely different from the culture of business?

Ownership concerns dignity as much as property

Writing in 1993, Andrew Wall had the following to say about ownership not of property, but of personal work and responsibility, in the new conditions introduced by imposition of the purchaser–provider split on the NHS, which laid the basis for commercialisation:

> The benefits of the Purchaser–Provider Split, now seemingly the gospel of the public services of the western world, are by no means self-evident. Organisations need to have the capacity to learn if they are to be flexible and adapt to circumstances. At a very fundamental level of work, anyone at any level of the hierarchy will have ideas about how their job could be done differently and better. The purchaser–provider split introduces something inherently unnatural because there is a forced division between those who do the job and those who plan the job.... People and organisations are motivated by the prospect of being able to have a significant say in their futures. Rob them of that, and they become lacklustre, unimaginative, and in the end obstructive, if only to attempt to recover some sense of power.[39]

Elsewhere he added a further important point:

> ... [this division] is unsound in that people (if they are to learn from experience) need to live with the consequences of their own actions.[40]

These words should be printed as a poster, displayed on every office wall and memorised by every administrator. They were written about the NHS, but Wall's conclusion applies to all organised production that cannot be wholly delegated to machines. They reach to the heart of Marx's most important and fundamental perception, the division of mind entailed in all production which makes satisfaction of human needs a byproduct of pursuit of profit. This division, which Marx called alienation, has undeniably raised productivity for commodities, both for goods and for services, to heights beyond anything hitherto imaginable. Now, stripped of the social frame which once preserved at least a paternal humanity, it is dragging creativity and self-respect down to unprecedented depths, filling our prisons with alienated youth, poisoning people's minds with fear of their neighbours and an inward contempt for themselves, and promoting every expression of egotism, including personal despair, as an opportunity to make money. In this sense – and only in this sense – all who operate any production process want and need to retain or recover ownership and control of their work, and thus regain status, self-respect and dignity.

Nobody has ever willingly forsaken control, and in that sense ownership, of their own work. When English, Scottish, Welsh and Irish peasants lost access to land and streamed into mines, mills and factories in the 18th and 19th centuries, they did so for the same reasons as peasants in nascent industrial economies throughout the world do so today. Unable any longer to make even a subsistence living on land shared with others or of their own, they have all had no other option. Corporate employment in industrial work has been their only means of escape from subsistence rural economies destroyed by free trade.

Nobody wants a boss, but almost everybody has been driven to accept one, because capitalism offers only a few niche alternatives for making a living. Providing they know and understand the product they are supposed to produce, how they produce it should be their own affair (so far as machinery allows), because people at points of production have the most effective ideas about how their work could be done differently and better. Only this exertion of their own imagination gives them dignity and status in their own eyes, and the eyes of their community. Doctors now fear loss of control over their work in the same way as the hand loom weavers of the 18th century, when machines suddenly degraded them from skilled craftsmen to unskilled labourers.

At the height of the BMS's dispute with Lloyd George in 1912, Sir Clifford Albutt, an eminent physician, described the work of contract GPs as 'perfunctory care by perfunctory men'. This was a just description of most GP care in most British industrial areas well into the 1980s. Most of the innovative general practice born in the 1960s was concentrated where it was easiest to do, in prosperous market or university towns and leafy suburbs. Where occasionally innovation occurred in industrial or inner-city ghettoes, it relied on socially committed evangelists trying to defeat the perfunctory tradition by lifetimes of often unsustainable struggle to create something better.

However, from Albutt to the GPs still clinging to independent contractor status today, all have been fundamentally mistaken in four ways:

(1) They have assumed that ownership of their work process as a personal responsibility was equivalent to ownership of health care as commercial (or, as they always prefer to call it, professional) property. There was and still is little evidence that, as property, professional ownership of any level of care can assure its quality. On the other hand, there is plenty of evidence from our own experience that, as responsibility, professional ownership of work processes is essential to motivation, and to effective, efficient and imaginative clinical judgement. These two kinds of ownership – of property, or of responsibility for work process – need to be understood as wholly distinct, and ultimately opposed to each other, if our aim is to serve whole communities. As property, ownership is at best irrelevant to progress. At worst, it is its greatest obstacle.

(2) They ignored the effect of fees-for-service in consolidating a transactional, provider–consumer model for care, inhibiting development of public health responsibilities, inhibiting development of a cooperative model for care through which patients could develop into co-producers, and suppressing healthy scepticism among both patients and professionals. However, though capitation methods of payment created stable registered populations, and therefore the possibility of planned and audited anticipatory care for whole populations, very few NHS GPs actually thought in these terms until government devised (QOFs) contracts that rewarded them for attainment of planned targets, and penalised them for failure. Piece-rated pay is certainly better than no funding at all for better work, but it does nothing to develop innovation beyond its own conceptual frame, or develop critical thought and initiative in its operatives.

(3) They ignored the positive consequences for professional motivation and public understanding of any system, however primitive, that included either more of the people through National Insurance, or all of the people through the NHS. The greatest difference between UK and US social attitudes (public and professional) is the determination of UK voters to retain a system that has eliminated the worst economic consequences of unforeseeable catastrophic illness, which they have themselves experienced. The two-thirds of US citizens who have some entitlement to more than crisis care have been made to fear that they may lose even what they have, if the other one third of their fellow citizens are somehow allowed to share in it. Lobbyists for insurance companies have bought enough senators and congressmen, enough broadcasting and press media, to create and maintain this fear of something which no US

citizens have experienced, unless they have lived in Canada, the UK, or other EU countries.[41] Having everybody inside a single system has been a hugely positive national learning experience, for both doctors and patients.

(4) Finally, they were wrong about lay control. They ignored the possibility that when it came to health care policies rather than individual clinical decisions, lay people might often see further, wider and deeper than doctors. With substantial lay input, health care might be more imaginative and wider in scope than in any medical monopoly. Public respect for medical and nursing science might be far more robust than they feared. No such input is on offer now by any political party anywhere near power, but this latent, untapped democratic power is still there. There may now be enough doctors who understand this to make its use possible for a braver government, loyal to socialising traditions.

Will primary care become big business?

As I write in early 2010, these issues have acquired a wholly new context. In 1997, New Labour leaders won a landslide election, with the following promise in their manifesto: 'Our fundamental purpose is simple but hugely important: to restore the NHS as a public service working cooperatively for patients not a commercial business driven by competition.'[42] That election was won with an implicit promise to end the Thatcher era of deregulated capitalism and privatisation of public services, and this explicit assurance that Kenneth Clarke's first steps towards merging business for profit with NHS public service would be rolled back.

In the New Labour government's first year, Health Minister Frank Dobson did his best to sustain this pledge, though even he accepted Prime Minister Blair's infatuation with the Conservative Party's Private Finance Initiative, and famously proclaimed that there was henceforth 'no other show in town'.[43] Dobson was then demoted to a humiliating role as New Labour opponent to Ken Livingstone as Mayor of London, after which he was cast out to the back benches, where he has done his best to undo the damage by becoming a merciless critic of New Labour's NHS policies. He was followed by a succession of health ministers who have driven the NHS ever deeper into divisive consumerism, promotion of corporate private sector providers, and virtually the entire programme of 'reform' advocated by the International Monetary Fund (IMF), World Bank (WB), and the numerous think-tanks from which the lobbying and public relations industries operate. The only criticism the Conservative Party has ever felt able to offer is that adoption of its policies has not yet gone far enough or fast enough, though New Labour has in fact done all this faster and further than any Conservative government had been able to do.

This 'reform' programme seeks to transform all public services into commercially competitive models, separating purchasers from providers, making all decisions into accounted transactions requiring a hugely expanded bureaucracy and incurring previously unimaginable transaction costs, managed by people experienced in commodity production and distribution, with every possible encouragement for penetration by transnational corporations. This process of 'reform' is being driven as far and as fast as professional resistance and public confusion allows, modified perhaps by mounting evidence that investment in these fields may be less profitable than was first imagined. Faced by the colossal competing costs of saving bankers from their gambling debts, government will be under even greater pressure to continue 'reform' not just to save money, but to withdraw so far as possible from responsibilities for care.[44]

Commercialisation depends on a huge assumption: that the public no longer cares who owns the NHS. All the main parties believe they have a new public, which cares only about what it consumes, not about who provides it, or why they provide it. This belief has always been natural to conservative parties. It is now shared by all centrist parties, as well as most health economists. As for what doctors believe, does this really matter to advocates of 'reform'? They seem to think consumers must learn that no providers can be trusted to serve any interests other than their own. Doctors are no longer portrayed as an exception to this, though the NHS itself provided them with an opportunity to rise above it, which growing numbers accepted. Exempted from social duty, why bother even to maintain an appearance of respect for it? Depending very much on how the question is posed, politicians may find growing support for these cynical views from public opinion polls, as consumerism pervades every aspect of society.

Government now seems determined in practice to encourage egotism throughout society. Young doctors entering general practice face prospects unknown in the UK since 1948, though long familiar in the US.[45] Young doctors now start with huge burdens of student debt. Few entering primary care can find employment as independent contractors, most have to work for established GPs. Many GP partnerships, run as businesses, have now become very profitable. In the first three years of the QOF contract, average gross earnings of established GP principals rose by 58% (from £73,000 in 2003 to £114,000 in 2006). Over the same period, the average pay these established GP principals gave to their salaried assistants rose by just 3%.[46] As workload rises, it becomes more profitable to employ young GPs as salaried assistants than to take on new partners, and more profitable still to delegate work to nurses, nurse-practitioners, or health care assistants. This process is producing both very rich GPs exploiting their colleagues, and a large and growing cohort of young doctors who can at last see that medical business is no better than any other business – its aim is profit, not service.[47] Despite the large fortunes now open to a few, judging by voting patterns for elections to BMA Council, a large majority of UK doctors see no future as entrepreneurs in a health care market.

As the 'reform' legislation intended, primary care in England (but not Scotland, Wales or Northern Ireland) is now open to large transnational corporations already experienced in providing care commercially on a very large scale, mainly for insured patients in the US and South Africa. Government and NHS administrations have leaned over backwards to ensure entry of these companies to primary care, particularly in industrial or post-industrial areas concentrating poor health, high demand and reputedly poor traditions of clinical medicine. Wherever retirements have created vacancies, companies have bid against established local GPs and would-be GP entrants for new contracts to supply services. Almost all of these have been successful.

Free trade in practice: two case studies

Advocates for liberal free trade like to talk about level playing fields, but they are now hard to find except in economic theory. The following case is of exceptional importance, in that it set a new course for New Labour primary care policy in one of the most challenging areas of England, in defiance of previous Labour traditions and expectations of Labour voters. Despite every effort to keep it quiet, it got sufficient public attention to ensure that no government minister or conscientious MP could have been unaware of it. Government persistence through two courts of appeal confirms that none of its consequences was unintended.

Dr Bess Barrett was an excellent, innovative GP in the former coalfield of North Derbyshire, who had long wished to develop much the same sort of service there as our Glyncorrwg team did in South Wales.[48] In 2005 an opportunity appeared when Langwith, a former mining village with big health problems, found itself without a GP. She proposed to form and lead a small team including a manager, a nurse, a pharmacist and a driver. Dr Barrett was a GP trainer, had special skills in diabetes and dermatology, had wide experience of planning and management at area level, and having set up a patient liaison group in her practice, was the lead GP for patient involvement on the local PCT. The pharmacist was an approved prescriber with links to Sheffield University. Three members of this team were governors of local schools, and all were well rooted in the neighbourhood. They proposed to work closely with social services and the local job centre, with which they had long-standing links. They proposed to build new premises at their own risk and keep them open from 8.30am to 6pm on land offered free by the local parish council, which had conducted a door-to-door poll showing overwhelming local support for a new centre. The elected council itself supported Dr Barrett's bid unanimously.

The only obvious weakness of this bid was the small size and intimate location of the team, against trends ever since 1966 favouring ever larger primary care units serving ever wider catchments. Against this was consistent evidence that, given a choice, most patients have always and everywhere preferred small units. In North East Derbyshire PCT, the two smallest practices always scored highest in all measures of patient satisfaction, a consistent finding in all research in this field. Aware of the risks of professional isolation, Dr Barrett's proposal included regular links with a larger practice nearby for participation in evaluation of work and commissioning.

Before New Labour politicians embarked on their crusade to marketise the NHS, few GPs would have wanted the harder work and lower earnings of such a practice. Dr Barrett's appointment would have been a formality. Her plan was submitted in outline for discussion and comment to Martin McShane MP, Chief Executive of the PCT, in August 2005. No comments had been received by October, when the PCT invited bids for the vacant practice. The Barrett team's fully costed bid was submitted in December. Later that month the PCT announced its choice of UnitedHealth Europe (UHE) as its 'preferred provider'. Dr Barrett's plan had not even been short-listed.

Some details of how this decision was reached were obtained under the Freedom of Information Act. Six bidders had been short-listed, five from companies operating for profit, only one from an existing NHS practice. Though described by the PCT as 'a young British company', UHE was in fact the European subsidiary of the largest single company in the US providing health care, with assets totalling $41,374,000,000. Its Executive Vice-President, R. Channing Wheeler, who has been appointed commercial director at the UK Department of Health overseeing purchase of care for NHS patients, is still under investigation by the US Securities and Exchange Commission over an alleged 409,000 illegal backdated share options between 1998 and 2002, with a civil action by public sector union shareholders seeking $5.5m damages.[49] UHE had no experience whatever of providing NHS primary care in the UK, and had not yet recruited any doctors for a clinical team. Despite this, UHE scored highest on having a 'proven track record of providing medical services', presumably in the US. Though UHE had apparently done nothing to ascertain local public opinion, and its bid had been unanimously opposed by the elected local council, it also scored highest on its 'record of engagement with public and patients'. Evidently these empty slots also were filled by experience of commercial care and managed public relations in the US. Asked at a public meeting what made UHE so clear a winner, Labour MP McShane said it was the company's strategic vision.

Ironically, UnitedHealth Europe, offspring of UnitedHealth America, had as its director Dr Richard Smith, one-time ardent exponent of Bevan's 1948 vision, and for many years an effective opponent of commercialisation of the NHS when he edited the *BMJ*.[50] However, UHE was ultimately unsuccessful. Dr Barrett's case went to appeal. A High Court judge ruled that the UHE bidders should not have been preferred, because they had not consulted the public they said they wanted to serve.[51] The PCT then appealed against this decision, and another appeal judge ruled that the local councillor who lodged the first appeal should have taken her case to a local Patients' Forum rather than to the High Court for judicial review. He remarked that the PCT had indeed ignored local opinion, including elected councillors, and he found specious the PCT's contention that selection of a corporate provider did not represent a material change in provision of primary care, but he still found himself bound to find in favour of the PCT because of this procedural error.[52] So the way was clear for the PCT to choose another transnational corporate bidder, which it immediately proceeded to do.

The government learned from this experience. Soon thereafter it imposed an auction for provision of primary care for 30 of the most socially deprived areas of England, many of them former mining areas, open to both corporate and traditional GP providers. Presumably it hoped that next time its policies would be less humiliatingly exposed.[53] If so, it failed. In 2008, in an exceptionally deprived area of the East End of London, two progressive established local GP partnerships were short-listed for a vacancy caused by retirement, together with a corporate bidder, Atos Healthcare, a subsidiary of a £4bn multinational corporation. One of the local bidders was a practice previously used in Labour election broadcasts as an example of the sort of excellent practice favoured by that party. The other was a practice attached to a major London teaching hospital, with a world reputation for its published research. It had to spend £35,000 in preparing its bid, because this now requires not only a business plan costed in detail, with a projected average cost per patient bound by contract, but also evidence of long-term back-up by accountants, lawyers, information technologists and all the other commercial advisers normally found only in large companies.[54] Experience is said to be important for selection. Apparently this doesn't mean experience of actually delivering care to NHS patients in similar neighbourhoods, but experience of running any large business profitably. Both these practices were passed over in favour of Atos, which had offered a 6% lower price per patient than the lowest GP bid, and greater resources for marketing and administration.[55] A few months after this decision, Atos was having difficulties in recruiting and retaining medical staff for this unit, and was trying (so far unsuccessfully) to renegotiate its prices to more realistic figures.

There are now many other examples.[56] Generally speaking, none of this is happening in the countryside or leafy suburbs, where NHS primary care has worked well enough for many years, and votes might be lost by forcing change, but new young doctors will enter these practices either at a high price to buy their share of partnership assets, including goodwill, or as salaried assistants at the mercy of their senior colleagues. As the same government also initiated university tuition fees, which now leave doctors with on average more than £22,000 of debt when they qualify,[57] salaried employment may eventually become as normal in affluent as in poor areas, but with colleagues rather than corporations as their employers.

This salaried service, either for giant corporations serving poor populations or for prosperous older GPs employing their younger colleagues, in no way resembles the salaried service in primary care pioneered in the South Wales coalfield, and defeated by the BMA in the early 20th century. Nor is it at all what the BMA now needs or intends as a trade union trying to represent all doctors. If the BMA wants to recruit the next generation of doctors, it must contemplate division of the profession three ways in NHS primary care: doctors exploited by companies to make money for their managers and shareholders, doctors exploited by their senior colleagues, and doctors salaried by the state. The BMA will probably continue to help rich doctors to stay rich, but as a mass-membership trade union, it is already subordinating this to majority needs, and doing so more vigorously than UNISON. its counterpart for all NHS staff other than doctors, more highly qualified nurses and technicians. How far and fast this development proceeds will depend on whether members start to take their union seriously. Progressive trade unions have never appeared spontaneously, they have to be built by their actively participant members who give their time, and usually lifelong commitment. The BMA has an essentially democratic structure, candidates for office openly committed to opposing industrialisation and commercialisation are now easily elected, so rapid change is certainly possible and probably imminent.

Another development, not anticipated by governments infatuated with market solutions, is that corporate investment in this field is proving far more difficult and much less profitable than was ever imagined, even before the 2008 financial crisis, which is now likely to dry up state funding for growth in the NHS. Doctors do not want to work for corporations if they can help it, so stable recruitment of well-motivated doctors to their projects has everywhere been difficult. Costs per patient offered in successful corporate bids have turned out to be unsustainable even as short-term loss-leaders, because though these companies know all about business, they know nothing about UK primary care. GPs never asked for the commercial providers of diagnostic tests and interval surgery (Independent Diagnostic and Treatment Centres) imposed by government to compete with NHS hospitals in England, so they have been grossly underused. In some areas, GPs are even being paid by PCTs to refer patients to ISTCs which have contracts guaranteeing payment even if their services are underused. To attract the first wave of investors to the new market in health care, these also were given guarantees that after five years, if they proved unprofitable, the NHS would buy back their facilities.[58] All these guarantees were originally concealed by prevaricating ministers in Parliament, and by commercial secrecy. Many commercial providers have consequently been paid millions for work they have not done, and for facilities built but redundant.[59] Many formerly eager investors are now withdrawing from the contest, fearing that they might eventually have to accept the risks of equal competition with public service.

Corporate islands may be maintained as obstacles to rational planning for the present, and potential competitors for the future, but they seem unlikely to take over the system as a whole. The entire promise to shift risks from the public to the private sector has been an illusion, first by the Conservative government which devised these 'reforms', then endorsed by the New Labour government and all main contestants in the general election of 2010. Equally absurd have been promises of a level playing field between competing providers. From start to finish, this quasi-market has been tilted to favour rapid growth of commercial provision and retreat from publicly accountable service.

Meanwhile, regional governments in Wales, Scotland and Northern Ireland, which have already got themselves off this path, will continue to seek their own solutions, which sooner or later may lead to salaried service for a direct NHS employer, and return to a centrally planned, unified service, itself responsible for providing care, and accountable to elected politicians.

Ownership of NHS hospitals

The central strategic decision of Nye Bevan's 1948 revolution was to nationalise virtually all hospitals.[60] This initiative was entirely his own, and contrary to the views and expectations of virtually everyone else in the post-war Labour government, all of whom had assumed that NHS hospitals would be built and controlled by local government.[61] Nationalisation was understood by Charles Webster, official and pre-eminent historian of the NHS, and by George Godber, its principal architect in the medical civil service, as the central feature of the NHS which ensured its success. By creating a single, unified workforce aiming at common standards and with centrally negotiated pay, Bevan also created a sense of collective participation in a civilising enterprise for the entire UK, and loyalty to a nationally shared idea. Because hospital-based specialists had a virtual monopoly of teaching and research and worked visibly at the leading edge of medical advance, GPs were bound to follow as best they could, and soon learned to thrive in the new service. This decision also greatly reduced the hostility of established hospital consultants, who regarded employment by local government with extreme mistrust.[62]

The fragmentation of work, demoralisation of staff, and failure of productivity to respond proportionately, or even at all, to a threefold rise in state spending on the NHS since New Labour was elected in 1997, has followed what amounted to creeping denationalisation of hospitals throughout the UK since the 1980s.[63] The dissenting regional governments in Scotland, Wales and Northern Ireland are having to find their own way back from this. Hospitals which were evolving functions complementary to those of their neighbours in the pre-'reform' NHS have seen their standardised, high-turnover, and therefore most profitable, functions (mostly routine elective surgery) lost to competing commercial units, while they are left with the most complex, difficult and least profitable work. Hospitals have been made into independent Trusts, competing with each other and with contracted commercial providers to attract patients. Trusts are led by centrally appointed trustees, willing to think and speak in the new language of business and accountancy, concerned with efficient production of a multitude of independent processes, rather than with comprehensive and balanced health outcomes. Trusts that perform well in commercial terms can qualify as Foundation Trusts, which are virtually free from central NHS control. They can sell their hitherto publicly owned and usually centrally placed land to developers, relocate to more peripheral sites and pocket the difference. They can raise their own loans in the finance markets, make their own investments, negotiate pay and conditions independently with staff unions, and take their own decisions about pay for senior managers or engagement of external business consultants. They can put whatever clinical functions they like in the hands of independent contractors. In sum, they can operate like any other business, except that so far they have no shareholders, and must put their profits back into the business.[64] They qualify for all this by achieving financial rather than clinical targets. Though enabling legislation was supposed to assure that quality of care would always have priority, experience has shown such assurances to be worthless. A large hospital complex, the Mid Staffordshire Trust, was given a 3-stars quality rating in 2003, 0-stars in 2004, and 1-star in 2005. In 2007, an external monitoring body drew attention to the Trust's exceptionally high mortality rates, but despite this and its declining quality ratings, it was given Foundation Trust status in February 2008. One month later, an investigation by the government's watchdog, the Healthcare Commission, began into its high mortality rates. The next year its chair and chief executive both resigned, and a month after that the investigator's report was published. The Chair of the Healthcare Commission concluded: 'This is a story of appalling standards of care and chaotic systems for looking after patients.'

Dr David Colin-Thomé, National Clinical Director for Primary Care and author of the report, drew special attention to the fact that though many patients' complaints and all surveys of patients' opinion pointed to serious failures, particularly in emergency care, no organised bodies of the NHS, staff, or appointed public representatives had expressed any concern over these 'appalling' outcomes of care.[65] So, if they were not paying attention to this, what were they attending to? To the solvency of the hospital, because, like every other hospital in NHS England, its first concern was economic survival by operating at a profit. Second, it was concerned to meet government output targets for process. The Trust seemed notoriously good at business, so it gained Foundation

Trust status and virtual immunity from government control just one month before its clinical failure was finally recognised.

The most obvious feature of this denationalising era has been an almost universal loss among NHS staff of any sense of ownership or personal control over their own work. The few exceptions to this have been those willing and able to profit from the incentive bonuses now applied to health care, in much the same way as they have functioned for speculative bankers. Staff who still struggle to preserve some continuity, to think not only about their immediate task but also about what may happen next, are being overcome by a sense of futility. Everyone has tasks to perform, but the aims they serve give priority to survival of each Trust as a competing business, not to clinical excellence or service to their now undefined catchment populations. *De facto* ownership has passed from clinicians to business executives. As for ownership by the people (never respected except in rhetoric), that has now been redefined as consumer choice.

Ownership of the NHS as a whole

Industrialisation and commercialisation of the NHS since Thatcher's accession in 1979 implies that ownership of medical care, for which doctors contended first with locally organised workers and then with the state, could end in the hands of neither doctors, nor workers, nor the state, but carved up among large transnational companies operating to maximise profit for their shareholders, with any contribution to health relegated to default, an unplanned and unplannable residue of unprofitable public health and emergency care for the indigent.[66]

All main established political parties have been converging towards agreement that, as consumers, patients may no longer care who owns the NHS. There are professional advocates for this view, but not many. Among the most vocal has been Dr Karol Sikora, a cancer specialist especially concerned with rapid approval for new treatments, a familiar voice in broadcasting. In 2007 he was reported as follows:

> as we all know, the NHS is hopelessly inefficient. The last bastion of communism in Europe, it is obsessed with political correctness, multiple and complex targets and inter-professional disputes about working practices, and it boasts a hugely over-bureaucratised management system ... Just like delivering an excellent pizza, cancer care is a global business ...[67]

This view won over our leading politicians years ago. New Labour has no quarrel with it, and the only difference offered by the Conservative Party is that transformation of the NHS into a brand label for commercial providers is not proceeding fast enough. Naturally, the implicit assumption that treating cancer might somehow resemble eating a pizza is attractive, so long as you don't know much about cancer. Dr Sikora knows about cancer, but he seems very ready to vulgarise his knowledge in the higher cause of economic correctness, as he understands it.[68] The huge bureaucracy to which he refers was largely caused by channelling greatly increased NHS funding on business lines.[69]

Creeping transfer of ownership of public services to commercial providers is a worldwide process, reaching every nation accessible to global investment. Its prime agents have been the World Bank, the International Monetary Fund (IMF) and the World Trade Organisation (WTO). Their policies have been imposed by international law through the General Agreement on Tariffs and Trade legislation, negotiated from time to time by governments, with virtually no discussion in parliaments, none at all with members of the parties represented in parliaments, virtually no media coverage, and no discussion with the public. Though created in 1946 as agencies of the United Nations, all three institutions have hitherto been controlled by the US. They represent the interests of transnational banks and giant corporations, extending their markets to occupy fields previously reserved for collective ownership through the state and accountable to elected representatives. In the UK in 1945, voters chose by an electoral landslide to create a National Health Service outside the market. They have never been consulted since about any of the steps taken to reverse this choice and push the NHS back into the market. Though different arguments have been presented to voters in different countries, the aim seems everywhere to have been the same: to expand the scope for profitable investment by multinational corporations (based mainly in the US) and transform national care systems from their traditional role as public service planners and providers, into bulk procurers in a health care market, capitalised from abroad.[70] The US government, which denies accountability of itself or its citizens before any international court and has unilaterally withdrawn from all international treaties limiting its weapons or how they are used, uses its command of these international economic institutions to replace traditions of public service by its own commercial ethics.

In the early 1990s, before many of the lay public understood what was happening, UK doctors, led by the BMA, the Royal Colleges (mainly the London Royal College of Physicians), the NHS Support Federation and the NHS Consultants Association, embarked on a public campaign to defend the NHS. The BMA drew public opinion to its side under the slogan 'Who do you trust, the government or your doctors?'. Guessing the limits of his enemy at that time, Kenneth Clarke stood firm. The Labour Party, even in opposition, was already evading joint action with doctors,[71] but public opinion overwhelmingly supported the BMA and so did many influential journalists. Faced with the imminent possibility of victory, the BMA and medical Royal Colleges seemed to have no idea what to do next.[72] Though the medical profession had wonderfully changed from opposition to the NHS in 1948 to its defence in the 1980s, to work with mass support in a popular alliance with patients and other NHS unions still seemed unthinkable for that generation of leaders. Instead, in November 1994 the BMA and Royal Colleges convened a summit meeting on core values, at which it announced the terms on which it was prepared to make peace. The keynote speech was delivered by Sir Maurice Shock, former Rector of Lincoln College Oxford, a pillar of the establishment (but not a medical doctor). He was reported in the *BMJ* as follows:

> British doctors were unprepared for the *Blitzkrieg* from the Right which overwhelmed them at the end of the 1980s ...They seemed to imagine that they were still living in Gladstone's world of minimal government, benign self-regulation, and a self-effacing state ... [but now] instead of the rights of man we have the rights of the consumer, the social contract has given way to the sales contract, and, above all, the electorate has been fed with political promises ... about rising standards of living and levels of public service ... Doctors cannot swim against the tide and must recognise that this is an age of regulated capitalism in which the consumer is courted and protected, encouraged to be autocratic, and persuaded of his or her power ... Doctors must be willing to get their hands dirty with making decisions on allocation of resources, must speak authoritatively and sensibly to the consumer ... If [doctors] organised themselves in these ways the government would have to work with doctors, because a *Blitzkrieg* can conquer, but cannot occupy.[73]

Sir Maurice's choice of metaphor reveals astonishing ignorance of its meaning to anyone aware of 20th-century European history, at least as understood by participants.[74] In Sir Maurice's view, the profession had somehow to regain its role as obedient servant to the few who rule, even after being dismissed as redundant to a capitalism no longer challenged by any credible alternative.[75]

An alternative strategy was obvious and, up to a point, had already worked. Had the doctors stood firm and made it clear that they were prepared to act jointly with the Royal College of Nursing (RCN), UNISON and other NHS unions, they would probably have had overwhelming public support, and quite possibly ensured the government's defeat at the next general election. The Labour Party might then have recovered its nerve, and regained some interest in developing democratic socialism, instead of providing red carpets for global billionaires. In fact, faced by a strong government determined to lead rather than follow public opinion, a retreat by an even stronger army – as the BMA, RCN, NHS unions plus majority public opinion plus the Labour opposition potentially were – became a rout. Sir Maurice Shock's proposal for abject capitulation and alliance with a commercialising government, against the public as excessively demanding consumers, signified exactly that. The *Blitzkrieg* has continued its advance ever since, and has consolidated its grip over Britain's intellectual and media establishment.

The plain fact, ignored by Sir Maurice and those who chose him as their mouthpiece, is that all health care professionals, from doctors and nurses to ward orderlies and cleaners, want ownership of their own field of action, the public wants some form of collective ownership of the NHS as a public service, and patients want joint ownership of decisions about their own diagnoses and plans for their own care, not as consumers but as participants. Ownership of those kinds is unrecognisable to managers operating an industrial or commercial model. The criteria for personal ownership (and therefore responsibility) set out by Andrew Wall cannot be met by staff operating as cogs in a managed machine, or by patients operating as consumers encouraged to believe that their only responsibility is to pay either fees or taxes, and then search the provider shops for their wants.

Ownership of that sort, ownership as personal and civic responsibility, is ultimately incompatible with private ownership of any part of the NHS system as personal property or small business. If specialists own the hospitals in which they work, or act as if they own them, this excludes all other staff from ownership, as well as patients. If GPs own primary care, this excludes all other primary care staff and patients from ownership. Doctors need to grow up, and they are rapidly doing so. For the NHS to survive as a public service, owned by the state on our collective behalf, all of us need to accept it as such, a step taken long ago by all staff other than doctors. If the BMA joined other staff unions, or if those other staff unions joined the BMA (which as I write they have done only verbally) to fight from that platform, they would have overwhelming public support. No government could then continue the process of commercialisation.

Summary and conclusions

Doctors in Britain have never owned hospitals, as personal or collective property, on a significant scale. Before the NHS, virtually all hospitals were built and funded either by the state or local government, or by various charities. Since 1948, virtually all hospitals have been owned and funded by the state, so the idea of ownership of hospitals by doctors as private property has become almost unthinkable.

On the other hand, the dominant medical culture has encouraged doctors to think and behave *as if* they owned the hospitals in which they work, and *as if* all other staff within them were their servants. From 1948 until the early 1980s, *de facto* ownership of this sort was an almost unchallenged reality, facilitated by absence of any effective local accountability.

Primary care followed a different path. Before responsibility for primary health care was accepted by the state, ownership of health care was a matter for contention between doctors as self-employed entrepreneurs, and representatives of the communities they served as potential alternative employers. This was most obvious in areas of heavy industry like South Wales. Developments in coal-mining areas before the Insurance Act of 1911 created models for local accountability and democratic control which the Act brought to an end by enlisting doctors as independent contractors to the state.

Contemporary ideas of ownership played a major role in disputes between doctors and the state, at the birth of both National Insurance in 1912 and the NHS in 1948. In both cases, doctors serving affluent populations, and therefore able to practise clinical medicine more or less as they had learned it in their medical schools, feared degradation of their work if it escaped their ownership and control. Though some of these fears were justified, state funding opened free access to care for all of the people, with virtually no loss of independence in taking clinical decisions between 1948 and the onset of NHS 'reforms' after 1983. State funding in fact expanded professional ownership as social responsibility, even though ownership as property diminished, with new possibilities for developing primary care further than anyone had previously imagined.

Remodelling of the NHS on commercial and industrial lines is now conscripting health professionals to essentially the same loss of control over the nature and purpose of their work as that experienced by hand loom weavers in the late 18th century, and other commodity producers ever since. Health professionals are in process of becoming industrial workers, valued according to their productivity not of health gain, but of commodity process to assure profitability and economic survival in competitive markets. This development is destabilising the work both of specialists in hospitals and of generalists in the community, as well as all other health care professionals.

Optimal creativity and productivity require a sense of ownership, in the sense of personal responsibility for those who do the work, with scope to use their judgement and learn from their own experience, without managers breathing down their necks. This cannot be provided either by the industrial model in which doctors become employed workers, or by the small business model based on private ownership of public service. Health care professionals cannot and should not own the parts of socially organised health care systems they operate, but they can and must aspire to regain responsibility for and control of their work within publicly owned and publicly accountable systems. They will fail unless they learn how to ally themselves with their own staff colleagues, their own patients, and with the communities they serve, to re-establish the NHS as a gift economy for all of the people, outside and beyond the world of business.

SIX

Justice and solidarity

Human biology and the practice of medicine are based on a belief that people are nearly enough alike that the secrets of disease in a king may be found by cutting into a pauper. Solidarity, a belief that humans are all of one species, that we are social animals who stand or fall together, whose survival depends on helping one another, and whose genetic diversity is a strength rather than a weakness, has sound foundations in human biology. To be understood, this must include scientific, evidence-based approaches to psychology, sociology, history and politics, because they all help to make our extraordinary species what it is.

Medical fascism

Despite this humane tradition of solidarity, doctors were in the front ranks of the imperial and eugenic movements in Europe and North America before the First World War. These laid foundations for fascism – the belief that our species is naturally ranked in league tables of worth and talent, created by eternal competition, rewarding the strong and punishing the weak. These movements rested on denial of shared human identity, on assumptions that differences between people were more important than what they had in common, and that positive or negative values of these differences were obvious, predictable and constant over time.[1] They celebrated primacy of intuitive feelings over evidence, of charismatic leadership over socially inclusive and participative politics, and power itself over the ends it pursued. All these features fitted well with the state of medical practice between the two world wars, when medical authority drew power from its still very loose association with science, but kept itself virtually immune from scientific criticism. Surgical practice particularly tended to follow an engineering rather than biological model, associated more with hopeful certainty than with measured doubt. Fascism readily accepted the idea of social surgery in a time of crisis, in which substantial suffering for some was a necessary price to pay to restore health to society, justifying suspension of customary laws.

Fascist ideas drew initially on social Darwinism, developed mainly in Britain and the US. These associated competition for means to live within and between species, with competition for means to live within and between societies.[2] In 1933 Germany had the world's most advanced research teams, its most innovative physicians and surgeons, and its most sophisticated university culture. None of these prevented reversion to mediaeval mysticism, persecution of opponents and scapegoated minorities, all organised by the state and backed by street violence, condoned by police and judges and supported by the new force of radio broadcasting. Its doctors provided simplistic biological justifications for these ideas. Doctors and nurses formed a higher proportion of Nazi Party membership than any other professionals.[3] In Germany, already by 1932, sterilisation legislation was prepared and accepted by a wide range of Catholic, Jewish and socialist eugenicists, though many in these groups would eventually be its victims. With organised opposition already imprisoned or murdered, the Nazi euthanasia programme met no serious contemporary resistance from professional or public opinion, or from leaders of the major religions.[4]

The ideas behind these developments were not unique to Germany.[5] In the US, following the same vulgarised quasi-scientific theories, at least 60,000 people were forcibly sterilised in the first half of the 20th century.[6] Similar measures were taken in Sweden in the 1930s.[7] They were contemplated by government in Britain, with similar widespread acceptance of simplistic assumptions about the nature of inheritance. Fortunately they were never implemented. By the mid-1930s scientists everywhere were beginning to recognise where all this was leading, and had some influence on liberal governments. This experience shows that in times of serious crisis, neither medical science, nor clinical practice, nor professional culture and traditional oaths provide inherent guarantees against even the most extreme inhumane thought and behaviour. As we have now entered what may well become a period of global crisis as serious as that of the 1930s, it is still relevant today.

People trained to cut patients up for their own good have a necessary ruthlessness which may easily slide into sadism. Wherever the full power of the state and media of mass communication have authorised violence by uniformed state servants or contractors, or by criminal sections of its population, against groups designated as enemies of society, as in the USSR, South Africa, from time to time in most of Latin America since the Second World War, and at present throughout the Middle East, only recently have medical professional organisations begun to organise serious resistance among their own members, though it has to be said they are now starting to make amends.[8]

Inhuman applications of humane science can occur only if our natural propensity for solidarity becomes concentrated on people of our own choice, or chosen for us, with others demonised and excluded.

These were the solidarities of our prehistory, when each tribe lived within its own small world, and every other tribe was a potential enemy. Tribal survival seemed all important, and human survival was not yet in question. Our answer must lie in refusing ever to accept such exclusions. Health professionals have a duty to serve everyone who needs their help, friend or foe. Doctors and nurses already have established institutional frames. Now, more than ever, they need to take these established conventions seriously, resisting pressure from both irresponsible journalists and populist politicians. In all wars there have been health workers who cared for their sick and wounded enemies, as well as for their friends. The Geneva Conventions may not have counted for much, but they still provide a foothold for progress.

Justice is never natural

More than other professionals, health workers face every day an inescapable truth: there is no natural justice. Three days after leaving school, an 18-year-old girl dies suddenly from a brainstem haemorrhage: fate, God, or developmental error gave her an aneurysm without warning symptoms. Among the mourners, one of her school friends has already silently received the gift of leukaemia, which will announce itself a few months later. We now understand this group of diseases well enough to cure it, in 8 cases out of 10, but only at the cost of multiplying the patient's risks of premature death from several other causes, and so eventually orphaning his or her children. For misfortune as for money – the more you have, the more you are likely to get. Disease, including propensities to addiction and other supposedly self-inflicted injuries, strikes indiscriminately.

Justice is a human concept. For justice to be brought into existence, people have to imagine it and then start to impose it on the natural world. Justice in health becomes possible to the extent that we understand not only how nature works, but also how society works. The task of advancing clinical medicine and medical science is a difficult but fascinating one, where discovery is its own most powerful reward, but this is never enough. To impose justice on the natural world, we must above all impose justice on ourselves, through rules governing relations between people, which we have ourselves designed. Property is, they say, nine-tenths of the law, and property is power – including power to design and impose laws, and to create cultures that accept them as natural and inevitable. Grossly unequal division of property and power has, throughout history, hitherto been a precondition for progress through rising productivity of labour. This has a paradoxical result: social justice, in material reality rather than imagination, has been made possible only through social injustice. Yet the idea of justice persists, the idea of a society where the rights of property must eventually be subordinated to the rights of people to enjoy healthy and creative lives. The NHS has given us enough of that experience to justify that idea as no longer a utopian dream, but an immediately attainable reality.

Who is my neighbour?

When I qualified in 1952, all NHS services were available free to anyone in my country who needed them. To include people who were not British citizens might at first sight seem to impose potentially limitless and unaffordable responsibility on the NHS, but in practice this never happened. If a Greek seaman or a French cook or an American lady visiting her sick grandmother happened to break a leg or get pneumonia, our first consideration was to help them, with no questions asked about who would pay. Though foreign visitors could have been made to fill in a lot of forms and pay for their care, in an already cash-free gift economy the costs of collection would have been close enough to potential revenues to make this a gratuitous act of meanness.

The definitive experiment was finally made by Margaret Thatcher's government in 1983.[9] Sheffield Health Authority staff were compelled to question 50,000 patients in the first three months of operation of her government's new procedure for charging overseas visitors. Among these they found a total of eight who were liable to pay. Their total charges amounted to £4,066, almost half of which was incurred by patients who never paid. The authority decided to resort to the courts only if this made economic sense, which of course it never did.[10]

Like unpaid doctors' fees in the era of pre-NHS trade, bad debts to the NHS generally cost more to pursue through the courts than the debts themselves are worth, but the idea that sick foreign visitors are 'health tourists', whereas our own sick nationals abroad are just unfortunate, is a lie too popular for our newspapers or populist politicians to leave alone. In 2008, NHS England introduced a system for charging foreign patients admitted in emergency to its hospitals, known as 'Stabilise and Discharge'. Such patients were discharged as soon as three consultants agreed they were stable, unless they paid with cash or a credit card. How did this work out? A middle-aged Indian man who had suffered a stroke was admitted to West Middlesex Hospital. He was told that he faced discharge within 48 hours unless he could pay for his care. The hospital's income generation manager (another new bureaucrat, created to satisfy newspapers that promote campaigns against bureaucrats, as well as xenophobia) said he did not believe the patient was a UK citizen, so he was not eligible for free care. This manager said this blunt approach had saved his hospital from £600,000 to £700,000 a year, and was enthusiastically supported by government. 'It is up to the Department of Health', he said, 'to see how brave they will be to use innovative ways to tackle health tourism.' In October 2008 the government abandoned this scheme in the face of widespread refusal by GPs to implement it.[11] British GPs evidently understood solidarity better than did New Labour politicians.[12]

Solidarity is simple and, broadly speaking, true. The simpler we can make it, the truer it can be. Health care is a field in which generosity is a natural behaviour tending to create generosity in return.[13] Despite many similar tales, the common experience of both staff and patients in the NHS has confirmed this optimism. For the most part, these stories are either tabloid fairytales, or based on exceptional incidents remembered precisely because they were exceptional.

Pooled risk

Solidarity has its origins in the survival advantages of reciprocity and pooled risk. If I help weak people when I am strong, then I may expect to find strong people to help me when I am weak; the principle of reciprocity.[14] All human societies have had this characteristic, which is even more obvious in the subsistence economies of hunter-gatherers and nomads than in more advanced economies with an agricultural or industrial surplus and some sort of evolved care system. Systems based on wholly inclusive pooled risk are immensely more efficient than contributory insurance systems of any kind. Above all, they are more efficient than the individually calculated risks of privately marketed insurance.[15] If everyone is entitled to care according to their need, a huge bureaucracy of risk assessors, premium collectors, fraud detectors and millionaire or billionaire directors leading an army of mostly corporate investors can all be released to do something more useful. All we need do is pay our taxes on a single assessment of income. These taxes then fund the cash-free internal economy of the NHS (or any other service we decide to transform from a commodity to a shared human right), and there is an end of it. The pre-'reform' NHS worked because few people wanted to be ill, and most were intelligent and civilised enough to understand that it made sense to pay throughout their lives for a service they hoped to use as little as possible themselves, because nobody knew when they might need it. Even though our press and approved experts constantly tell us otherwise, this was and still is how most people seem to think most of the time. This view is reinforced by common experience of the NHS, even in its now mutilated state. The great weakness of the US is that neither its people nor its health professionals have ever had that experience, and both lack confidence that other people share the generous beliefs most of them still dare to possess.[16]

Solidarity is not altruism

Solidarity should not be confused with altruism. This is an area of thought which requires rigorous clarity and realism, not sentimentality. Adam Smith's opinion expressed in *The Wealth of Nations*, that most people most of the time act in their own interest, was correct. Sustainable economics deals not with exceptional people in exceptional states of moral uplift, but with ordinary people in their everyday behaviour.

The concept of altruism, motivation to act not for oneself but for others against one's own personal interest, is natural and appropriate for liberal academics, whose own experience continually reinforces their belief that a large social conscience is an economic burden, and that to act generously is usually against their own material interest. For generations of organised industrial workers this was simply not true. They thought in terms not of altruism, but of solidarity. Experience taught them that their personal interests, or those of their families, were almost always best served, in the long run, by acting in the interests of their entire working community. Institutions outside the market, like the NHS and public education, were created as expressions of that solidarity, and by the response of rulers to the threat which organised labour posed to their privileges, not by the altruism of either group.

The concept of solidarity as a guiding principle for health care has its diametrical opposite in the view that health care can most effectively and efficiently be provided as a commodity traded for profit. Fully developed free-market society compels everyone to become either a winner or a loser. Both of these states distort or destroy human creativity, our means to reach any better future. Even if some losers somehow obtain more crumbs from the winners than they can produce from their own subsistence production, eventually even the winners will lose – first their integrity and self-respect, then our planet as a shared habitat.

Motivation

Does anyone really believe that advances in medical science or innovations in care can be driven faster and more efficiently by greed than by ambition to serve society? Does anyone really believe that the great pioneers of medical and nursing science would have worked harder for profit, either for themselves or for an employer, than for the dignity and honour of having achieved something real to make the world a happier place?[17]

In a public service frankly committed to meeting human needs rather than making a profit, motivation is rarely a problem. Overwhelmingly, NHS staff love their work, and ask only to be allowed to do it to the standards they have learned. When some of them seem to hate or fear their work, serious questions need to be asked, usually about wages, workload, or bullying in the still persistent staff hierarchy, but, above all, whether the service is in fact devoted to meeting human needs rather than business-oriented management targets, and whether staff really have control of their own work.

Undeniably, profit provides powerful motivation, and competition soon drives idlers out of the market. Undeniably, many units in public service become stagnant, their staffs content to meet the letter of their contracts, without imaginative commitment to proclaimed goals. The cure for this common collective disease is not profit for an employer and tight management for employees, but inclusion of research, teaching and team development as essential functions for all service units without exception. Participation in research, teaching and team development ensure that staff continue to learn through their own experience.

Solidarity works both ways. The NHS also depends on patients and communities helping NHS staff. When society itself begins to fall apart, into a war of every man against every man, a lifelong battle between consumers where disciplined queuing has become a lost social skill, and personal demands have become an irresistible force (as they do, for example, in drug dependence), solidarity may seem almost impossible to regain. However, there seems to be no other way back to a stable, evolving society. To accept that we have lost solidarity is an unconditional surrender to greed, and betrayal of the future. Units of the NHS itself must then provide spaces in which to rebuild solidarity where it has been lost.

Internal inequalities in health and health care

My mother, Dr Alison Macbeth, qualified in medicine just after the First World War and was in the first cohort of specialist endocrinologists. When she was 12 years old she had acute rheumatic fever, then a common disease among the poor, but often seen also in affluent professional families like hers. At 52 she had a dense embolic stroke from mitral stenosis, a late consequence of that childhood event. Five years later she had another embolic stroke and died.

Today, acute rheumatic fever has virtually disappeared in Britain. Working as a GP in relatively poor communities, I saw three new cases between 1953 and 1963, the last I ever saw. Students seeking experience of this now rare but formerly common disease will still find plenty in West Africa, Rio de Janeiro or India, and occasionally in Chicago, Washington DC and Harlem.[18] Acute rheumatic heart disease and other disorders related to streptococcal infection, like acute nephritis, are causally related to poverty, chiefly because of domestic overcrowding. Material poverty of that degree has become rare in Britain, except in neighbourhoods of recent immigrants and our many areas of high unemployment.[19] The lesson is that where affluent people live in the same cities as poor people, some of their children will share the diseases of the poor.

The reflex *Daily Mail* answer to this is social segregation. Those who can afford it retreat to suburbanised countryside or gated urban communities, those who can be imprisoned or expelled from the country are thrown out, and those too poor and too British to do either of these are expected to shut up and behave themselves. Experience of drug addiction and AIDS shows that all gates fail and all frontiers are porous. Fortunately, so long as the poor exist, their diseases will threaten the offspring of the rich, and problems will not go away until they are solved for the whole population, as public health doctors have observed:

> The belief that subpopulations in one country are separate and do not operate as a single ecosystem affecting each other has propelled the US into a crisis of social and economic structure and of public health and public order which is so severe that even such crude measures as life expectancy show deterioration. It reflects a profound error: concentration is mistaken for containment.... Public policies or economic practices which marginalise vulnerable communities within Europe may be expected to create a crisis similar to that now raging in the United States.[20]

Large mortality differences between social groups, and the even larger morbidity differences they approximately represent, are a danger to everyone. Though technical repairs later created personal clinical solutions to my mother's problem (mitral valvotomy, valve replacements, atrial embolectomy and continuous anticoagulants), these remain inefficient and costly compared with preventive measures easily available for at least the past two centuries, if there were the political will – rehousing poor people in the conditions we all want for our own families.[21] No serious national programme for social housing existed in Britain until after the two World Wars, and even then they were not sustained.[22] The parallel between rheumatic heart disease and coronary heart disease is almost exact – both were social epidemics for which there were two sets of answers: either extremely clever but costly and socially inefficient surgical repairs, or mass changes in planned social housing, education and our food economy to develop people as intelligent citizens rather than passive consumers, and provide conditions in which intelligent choices could be made.[23] That is no more impossible now than was decent housing for everyone in the first half of the 20th century.

We also have consistent evidence over long periods of time, mainly from studies in California and Sweden, that people who live within larger, more integrated, sustained and participative personal networks of family, friends, neighbours and workmates live longer than those who are isolated. Active, participative community is important for health. This is probably linked not to specific disease pathways, but to more general factors related to rates of senescence and resistance to disease.[24] Close, mutually supportive relationships are for most people a necessary part of healthy life. The grossly unequal, destabilised, acquisitive society created by the unregulated operation of market forces is therefore inherently unhealthy.[25] Richard Wilkinson has presented overwhelming evidence from all over the world confirming that inequality itself, not only absolute or relative poverty, operates as a cause of ill health. So potent is it that even the richest people in the most unequal countries tend to be less healthy than the richest people in the least unequal countries.[26] Market forces propagate ill health, above all mental ill health, just as they propagate crime and every kind of selfish behaviour, by dividing people from one another and compelling them to compete rather than cooperate. Within established modes of thought that perceive health only as absence of specific disease this is easier to understand than to prove, but it remains a stubbornly held popular belief because it confirms common experience, as well as being the consensus view of most sociologists.

Global inequalities in health and health care

The dangers presented to national health by socio-economic ghettoes have their obvious counterpart in dangers to world health presented by pools of uncontrolled disease in virtually all countries outside Europe, North America, Australia and New Zealand. This used to be the main agenda of the World Health Organization (WHO) when it was a respected independent agency of the United Nations with perceived responsibility for advancing world health, not a poor relation of the World Bank (WB), as it has now become.

The WB started taking an interest in global health policy in the late 1970s, when health care began to interest investors. From 1984 to 1989 WB loans related to health care trundled along at a steady US$0.25bn a year, about half as much as the WHO budget. In 1996 WB loans for health care began an escalating rise still continuing today, taking WB investments in health care to more than double the entire WHO budget by 2000.[27]

This reflected changing patterns of US investment. In the US, more than one third of economic growth between 1994 and 1999 was in service exports. The WB calculated that in less-developed countries alone, infrastructure development with some private backing rose from US$15.6bn in 1990 to US$120bn in 1997. About 15% was direct foreign investment in public schemes, with loans or aid conditional on new policies of privatisation, direct patient charges, and a free hand for imported pharmaceuticals.[28] Effective socialised care services, which had once provided splendid examples of successful best practice, for instance in Kerala and Sri Lanka, were broken up and privatised under WB pressure, with predictably dire consequences for public health.[29] A struggle has been going on since November 2004 in the European Union between its Competitiveness Council led by Fritz Bolkestein, which wants a single market for all service industries, and defenders of EU Treaty Article 52, who insist that member states must each retain responsibility for their own public health services.[30] This struggle included politicians concerned to get re-elected, and 60,000 trade unionists who demonstrated in Brussels in March 2005 to remind them of that fact (unreported by mainstream British news media).[31]

Effectively, bankers have replaced health professionals as directors of global health policy. Together with the World Trade Organization (WTO), they have reversed the consistent general direction of WHO policy from 1946 to 1990 favouring socialisation of health care. This was not because WHO was wedded to a socialist ideology, but because public service was so obviously more cost-effective than private trade.[32]

All the most powerful global institutions, the United Nations and its satellite organisations like UNICEF and WHO, date from the end of the Second World War, when the US economy emerged with its manufacturing capacity doubled and every other combatant nation was either devastated or bankrupt. These institutions all depended chiefly on US funding. All except WHO (which went to the old League of Nations building in Geneva) were sited in the US, mainly to ensure that isolationism would not blight the first shoots of world government, as it had in 1919. Ever since then, continued US support for the UN has been conditional on support for US policies. When the UN refused to endorse US aggression against Iraq, the George W. Bush presidency came close to discarding the UN and its satellite agencies altogether.[33] Despite all evidence to the contrary, the idea that the US is so large, so wealthy and so mightily armed that it can ignore what happens to the rest of the planet has too firm a grip on the American imagination to disappear quickly. Essentially the same idea still thrives in Europe, which gave birth to every modern empire, and with it, the conviction that Europeans, together with their US descendants, are the natural rulers of the rest of humanity. Past memories and present illusions of empire underlie every denial of our need for solidarity simply for civilisation to survive.

Yet such beliefs will certainly fail. The planet is indivisible, and so is the damage done to it by two centuries of reckless industrial expansion, without regard even to physical consequences, let alone the consequences for human relationships, culture and self-respect. The global institutions created in 1945, jointly by naïve idealists and hard-nosed statesmen, could still provide the beginnings of democratic world government. Indeed, they will have to. Global solutions will have to be found for the global problems created by climate change. As European and North American cities begin to experience devastation similar to what has long been familiar to the rest of the world, people will begin to think more in terms of solidarity with the entire human race.

Or the end of solidarity?

Is such optimism justified? Ever since the Second World War, virtually all mainstream experts on social change have agreed that the social base for solidarity is diminishing, at increasing speed. Employment in heavy industry and manufacture has declined, consumer choice appears to replace trade union and political organisation as a way for people to improve their lives, and most of what used to be called the working class is now said by these experts to have become middle class. As for everything else, we tend to adopt US terminology, in which the working class is in practice defined as people at the margins of the economy, mostly without work – the reserve army of unemployed.

Two years after he became Prime Minister, Tony Blair said that he had

> a 10 year programme to tackle poverty and social exclusion. At the end of it I believe we will have an expanding middle class ... which will include millions of people who traditionally saw themselves as working class, but whose ambitions are far broader than their parents and grandparents.[34]

Along with all those who have built careers on his patronage, he believed that the natural ideology of this aspirant middle class was consumerism. He and his fellow inventors of New Labour and the 'Third Way' were trying to give the one-nation conservatism of Benjamin Disraeli a broader mass base, adding millions of people who voted for the Liberal Party in the 19th century and for Labour in the 20th century to Disraeli's jingo imperialists and deferential servants, to bring virtually the whole of society within a single ideology – as sometimes appeared to have been achieved in the US, under the presidency of his friend George W. Bush. This New Labour might be more attractive than the Conservative Party to those who owned almost all of the UK economy. It presented no real threat to their control, yet was still sufficiently associated with the founders of state welfare and egalitarian rhetoric that it might still hold the loyalty of its traditional working-class electorate. It might then bat the Conservative Party into the long grass for a very long time, and perhaps even replace it as the natural party of UK government.

Defining social class

Changes in the class structure of advanced capitalist economies are undeniable. They have greatly weakened the social groups which originally created socialised health care in the UK and its equivalents elsewhere in Europe, and only just failed to do so in the US.[35] However, there are now new social groups. The old class divisions remain, between people who live from what they own and people who live from whatever work the owners of capital find it profitable to give them, but the social composition of this working class has changed. Whether this new composition favours continued development of the NHS as a gift economy, or its disintegration into a residual safety net for victims of market failure, is the question we need to consider.

Social class may be defined objectively, by observed status, wealth or income, or subjectively, by the groups with which people themselves choose to identify. Considering social classes as agents for social change, these subjective self-definitions are important. If people do not think of themselves as members of a class, they will not act as members of that class. Marx used social class to analyse the power structure of societies. He believed that in every society control of production of means for existence was the foundation for all power. He defined social classes not in terms of their wealth, gender or race, but entirely in terms of the nature and extent of their control over the processes of production. I share that view. Unlike almost everything else associated with Marxism over the 160 years or so of its existence, I believe this survives unchanged.

In advanced industrial economies with little or no peasant class, significant independent subsistence production has become virtually impossible. Marx's perception of two great social classes, a small class of powerful owners and a large class of powerless and propertyless operatives who depend on owners to employ them, is therefore more obviously valid now than it was when he launched this idea in 1848.[36]

Though this is a powerful device for social and historical analysis, there is no evidence that Marx ever intended it as a precise statistical tool. He set out not a detailed anatomy of the form of society, but a broad analysis of its functions, its physiology, how it worked, and from the point of view of those wanting to change it. Analysis by people wanting to defend the rules of society rather than to change them is naturally different. Starting from where most people are now, and from available data, we find only categories useful to business, government and social policy as agreed by conventional wisdom.

The following subjective data came from the Centre for Elections and Social Trends in 1999:

	1966	1979	1987	1997
Percentage of UK adults describing themselves as:				
Middle class	30%	32%	34%	36%
Working class	65%	63%	62%	61%
Don't know	5%	5%	4%	3%

By 2007, the BBC reported that a British Social Attitudes survey had found that 57% of people still described themselves as working class.

We can compare these data with UK census rankings in 1951, based objectively on occupation. If, as was formerly customary, we accept that Registrar General's Social Classes I, II, and III non-manual were the Middle Class, these jointly formed 27.8% of the population in 1951. Social Classes III manual, IV and V, then described as Working Class, together formed 72% of the population. By 1995, the Middle Class thus defined had grown to 51.2% of the population, and the Working Class had declined to 48.9%.

This confirms that, as a cultural group, the Working Class (as thus defined) is diminishing, with corresponding recruitment to the Middle Class. However, it does not support widespread adoption by UK media of US media terminology, which describes virtually everyone in employment as middle class (the 'middle America' wooed by presidential candidates, corresponding to the 'middle Britain' which has become the pivot of all political discussion for UK media). In fact this terminology seems doubtful even in the US, where a high proportion of industrial workers still seem to describe themselves as working class, whatever media discussants may think. One sociologist has estimated their number as over 60% of the population.[37]

Market researchers target various social groups as consumers with different spending capacities and preferences. As usual, they allocate most white-collar workers above the lowest grades to the middle class, and all manual workers, however skilled and well paid, to the working class, together with people without work but competing for the lowest-paid employment. Using their definitions, these researchers confirm a rapid fall in the proportion of working-class people, from about 64% of the UK population in 1975 to about 52% in 1997, and a corresponding rise in the middle class from about 36% in 1975 to about 48% in 1997. This corresponds with the decline in UK manufacture which continues today.[38]

This conventionally defined industrial working class has provided bedrock voters for the Labour Party ever since it overtook the Liberals as a popular mass party after the First World War, and bedrock support for shared risk in an NHS gift economy. However, there has always been a substantial minority working-class vote for the Conservative Party, rarely falling much below 20% even in Labour strongholds of heavy industry. This provides stable support for consumerism – every man for himself. Nevertheless, though there has been a catastrophic fall in the number of workers employed in mining, fisheries, agriculture, manufacturing and heavy industry, the British industrial working class would still be a huge social, cultural and political force if it had confidence in itself, defined itself in contemporary terms and had political leadership. Allied with the new kinds of worker generated by new kinds of commodity in a knowledge-based economy, such an alliance is potentially larger than ever before. The actual composition of the 'middle class' seems extremely suspect. It certainly contains many white-collar workers with no more power, property or security than blue-collar manual workers. Though white-collar workers mostly lack the traditions of militant solidarity typical of workers in mining and most industrial manufacturing, they have in fact provided most new entrants to trade unions over the past 30 years, a development always requiring real personal leadership and sacrifices to achieve.

A middle with a bottom but no top?

The term 'middle class' implies that it has some higher class above it, and another class below it: or, if we prefer the North American myth of classlessness in a mobile society without significant inherited wealth or power, above or below these middle rungs on the social ladder. Either way, it implies three layers of society. The people beneath are the working class, whose size depends on how many white-collar workers are allocated, or allocate themselves, to middle-class status. However, a working class as defined by Marxists (people who do not themselves own or control the organisation and material resources for production, and must seek employment from those who do) obviously still exists, comprising up to 80% of whole populations in mature economies. The great statistical mystery is the hypothetical class above the middle class, presupposed by this terminology, but ignored by population censuses or surveys. According to market research, both in 1975 and in 1997, the middle class and working class together formed 100% of the population. This middle seems to have something below it, but nothing above it. Even the Registrar General has no category for the super-rich, the top executives whose annual incomes can be measured in millions. They are included in Social Class I along with other higher managers and all professionals except teachers (relegated to Social Class II because they are so badly paid). Apparently no upper class is perceptible.

Unlike in any previous era, few now wish to admit they belong to a class whose wealth and power are by orders of magnitude greater than those possessed by anyone else. It is now hard to find anyone too rich or too powerful to find refuge in the ubiquitous middle class, at least when the nature of society is being discussed. The English queen, with one of the world's largest personal fortunes,[39] has been described on the BBC as the embodiment of English middle-class values, though even middle-class life is completely outside her personal experience.

No candidate for high office, in either Britain or the US, can afford to appear anything other than middle class, even if massive funding from billionaires is already a precondition for election to the presidency in the US, and is becoming so for increasingly presidential prime ministers in Britain. In fact, the super-rich and powerful are so few, as a fraction of the whole population, that no census categorises them.

Suddenly, in the global economic crisis of 2007–08, the super-rich owners of the global economy lost their invisibility. Even media commentators began to question why people who had created a mountain of illusory wealth by gambling in the global finance market should be allowed to pay themselves astronomical incomes, be rescued by government when their bets failed, and then write their own cheques for themselves.[40] Even among people close to the top of the business world, fundamental questions are now being asked about the risks to capitalist society posed by reckless, unregulated pursuit of profit by the people who control global investment of wealth. According to the Office for National Statistics, by September 2009, UK total net debt had risen to £824.8bn, 59% of GDP. Of this total debt, £142bn was incurred by bank salvages. Without it, total debt would have been only 49% of GDP. Government policy had formerly aimed at a ceiling of 40%. Speaking to business leaders, the Governor of the Bank of England warned that UK national debt was

> rising rapidly, not least because of support to the banking system. We shall all be paying for the impact of this crisis on the public finances for a generation.... To paraphrase a great wartime leader, never in the field of human endeavour has so much money been owed by so few to so many.[41]

Despite such warnings from within its own ranks, casinos in the City of London and Wall Street are already returning to the policies which caused the crisis. Only 12 months after the UK banking sector was rescued by public money, the Centre for Economics and Business Research predicted a resumed annual 50% growth rate for bonus payments to top bankers, a forecast now being fulfilled.[42]

The ruling class is frightened, and with good reason. Capitalism is not our only possible economy or society. At least some of its more intelligent advocates realise that fundamental change of some kind is necessary. On 9 August 2009, almost exactly two years after the global financial crisis erupted, a group of people gathered in London: a former deputy governor of the Bank of England, Sir John Gieve; Paul Woolley, fund manager and academic; and Lord Adair Turner, chairman of the

Financial Services Authority (FSA) and former director-general of the Confederation of British Industry. There were also a couple of journalists, who reported their thoughts in *Prospect*, a magazine for such people. Turner had been unguarded in his comments. It was not, he said, part of the FSA's job to champion the City, it had to be 'very, very wary of seeing the competitiveness of London as a major aim'. The financial sector, he said, had become 'swollen' and swallowed up too many of Britain's 'highly intelligent people from our best universities'. Parts of it had grown well beyond 'socially reasonable' size, and carried out activities that were 'socially useless'. The authorities, he said, should not succumb to arguments claiming that activities that increased the size of the financial sector were necessarily good in themselves. Not everybody round the table agreed. 'I don't think it's very helpful to try to define the right size for the financial sector any more than trying to define the right size of the cosmetics industry,' said Gieve. Turner replied, 'Higher capital requirements against trading activities will be our most powerful tool to eliminate excessive activity and profits, and if increased capital requirements are insufficient, I am happy to consider taxes on financial transactions — Tobin taxes ... The problem is that getting global agreement will be very difficult. But at least proposals for special financial sector taxes, with increased capital requirements, address the issue of excessive remuneration.'

Turner's remarks had no support from the Treasury, nor from New Labour Chancellor Alastair Darling,[43] nor from any other leading politician from any of the UK's major political parties. Nor should we expect it. Social progress does not descend from boardrooms, or even from heaven, it is either built by the daily struggle of working people or it does not happen at all.

Turner's remarks call into question the very root of classical economics, supremacy of the profit motive. Though the UK New Labour Party no longer dares to say it, there are some even among the ruling class who do. We have reached a crisis in which everyone, without exception, needs to reconsider where they stand. Social class loyalties are real, but in the end they depend on circumstances, and circumstances are changing.

Transition from industrial to intellectual economy

In every mature, developed economy, we are now seeing a painful transition from manufacture to services, and to intellectual production of new knowledge.[44] Transition of workers from manual to intellectual work does not necessarily imply a parallel transition from defining themselves as producers to allowing others to redefine them as consumers. The solidarity of coal miners, steel and tinplate workers, and their families who stood together with their breadwinners to compel capitalists to concede socially funded and organised health care systems, did not appear spontaneously, painlessly or inevitably. Though South Wales eventually became an area of industrial militancy matched only by the Clyde, and eventually employed a higher proportion of people in nationalised industry and public services than any other part of Britain, it took more than a century of bitter struggle to get there. The social base for solidarity has indeed changed, but the need for it is greater than ever. Without it, the gains it made for us all will soon be lost. The real question is how to reconstruct something like it, but from new social ingredients in the fundamentally different conditions of an increasingly knowledge-based economy. This expanded concept of the working class could become a more powerful political force than anything in the past.[45]

The spontaneous and self-propogating nature of consumerism makes it an extremely powerful force, but central to it lies a self-limiting contradiction. Market capitalism promotes people as avid consumers, but simultaneously degrades them as socially responsible creators of value. In exchange for fantasy worlds they can buy as commodities, it creates a real world of greed, selfishness, the death of fellowship and community, and a mass philosophy of hedonism. Self-respect is essential to health. How can we respect ourselves if we allow such a world to become our children's inheritance? Creation of a new social base for solidarity, with the NHS gift economy as its spearhead, is the theme of the next, and final, chapter.

Summary and conclusions

Humane development of science depends on including the entire population within its scope, on an equal footing – all for each and each for all. Internal equivalence of our species provides the foundation for medical science, and social inclusiveness is the foundation for effective care systems. Solidarity created state care systems, and their shortcomings are largely attributable to a lack of it.

Consumerism stands opposed to this, with every man for himself and every woman for herself as its philosophy. It tells us that as we become richer, we become less able to afford the former generosity and fellowship of the poor. Though this set of ideas now dominates people at the top, hopefully it may fail to take a majority of people with it. Public belief in solidarity, at least for health care in the UK, has so far generally withstood almost three decades of sustained assault from those with the power to form public opinion.

The philosophy of consumerism ignores the real world even more than the most romantic concepts of solidarity. It assumes we still live in an economy of small entrepreneurs, so self-reliant that they have little need of the state. No such economy in fact exists, or ever has existed. Small entrepreneurs sink as fast as new ones set sail, and the state and unelected bureaucracy continues to expand under both New Labour and Conservative administrations, whatever their rhetoric. Attempts by the Liberal-Democrat Party to create yet another centrist party somehow squeezed in between Conservatives and New Labour cannot provide any coherent alternative set of ideas.Before 'reform' of welfare economies, the state-funded and organised ventures were too large, and entailed risks too great, for any prudent investor to bear. The wave of privatisations of state industries, services and utilities has not reduced state funding. It has generally increased it, but diverted the money from direct investment in state property, with at least some public accountability through Parliament, into colossal subsidies to giant corporations now operating for profit where once the state operated only to break even, and to colossal spending on the police and prisons required to contain the losers in an infinitely competitive society. The new pattern for state enterprise is partnership with big business, where business takes the profits and the public, through the state, takes the risks.[46]

Assumptions that solidarity is natural to the declining industrial working class but not to the rising middle class are illusory. Neither justice nor solidarity were ever natural, they had to be built through experience and struggle by those with most to gain from them and least to lose. Most of the so-called middle class is the working class in new conditions. This expanded working class will have to struggle to build and maintain solidarity, in new ways and in a new culture of its own. Class analyses proclaiming a new era of peace based on a middle class to which almost everyone belongs, with the working class marginalised to vanishing industries or permanent unemployment, are based on superficial assumptions. The reality continues to be nations divided between a minority who live from what they own, and a majority who live from what they do. The future of the NHS depends on this majority.

SEVEN

A space in which to learn

This book has provided evidence, derived from actual care processes, that commercial patterns, no matter how modified, are inappropriate for any health care system aiming to cover the whole lives of whole populations, at optimal efficiency. Health gain for whole populations cannot be produced efficiently as a by-product of investment for profit. Under present UK and EU company laws, wherever responsibility for service is contracted out to private sector providers, they are compelled to ignore such evidence, and subordinate the needs of society to commercial ambitions. The consequences are concealed by laws guarding commercial secrecy, and by politicians and media commentators apparently incapable of thinking outside a provider/ consumer box or of imagining any cooperative rather than competitive society in practical terms.

Fully rational development and use of medical knowledge for all who need it requires a gift economy, congruent with the shape of continuing clinical decisions in continuing real lives. In such an economy, staff and patients could learn together, from their own successes and errors. They could learn to work in new ways, harnessing the reserves of motivation and goodwill that are now frustrated or wasted by confining patients and communities to consumer roles, magnifying wants and ignoring needs. Such an economy would depend on levels of personal trust which are unsustainable in commercial transactions. Its own cooperative processes could build that trust, instead of eroding it by pillorying staff for unexpected outcomes.

A gift economy in health care is justified not only because it could be happier, more imaginative and more human, but because it would probably be more efficient. It would probably promote sustained commitment by staff and intelligent participation by patients, thus expanding resources at little or no additional cost. Because it would support sceptical appraisal of claimed innovations, rather than credulous acceptance of promoted wants, it could expand at a sustainable pace, similar to that of experimentally proven advances in science. Because its processes would be open to public scrutiny, not cloaked by commercial secrecy or falsified by promotion, we could see the negative as well as positive consequences of our decisions, and learn from them.

This book has also provided evidence that from 1948 until the early 1980s, when the NHS was allowed (often grudgingly, and always with insufficient funding) to pursue the needs of our whole population as then understood, we developed the beginnings of this NHS gift economy. Despite its many paternalistic faults, it was more cost-effective, more popular with our public, patients and professional staff, than anything previously experienced in the UK.[1] The NHS began to develop a new culture, shifting profit motivation from the centres of hospital and specialist practice to a marginalised periphery, increasingly despised by advancing medical education and research. Though profit motivation persisted in primary care through GPs' private contractor status, there too there was a similar shift. A growing proportion of GPs learned from their own experience to accept continuing and personal responsibility for public service to all within their registered populations. Added together, these populations included virtually everyone – as citizens in communities, not episodic customers shopping around without a home.

Paths are made by walking[2]

This nascent new economy and culture was no more than a beginning. Professional interest in business rather than public service never disappeared. Initial political leadership allowed the NHS to take first, uncertain, tentative steps towards a possible future economy and culture of more equal relationships, in which traditions of medical trade could diminish and new traditions of shared responsibilities within public service could grow. Nowhere did this learning process come anywhere near completion, nor did anyone with practical experience expect it to. The ideas of patients and communities developing as co-producers of health rather than consumers of care, and of health professionals thinking and acting as though they not only used the conclusions of science, but could themselves become contributors to scientific development as a social process, following its own rigorous ethics rather than the fundamental brutality of business, have never been fully accepted, developed or understood, even by a majority of NHS staff, let alone the politicians elected to lead it.

Even in the favourable conditions provided by the NHS Act of 1946, implemented in 1948, it took about four decades of experience before any of these ideas began to be clearly articulated even by innovators. Even if governments had led rather than trailed behind and finally opposed this process, we would have needed several generations to create the entirely new culture we need to apply the full power of scientific thinking to all our health problems. In my experience, few if any innovators in care can ever bring about real change within less than five years of practice. Experiments in new forms of delivery designed to provide significant answers in less than that time are almost always doomed to fail, because that is the least time it takes for any real community to believe such innovators are seriously committed to change, rather than to the next step in their own ascending careers. People are accustomed to being deceived. To regain trust, they must first see evidence that the walls around professional and institutional power are falling.

So I don't want to imply that we ever enjoyed a golden age we are now losing. Many of these ideas are indeed golden, but ideas advance and recede faster than acts. Routine practice was bound to change slowly and hesitantly, groping through the ordinary chaos of wants which every day threaten to drown frontline staff, facing the realities of always understaffed and underfunded care for those most in need of it. Staff in both hospitals and primary care mostly work very hard indeed, above all in areas of social hardship. They did in 1948, and they still do now. The content and responsibilities of care have changed, but the intensity of work is even more demanding, because so much more is now possible. This still makes it hard for staff to accept that there is even more work which needs to be done, over and above what they are already doing.[3]

I hope also that I have not given the impression that over this period advances in medical science have not been applied at increasing speed. On the contrary, knowledge has generally expanded ever faster as time has passed, simply because every answer poses more questions, in new ways that may make them potentially soluble for the first time. This progress may be impeded by institutional change and state policies, but probably nothing can stop it. This in itself proves the motivational power driving pursuit of new knowledge to be immeasurably greater than that which drives pursuit of profit. Generally speaking, knowledge of human biology has expanded faster since marketisation of the NHS began in the early 1980s, than it did before the NHS gift economy faced serious challenge. There are many reasons for this, but the main one is simply that scientific knowledge expands exponentially, whatever governments do or think. The market accelerates scientific advance in respect of marketable commodities, but impedes development of social products.[4]

We need to be extremely cautious when evaluating supposed progress or decline over time in the quality of care in national systems. Wherever clinical performance has been evaluated comprehensively and critically for the first time, results have initially been shocking, far worse than even the least optimistic professionals ever expected – usually less than 50% of consensus views of whatever contemporary experts believed to be tolerable in a developed economy.[5] In this sense, of course the NHS in 2010 is far better than it was in 1948. Evaluation should be cautious, but measure we must. Apart from the excessive accounting incurred by market relationships within any public service invaded by business culture, a huge expansion in measurement and monitoring at all levels was long overdue by the 1980s. Much of the expansion thereafter was useful for rational policy decisions (or could have been if it had been released from commercial secrecy). The Quality and Outcomes Framework (QOF) in particular arose from just such experiences as I had myself, together with other pioneers of proactive primary care. Its misuse by governments, using routine measurement and information technology as a means to subordinate primary care to business requirements, has not destroyed its potential positive value for introducing more systematic approaches to care. The innovatory practice and research required for initial and subsequent development of care will be useful long after public service has again become properly distanced from business.

As we know more we can do more, so public expectations rise. If the gap between what could be done and what actually is done becomes intolerably wide, policies which limit what is done to whatever is profitable for business will eventually lose public consent. This process is already far advanced in every country with an economy developed sufficiently to sustain a publicly funded health service. Exponential expansion in medical knowledge will continue, even if research and education are mutilated by ignorant governments, because the more we know the more inquisitive we become. Motivation to know more is more powerful than greed. Exponentially expanding knowledge will lead to exponentially expanding and better informed public expectations. These will eventually begin to replace sometimes infantile consumer wants by insistent expression of needs, backed by professional carers. Such understanding does not depend on formal education.[6] Even in the worst circumstances, this process provides sound grounds for optimism. The capacity of any developed economy to produce enough to meet basic human needs, and to expand more or less indefinitely by at least 2%–3% a year, cannot forever be held back by competition to maximise profit. Its only true rate-limiting factor is sustainable use of materials. That factor would be much easier to control if the main purpose of production were to meet human needs, for future generations as well as our own, rather than to maximise profits and capital accumulation. Given this rate of growth, and including useful work as itself a human need, there is virtually nothing worthwhile which we could not afford.[7]

Recognition that health care is a production process, with measurable inputs, outputs and efficiency, was a colossal step forward. For this we should thank Margaret Thatcher, if nothing else. However, her assumption that the only way to create national wealth was through production of commodities to sell for somebody's profit, now apparently shared by the leaders of all major political parties, revealed an ignorance of how national wealth was already being produced in the NHS, through a nascent gift economy to which she and they were, and still are, apparently blind.

In the 1948–80 NHS, we had a space to learn how to behave and work in a higher, more civilised society for our descendants, rather than the in many ways empty inheritance we now leave them. That space is what we are now in imminent danger of losing, if consumerism continues to make headway among the public, and if we fail to develop its alternative as the core agenda of a renewed social and political movement towards an expanded democracy, where we do not merely assent to whatever fait accompli our ruling classes have agreed on, but participate as active builders of a progressive society.

The people's war precipitated birth of the NHS

Foundations for the NHS were conceived by mining communities in the 19th century. That idea developed all its main features in embryonic form, but it took a second world war to bring it to nationwide birth.

Experience of mass poverty and unemployment, side by side with immense wealth used only to expand itself, and followed by experience of ability to use all our human and material resources fully in war, taught us that we did not need to tolerate an economy in which all major decisions were taken by a few very rich families in their own interest. This was the issue dividing left from right in politics, and had been so ever since ordinary people began to win even a small voice in their government. So politics then was real. Voting seemed to make a big difference to us all, not just to the careers of politicians. It concerned personal and family relationships, relationships at work, our interests in what we produced or helped to produce for ourselves and for others. Most of all, it concerned how we shaped our future, using our rapidly expanding productivity of labour to do first what was most necessary and for more people.

Roughly from 1940 to 1945, this became the national mood, particularly in our armed forces, and among people thinking ahead about what we had learned from total war, and how this might affect the shape of post-war society. Pioneering studies in nutrition, epidemiology and health services organisation in the 1930s were at the time ignored by government. In 1940, when all continental Europe from North Cape to Gibraltar to the Bosphorus fell under fascist control, Nazi invasion seemed imminent, national survival was at stake, and every man and woman became a potential defender of what remained of enlightenment, these studies became finally recognised as urgent, relevant and requiring only political will to apply them. For the first time, virtually everyone was enabled to perform some at least supposedly useful function in society. Where the market had failed to develop a necessary sort of production, the state stepped in, on behalf of us all.[8] For the first time, everyone had a job. A national minimum diet was assured for everyone, so that there was in fact less hunger and malnutrition in conditions of scarcity than there had been through 20 years of surplus production by farmers unable to sell what they produced. For the first time, all our children were immunised against diphtheria, which had killed about 3,000 children a year in ordinary times of inertia.[9] For the first time, all existing health care resources were identified and pressed into use. They were found to be grossly inadequate, unplanned and irrationally distributed, depending on capricious charity rather than planned and equitable taxation. For the first time, in anticipation of mass casualties from enemy bombing, nationwide services were created for blood transfusion and emergency hospital care, backed by bacteriological and biochemical laboratories and diagnostic X-rays.

The material and political foundations for a people's NHS were laid in the people's war.[10] Self-interested motivation was forced into eclipse, all national effort was officially devoted to collective survival, and risks were taken wherever still stubborn bureaucratic and hierarchical defences had to be overcome.[11] The 1945 general election, and its landslide victory for Labour, were a triumphant expression of that mood, before the old order could recover from its astonishment, mobilise its counter-attack, and adopt new disguises for its long road back to unregulated capitalism. So now once again a few rich men take all major decisions on what work we do and where and how we do it, leaving elected governments powerless and in public contempt, and the very idea of democracy again in question. Adding a few rich women to these is a strange notion of progress.

That period, from 1940 to 1948, was a space in which we learned what was really important, in the world and in our lives. It spawned many new or refreshed public services, partly recognised as 'the welfare state', but also including creative and cultural services with a far wider social base than ever before. All these developments were outside the world of business. In these spaces people could think and act without concerning themselves about anyone's profit. Yes, we had to balance the books – in nothing could we consume more than we produced for long – but we could devise our own means to reach our own ends, without regard to profit for managers or shareholders, because through the elected state we could begin to imagine ourselves as collective owners, our work funded from collective taxation. Sporting, cultural, educational, mutually entertaining and recreational spaces provided at least some part of our lives that did not depend on making more profit for a boss. People could do what they did and say what they said, outside and beyond the limits set by the mean, self-important and self-serving world of business, where everything began and ended with the bottom line.

Of course, this was only what some people thought, some of the time. It was vaguely defined and still full of ambiguities, but its enemies recognised well enough the reality and strength of this set of ideas, which broke loose in May 1945. Those enemies did not find their feet again until 1956, when Harold Macmillan managed to redesign the Conservative Party, no longer with a few thousand coaches and horses, but with millions of family cars. By then, the welfare state seemed irreversible.

Since the 1980s, and the 'new' economics of Ronald Reagan and Margaret Thatcher, those learning spaces have, step by step, been restored to business, opened to competition, and closed to any imagination that cannot contribute to commerce.[12] As we lose these spaces, we enter a new sort of totalitarian society, where every conceivable human need must be expressed as an individual want, to be satisfied by some individual material good or service, sold by some profit-seeking business. Conformity to this set of ideas becomes the test of loyalty. Anyone who suggests that there may be any other way to organise work can be howled down by a 'silent majority' apparently defined by people rich enough to own or control newspapers, television or radio broadcasting.

Today, we could hardly be further from the socially hopeful situation we had in 1945, when we had the collective courage, generosity and imagination to create the NHS. That was the end of an almost unimaginably painful 36 years of wasted human ingenuity and effort, starting in August 1914. Do we really have to go through all that again, to recreate such a national or even global mood of optimism and impatience? We have learned a lot since then, above all from the gross errors of initial attempts to build more human society, always in societies where capitalism had scarcely even begun to develop, let alone reached maturity, and which therefore lacked the social institutions required to create a democratic socialist society, depending on mass participation rather than coercion and providing means for everyone to participate actively and imaginatively in production of wealth in its widest sense. We in Britain were first into the tunnel. Why should we not be first to find a way out of it?

We need again to create and legislate for more spaces outside business, where we could produce wealth differently, according to social consensus priorities. Everyone participating in production within these spaces should be able to contribute their ideas, derived from and tested by practical experience, learning from their own achievements and mistakes in their own work, weighing themselves and each other according to what they produce and create, not what they consume.

The axe will fall

Virtually the entire UK print and broadcast media have agreed that the axe must fall, not on those who own and control most of our economy, whose speculation and reckless sales caused the crisis, but on everyone else, and every social institution not devoted to profit. Public services as a whole have already been condemned to anticipated cuts averaging 25% of their budgets, with official forecasts that some sectors may reach 30%, and some government departments 40%. Most of this will fall on welfare budgets, on which millions of new unemployed will have to depend. 'Incentives to work' (that is, penalties for being without work) are to be increased, while government will cut public sector jobs. This will strike most of all at the old areas of heavy industry such as Wales, Scotland, Northern Ireland and the Midlands and North of England. Work for private employers will have to depend on exports to a world in which every nation is now trying to export more and import less. It is a formula virtually guaranteed to repeat the horrors of the 1930s.

Of course we need fundamental change, but what sort of change? To eliminate this disease, rather than put whole societies on life support every few decades, we should address causes, not just effects. The poor have always bailed out the rich, but it's time to stop. We are descended from people who have seen and endured all this before. We know where it leads. The deniers and fools are those who want to repeat the same follies, just to sustain the same set of illusions, until the next crisis – above all, illusory wealth, representing not real production of useful things and services, but gambling, overproduction of anything and everything that can be sold, without investment in production of necessities which millions of people are too poor to buy. The realists are those who finally stop looking only for lifebelts, and try instead to understand why our ship is sinking, and what can be done about it.

This crisis needs surgery – social change more profound than anything we have seen since the 19th century. Even among economists, a few have learned something since that last great crisis of global capitalism in the 1930s, with all its appalling consequences, not least the rise of fascism and the Second World War. Here in Wales, Professor Alan Lovett, Dean of University of Glamorgan Business School, offered this advice:

> ... the singular shareholder wealth-maximising objective must be removed from company law to prevent executives hiding behind the law as an excuse for their own lack of commitment. *Profit would thus become a constraint, not an objective.*[14] (My emphasis)

Coming from a business school, this is a revolutionary conclusion. It goes right back to Adam Smith, who rightly perceived that useful objects can be produced more efficiently with profit rather than human needs as the objective of production; by workers functioning as machines, rather than as creative human beings, producing not what is most needed, but what is most profitable. But there are limits, among them the appalling effects of first turning people into cogs for a profit machine, then binning them when primitive machines are superseded by something producing even more, even faster, with even less human input, for whatever people can be induced to want. Adam Smith analysed an evolving society. It has now reached a point where the motivations needed to produce pins or loaves of bread are irrelevant to a far more sophisticated product – health gain through medical care.

Regardless of stock markets, medical knowledge will go on expanding. For that knowledge to be applied, the NHS must get larger, not smaller, employing more people with more education and higher skills. None of our labour-intensive human services can afford to lose a single job, without more damage to our sick society, so the NHS cannot grow at the expense of its workforce.

If we in the UK were to act, our signal to the rest of the world would find a mass response. Britain is no longer a great power, either through what's left of its real economy, or less still through its military status.

But ideologically and historically it still has immense potential force. Because Britain was the birthplace of modern industry and concepts of political economy, we still have an influential global platform. In the NHS, if it returned to the direction in which it set out in 1948, we have a potentially influential international institution, which could be producing new knowledge and ideas more useful and instructive to the world than any army. In the historical traditions of the British labour movement, before it tried to pass itself off as the bankers' best friend, we still have foundations on which to build the new, broader, mightier movements possible through shared information technology. The labour movement made the NHS and conceived its precursors. Only an expanded and renewed labour movement, incorporating a larger proportion of our whole population than ever before, can defend and extend it.

The first step in rebuilding that movement must be recognition of its own errors. For people who believe that is too difficult or too dangerous to be feasible, it might help to consider the experience of every clinician I know and respect. At one time or another, everyone responsible for other people's lives finds that they made a wrong decision. It seemed the best choice at the time, but subsequent events showed it was not. As a result, a patient died. Your colleagues assure you that you are not really to blame. They would have done the same, they say. It was inevitable. And so on. But really what they are saying, to themselves, is 'There, but for the grace of God, go I. If I blame him now, somebody one day will blame me.' So their comforting words don't help. You know you got it wrong, with catastrophic consequences. In those circumstances there is only one intelligent course available: go to the bereaved relatives, tell them the truth, and let them judge your actions for themselves. Forget legal advice, or the terms of your contract. There is no other honourable course. If you don't take it, not only will you be guilty in the eyes of all who have been directly involved, you will remain guilty in your own eyes, and for the rest of your life. So that's what you do, and in almost every case, when your story has been told honestly, and you have shown that you have learned from the experience, the bereaved relatives don't go to a lawyer and smash your life in revenge. You are far less likely to be crucified for telling the truth than for trying to evade it, but even that is better than living with your own contempt.

It is perhaps unrealistic to expect such honourable conduct from people who initiated an illegal war, defying two million of their fellow citizens who marched through London streets, imploring them not to. But for the UK labour movement to recover, the mass of its supporters, and those who in the past looked to the labour movement for social progress, must admit the colossal mistakes made through trying to make it what it was not, and what nobody needed – just another party which leaves all real decisions to those with wealth and power in the global marketplace.

Let's not wait till we have nothing left to lose.

Notes and references

Preface to the second edition

[1] There is just one important piece of evidence comparing performance of the entire NHS with just one chunk of the hugely variable market in health care in the US, the Kaiser Permanente (KP) health care programme in San Francisco (Feachem, G.A., Sekhri, N.K., White, K.L., 'Getting more for their dollar: a comparison of the NHS with California's Kaiser Permanente', *British Medical Journal* 2002; 324: 135–43). According to Prof Feachem, KP provides a higher quality service than the NHS at a much lower cost. Surprisingly, he has as one co-author, Prof Kerr White, formerly a lifelong advocate for a national health service covering the whole US population. KP is not representative of the whole US care system. It is nominally not for profit. Profits are listed in its balance sheets, but they are apparently mostly shared by its medical staff and administrators. It is generally recognised as the most enlightened large unit so far developed in the US. However, even as a comparison not between two national systems, but between the NHS as a national system and KP as a single large corporate unit, like was not compared with like, and many other aspects of this study make its conclusions extremely doubtful. Its methodology falls far short of the standards normally required for research papers in peer-reviewed journals.

Unlike the NHS, KP does not cover any whole geographically defined population. It has responsibility only for people who can afford to be its customers, or are entitled to its care through an employment contract, or a government programme such as Medicare or Medicaid, whereas the NHS has responsibility for continuing care (not just emergencies) for every UK citizen, regardless of their wealth or circumstances. KP does not provide care for mental illness, or for chronic illness in dependent elderly people. By its own admission, Feachem's paper includes no comparison of case-mix data, which might have gone some way to show that, despite all these serious exclusions (all of which put much greater burdens on the NHS), like was being compared with like, or at least that this difference was somehow allowed for in comparisons. Data on case-mix were available both for the NHS and for KP when this study was done, so why were they not used? Most seriously of all, its cost comparisons are invalid. As everyone knows, the cost of all medical, nursing and other staff procedures, and of all medications, is very much higher in the US than in the UK, precisely because in the US their prices are set by market competition, whereas in the UK both NHS staff and commercial suppliers relate to a state monopoly which must minimise costs and is in a much stronger bargaining position than KP. This is an important advantage inherent in the NHS as a state-organised gift economy designed to meet needs, rather than a commodity economy designed to maintain profit. International price differences of this kind, largely determined by the strength of public care systems as market negotiators, are the main variable determining their comparative efficiency (Parkin, D.W., McGuire, A.J., Yule, B.F., 'What do international comparisons of health care expenditure really show?', *Community Medicine* 1989; 11: 116–23). Feachem deletes this difference by adjusting all NHS data to US prices, comparing the NHS with KP not according to its actual costs, but according to notional costs it would face if it were operating in the US. Apparently an aim of this paper was to show greater cost-effectiveness in a market system than in a system of profit-free public service, and that is how it was been interpreted by all media commentators. The study design assured that this conclusion would be reached.

Feachem showed his first draft of this study to an eminent colleague, Prof Clive Smee, who advised him not to publish it, for the following reasons:

> Kaiser is indisputably much more expensive than the NHS *per capita*. At the currency conversion rate used by the authors and after their adjustments for differences in service and population coverage the *per capita* cost of the NHS is barely 60% of Kaiser – $1161 compared with $1951. If we are looking at the total costs or macro-efficiency of two systems it is simply wrong to adjust for differences in healthcare prices, over and above adjusting for general differences in prices. But to suggest that NHS *per capita* costs are 60% of those in Kaiser is to give the comparison a spurious accuracy that is not warranted by the data presented ... Alternative (and arguably more defensible) assumptions – e.g. about treatment of Kaiser's profits, their 'considerable' administrative costs, and the currency conversion rate – would reduce NHS costs *per capita* to barely half those of Kaiser ... The NHS has equity and universal coverage objectives that are irrelevant to Kaiser. The NHS also aspires to provide a range of health services that is significantly more comprehensive than is available under Kaiser ... from the data in this paper there can be no doubt at all that in terms of total costs *per capita* or macro-efficiency, Kaiser is far more expensive than the NHS. (Smee, C.H., 'What have we really learned from the NHS v Kaiser comparison?', *BMJ* website, Letters, accessed 31 January 2002).

This paper could be used to illustrate all the most serious errors of biased design and statistical casuistry. Had its authors been less powerful, and its peer-reviewers applied normal standards, it is hard to believe it could have been published in any reputable peer-reviewed journal. Its only importance lies in its status as a publication in an authoritative and normally objective peer-reviewed international journal of medical science, the *British Medical Journal* (*BMJ*), which has been quoted over and over again by advocates of marketed care. *BMJ* website correspondence, almost all of it critical and from experts in the field in both Britain and the US, had reached 70 pages by 20 February 2002. Shortly after it was published, the then *BMJ* editor resigned, to take up a new post as director of the UK branch of the largest health care corporation in the US.

[2] Gannon, Z., Lawson, N., *Co-Production: The Modernisation of Public Services by Staff and Users*, www.compassonline.org.uk, accessed 1 January 2010. The idea of co-production in public services seems to have originated from Gail Wilson ('Co-production and self-care: new approaches to managing community care services for older people', *Social Policy & Administration* 1994; 28: 236–50).

[3] Webster, C., *The National Health Service: A Political History*, Oxford: Oxford University Press, 1998. I had already read Webster's excellent official history of the NHS, but those volumes naturally compelled him to restrain so far as possible his own opinions to what the civil service would tolerate. In this short history he combines inside knowledge of how government policies were made, or more often allowed to drift along making themselves, with refreshing expression of his own exasperation with drifters or, occasionally, admiration for rare examples of imagination and leadership.

[4] Adam Smith held more enlightened views than most of the people who now claim him as a founding father of classical economics. Here is what he had to say about the state:

> Civil government, so far as it is instituted for the security of property, is in reality instituted for the defence of the rich against the poor, or of those who have some property against those who have none at all. (Smith, A., *An Enquiry into the Nature and Causes of the Wealth of Nations* (1762), Oxford: Oxford University Press, 1993, p 413)

And about how it should be funded:

> The subjects of every state ought to contribute towards the support of the government, as nearly as possible in proportion to their respective abilities; that is, in proportion to the revenue which they respectively

enjoy under the protection of the state. (Smith, A., *An Enquiry into the Nature and Causes of the Wealth of Nations*, p 451)

We now call this suggestion income tax.

[5] The book most relevant to my argument is Naomi Klein's wonderful *Shock Doctrine: The Rise of Disaster Capitalism*, New York: Metropolitan Books, Henry Holt, 2007.

Chapter One

[1] A commodity is a good or service produced for sale in the market, at a price determined by demand and competition. A good or service produced as a gift, just to help somebody, perhaps in your family, is not a commodity. The cobbler who makes a pair of shoes to sell has made a commodity. The same pair of shoes, but made as a gift for his child, is not a commodity. As my argument proceeds, this apparently simple difference will turn out to be critically important.

[2] Dental care was the first bastion of the 1948 NHS gift economy to fall, essentially because it has always been taken less seriously than care for every other part of the body, and because NHS dentists were paid by fees for each item of service in a shop-around market (easily translated into direct patient charges), rather than as GPs originally were, by flat rate capitation for registered populations. Oral health deserves as much respect as any other kind of health. In many areas, NHS dentists are now hard to find, because private practice, especially for cosmetic dentistry, has become so much more profitable than NHS work. However, in Wales at least, dentists as an organised profession are opposing this trend. Stuart Geddes, Director of the British Dental Association in Wales, says dental charges are inequitable, deter people from seeking necessary treatment, and violate the basic NHS principle of free care at time of use. At present, 45% of adults in Wales have to pay dental charges, ranging from £12 to £177 for each treatment. Based on 2007 data, free NHS dental care in Wales would cost government about £26.7m a year. NHS dental charges in Wales have now been frozen at £12 for a check-up between ages 25 and 60 (they are free above and below this age range); in England these charges have now risen to £16.20 (Brindley, M., 'All patients in Wales should receive free NHS dentistry in a bid to improve the nation's oral health, a dentists' leader urged last night', *Western Mail*, 25 August 2008).

[3] English readers usually have two problems about Aneurin Bevan. First, they don't know how to pronounce his name. The Welsh name Aneurin is

pronounced 'an eye rin' not 'an urine'. It is often shortened to 'Ni' or, more often, to 'Nye'. Secondly, they often confuse him with one of his greatest enemies in the Labour Party, the powerful right-wing trade union bully and darling of the Conservative press, Ernest Bevin.

[4] The campaign of lies launched in 2009 against President Barack Obama's extremely timid health care reforms by the Republican Party and by lobbyists for insurance companies is only the most recent in a long history of demonisation of the NHS in the US. Among the first instances of this was the lie that UK citizens could no longer choose their own personal doctor. Free choice of GP has always been available and was never under threat.

[5] Webster, C., 'Overthrowing the market in health care: the achievements of the early National Health Service', *Journal of the Royal College of Physicians* (London) 1994; 28: 502–7.

[6] Titmuss, R.M. (Oakley, A., Ashton, J., eds), *The Gift Relationship: From Human Blood to Social Policy*, original edition (1970) with new chapters by Virginia Berridge, Vanessa Martlew, Gillian Weaver, Susan Williams and Julian Le Grand, London: London School of Economics and Political Science, 1997. Titmuss provided a comparative analysis of the economics of blood for transfusion in Britain, where blood was available only as a free gift from volunteer donors, and the US, where almost all blood for transfusion came from paid donors through commercial enterprises. The UK National Blood Transfusion Service (NBTS) was a government service created during the Second World War, organising and recruiting on a mass scale in peacetime as a natural development parallel to the NHS. Using data from the 1960s, Titmuss found good evidence of greatly reduced costs and very much higher quality in the UK programme, with much lower risks of the then known contaminants, mainly hepatitis viruses (this was long before the AIDS pandemic). In Britain at least, few then challenged his conclusions (Darnborough, J., 'What price blood?', *Lancet* 1974; 1: 861). By the 1980s, commercial providers were hammering on the door everywhere, and illicit insider trading in high-value blood products (not blood for transfusion, but plasma derivatives) was becoming a serious problem within state services. In New Zealand, where government was about to impose market competition on its hitherto gift economy in blood for transfusion, 345 consecutive donors were questioned, with a 98% response. Over half were opposed to profits being made from blood, 71% were concerned about blood quality in a commercialised service, 41% would no longer give blood if profits were made from selling blood products, and 10% were reconsidering giving blood in future (Howden-Chapman, P., Carter, J., Woods, N., 'Blood money: blood donors' attitudes to changes in the New Zealand blood transfusion service',

British Medical Journal 1996; 312: 1131–2). Since then blood products derived from blood for transfusion have become an extremely profitable byproduct for the NBTS, creating fears that the UK system will soon be indistinguishable from that in the US (Oakley, A.,'Blood donation – altruism or profit?', *British Medical Journal* 1996; 312: 1114). Human body organs are now being seriously proposed by some health economists as commodities in an effective or even morally superior legal market (Taylor, J.S., *Stakes and Kidneys: Why Markets in Human Body Parts are Morally Imperative*, Aldershot: Ashgate, 2005; Cherry, M.J., *Kidney for Sale by Owner: Human Organs, Transplantation and the Market*, Washington, DC: Georgetown University Press, 2005). So far as I know, Titmuss never advanced his 'gift relationship' as a more general economic alternative, but clearly it had such possibilities, which were considered seriously at the time by some US economists – and, of course, rejected.

[7] Ching, P., 'User fees, demand for children's health care and access across income groups: the Philippine case', *Social Science & Medicine* 1995; 41: 37–46; and Mocan, H.N., Tekin, E., Zax, J.S., 'The demand for medical care in urban China', *World Development* 2004; 32: 289–304. Both studies confirm low elasticity of consumer demand for medical care in fee-paid market systems. Poor people regard medical care as a necessity, overriding all other needs, with low income elasticity, around 0.3.

[8] Notably by Ffrangcon Roberts (*The Cost of Health*, London: Turnstile Press, 1952) and Enoch Powell (*A New Look at Medicine and Politics*, London: Pitman Medical, 1966).

[9] In the first few years of the NHS, leaders of all major political parties believed newspaper tales of runaway costs in the free service. A Conservative government set up a Royal Commission (the Guillebaud Commission) to look into the matter, confident that huge excess costs would be confirmed. The consequent report published in 1956 (*Report of the Committee of Enquiry into the cost of the National Health Service*, Cmd 9663, London: HMSO, 1956) reached an exactly opposite conclusion: evidence showed gross underfunding, but remarkably economical use of such funds as were available. Largely for this reason, the Conservative minister who received this report, Ian Macleod, had little difficulty in persuading his party to accept the principles of the NHS, starting a political consensus that lasted more than three decades. Again, in 2001, the Wanless Report, commissioned by government and chaired by a banker, estimated a £267bn shortfall in NHS investment compared with average EU investment in health care over the previous 26 years (*Lancet* 2001; 358: 1971).

[10] Though US health economist Alain Enthoven has always been a strenuous and effective advocate for return of the NHS to the market and redefinition of UK health care as a traded commodity, he readily conceded that European public systems generally, and the NHS in particular, were more inclusive and more efficient than the US marketed care system when it was dominated by medical ownership (Enthoven, A., 'International comparisons of health care systems: what can Europeans learn from Americans?', pp 57–71 in OECD Social Policy Studies 7, *Health Care Systems in Transition*, Paris: OECD, 1990). He believed, and still asserts, that now that it is dominated by large corporations, the US market in health care will be more cost-effective than the NHS gift economy he and his supporters have so largely disrupted, but nobody has so far provided any evidence that his faith in this new market will be justified by experience.

[11] First steps in this process of indoctrination were set out clearly in an excellent collection of papers, OECD Social Policy Studies 7, *Health Care Systems in Transition*, Paris: OECD, 1990. This includes both the main advocate for market competition, Alain Enthoven, and the initial scepticism of most other contributors.

[12] The specialists were attracted to the NHS because only state funding could provide the expanded hospital service they needed to support their work. I have given a full account of this complex story in my book *A New Kind of Doctor* (London: Merlin Press, 1988).

[13] For initial advocacy, see Enthoven, A., *Reflections on the Management of the National Health Service: An American Looks at Incentives to Efficiency in Health Services Management in the UK*, Occasional Papers 5, London: Nuffield Provincial Hospitals Trust, 1985; and Enthoven, A., *Theory and Practice of Managed Competition in Health Care Finance*, New York: North Holland Publishing, 1988. For an initial academic critique, see Fairfield, G., Hunter, D.J., Mechanic, D., Rosleff, F., 'Managed care: origins, principles and evolution', *British Medical Journal* 1997; 314: 1823–6.

[14] One example of these public–private partnerships (PPPs) is typical of many others. Guy's & St Thomas' Foundation Hospital Trust, a major NHS university hospital complex in London, has set up a 50:50 public–private partnership with Serco, a private company, to run all its pathology services, GSTS Pathology. The company apparently aims to win a 30% share of the entire market for pathology services in England (Davie, E., 'Consultant voices fears about ambitious private partnership', *bmaNews*, 14 November 2009).

According to Wikipedia, Serco was founded in 1929 as the UK branch of the Radio Corporation of America. It now provides management services at NHS hospitals for Norfolk and Norwich, Leicester Royal Infirmary and Wishaw Hospital Trusts, manages and operates Bradford, Stoke-on-Trent and Walsall Local Education Authorities, operates the UK National Physical Laboratory, four prisons, two immigration removal centres, electronic tagging systems, the Docklands Light Railway, the Ballistic Missiles Early Warning system at RAF Fylingdales, RAF bases at Brize Norton, Halton, Northolt and Ascension Island, is one of three companies operating the Atomic Weapons Establishment at Aldermaston, and shares with another company operation of Royal Navy bases at Portsmouth, Devonport and the Clyde, and many other formerly public service ventures in the UK, as well as many others in Canada, Australia and elsewhere in the EU and Middle East. All these operations, including those for the NHS, and all the contracts setting their terms and conditions, are covered by commercial secrecy and are virtually immune from public scrutiny. This seems to typify the relation between business and elected government now tacitly or overtly endorsed by all main UK political parties.

[15] This offensive took many forms, more or less appropriate to anticipated resistance, but often violent, particularly in Latin America. The piecemeal approach adopted in Britain was very effective, mainly because it faced little effective resistance within the Labour Party or its affiliated trade unions.

[16] Charges were gradually introduced after 1952, in a stepwise retreat from the principle of a free service led by Hugh Gaitskell as Chancellor of the Exchequer, stoutly resisted by Bevan. The detailed story is well told by Charles Webster in his official history of the NHS, *The Health Services since the War. Vol. 1. Problems of Health Care: The National Health Service before 1957*, London: HMSO, 1988.

[17] In North American usage, a consultation is a meeting between two doctors to discuss a problem. In British usage, a consultation is a meeting between a doctor (or other professional) and a patient. In North American usage, that is called a 'visit'. In British usage, a visit is a house-call – a consultation in the patient's home. I shall use British usage throughout this book.

[18] The assumption that user charges are necessary and effective for controlling health care costs depends on the validity of the provider–consumer transaction as a model for health care. As Evans and Barer pointed out in 1990, it was in the US, where user charges were highest and most prevalent, that costs were (and still are) most obviously out of control (Evans, R.G., Barer, M.L., 'The American predicament', OECD Policy Studies 7, *Health Care Systems*

in Transition, Paris: OECD, 1990, pp 80–5. Even relatively low user charges impair uptake of necessary prescribed medication, both in rich countries like Britain (Beardon, P.H.G., McGilchrist, M.M., McKendrick, A.D. et al, 'Primary non-compliance with prescribed medication in primary care', *British Medical Journal* 1993; 307: 846–8) and even more so in poor countries, with sometimes appalling consequences (Editorial, 'Charging for health services in the third world', *Lancet* 1992; 340: 458–9). Levels of user charges in different European countries reflect differences in the political balance between popular pressures for solidarity and politicians' susceptibility to the transactional model for care. Studies in 1987 showed user charges as percentages of total medication price as about 34% in France, about 30% in Belgium, about 27% in the UK, about 25% in Italy, about 9% in the Netherlands and about 10% in Germany. These differences are probably stable (Mossialos, E., 'Tables of data on the EEC pharmaceutical industry, prescribing and co-payments', Paper read at International Association for Health Policy Conference, Bishop's Stortford, October 1993).

[19] Hart, J.T., 'Two paths for medical practice', *Lancet* 1992; 340: 772–5.

[20] A UK typical public opinion poll in 2005 showed 89% opposed to commercial provision of health care (Lister, J., 'The reinvention of failure', *Guardian*, 20 July 2005). So far there is no more recent evidence that this has changed. Among GPs in 2009, only 7% thought provision of services by commercial companies was a good idea, 86% thought it was not. Asked if they would be worried about the future of local NHS services if they were left to market forces, 94% said yes, 6% said no (*GP Magazine* readers' survey, June 2009).

[21] This has been true most of all of the Labour Party, most of whose members have always regarded the NHS as the embodiment of their concepts of socialism, with public ownership and accountability as central. Since the early days of the Labour Party, votes at its annual conference were supposed to be its ultimate authority. In 2001, Labour Party leaders planned to evade discussion of privatisation policies at annual conference by convening a meeting of the National Policy Forum on 28 July. This created enough new policy forums (where delegates had advisory functions at most) to exclude the whole privatisation agenda from discussion at the conference. By then party membership had declined from 420,000 in 1997 to 254,000 in 2001, a fall of at least 166,000 (*Tribune*, 29 June 2001). This fall has continued ever since, to about one third at most.

[22] Speaking of Margaret Thatcher's government soon after his retirement, former Chief Scientist at her Department of Health Dr Peter Woodford said: '... what I deprecate above all is this government's apparent belief that the only incentive for anyone to work hard and well is money and material greed', *Guardian*, 31 January 1994, reported in *LRD Fact Service* 1994; 56: 17–18.

[23] Menendez, R., *New England Journal of Medicine* 1999; 341: 1769. He was responding to three key papers: Silverman, E.M., Skinner, J.S., Fisher, E.S., 'The association between for-profit hospital ownership and increased Medicare spending', *New England Journal of Medicine* 1999; 341: 420–6; Woolhandler, S., Himmelstein, D.U., 'When money is the mission – the high costs of investor owned care', *New England Journal of Medicine* 1999; 341: 444–6; and Himmelstein, D., Woolhandler, S., Hellander, I., Wolfe, S.M., 'Quality of care in investor-owned *vs* not-for-profit HMOs', *JAMA* 1999; 282: 159–63.

[24] Richard D. North has written a whole book in this vein, given prime space for discussion by the BBC (North, R.D., *Rich is Beautiful: A Very Personal Defence of Mass Affluence*, London: Social Affairs Unit, 2005).

[25] Kassirer, J.P., 'Managed care and the morality of the marketplace', *New England Journal of Medicine* 1995; 333: 50–2.

[26] Jolly, R. (ed), *United Nations Report on Human Development*, 1996. According to a report from the Helsinki-based World Institute for Development Economics Research, part of the United Nations University, released on 5 December 2006, the richest 1% of the world population own 40% of total household wealth. The bottom 50% own just over 1%. The threshold for reaching the top 1% was $500,000. The bottom 50% owned less than $2,200. Household wealth was defined as the value of physical and financial assets, minus debts. Almost 90% of the richest 1% lived in North America, Europe or Japan. Six per cent of adults lived in North America, but they owned 34% of the world's household wealth. Average net wealth in the US was $143,867 *per capita* in 2000, but it was higher still in Japan at $180,837. James Davies, Professor of Economics at the University of Western Ontario, and an author of the report, said global income inequality had been rising for the past 20–25 years, and this was probably true also of household wealth (*CBC News*, 5 December 2006). In 2008, an estimated 40% of the world population still had no access to a toilet or latrine, and 90% of the world's sewage was still discharged to soil, sea or fresh water (George, R., *The Big Necessity: Adventures in the World of Human Waste*, London: Portobello, 2008). Net effects of aid from rich to poor countries have been aptly summarised as: '... largely a matter of poor people in rich countries giving money to rich people in poor countries' (Caulfield,

C., *Masters of Illusion: The World Bank and the Poverty of Nations*, London: Macmillan, 1996), a desperately sad story completed by Sebastian Mellanby (*The World's Banker: A Story of Failed States, Financial Crises, and the Wealth and Poverty of Nations*, New Haven: Yale University Press, 2005).

[27] None of the horror stories approaching those spread by extreme Republicans in their campaign against President Obama's modest plans to extend health insurance to 47 million US citizens outside the care system has been substantiated; but they have plenty closer to home. According to the *Los Angeles Times*, reported by AP in the UK *Guardian*, 10 February 2007, a hospital van drove to the Los Angeles Skid Row district and dumped a paraplegic man, leaving him crawling in the street with only a soiled gown and a broken colostomy bag. Witnesses took the van's details and the police traced it to Hollywood Presbyterian Medical Center. The city government was already prosecuting the Kaiser Permanente health group over a similar alleged offence.

[28] Speaking at a Socialist Health Association fringe meeting at the Labour Party annual conference in 2009, Chairman of BMA Council Dr Hamish Meldrum said that NHS market 'reforms' were not working. This was the driving force behind the BMA's Look After Our NHS campaign. Market reforms had led to spending more on measuring operation of the market system, making less available for patient care, and were corrupting and fragmenting the service (*bmaNews*, 3 October 2009). In the BMA, Dr Meldrum held the same position in 2009 as did Dr Charles Hill when he led doctors to defeat in 1948, opposing the birth of the NHS.

Chapter Two

[1] The concept of healthy death, not just its timing but the nature of terminal experience, has been familiar to experienced clinicians for generations. It is still neglected as a clinical function and grossly underfunded (Murray, S.A., Boyd, K., Sheikh, A., Thomas, K., Higginson, I.J., 'Developing primary palliative care: people with terminal conditions should be able to die at home with diginity', *British Medical Journal* 2004; 329: 1056).

[2] Crude measures though they are, infant mortality rates and average expectation of life at birth do demonstrate the gross inefficiency of marketed health care in the US, the original driving force behind privatisation of public health care services throughout the world. Though the US still holds first place in the world for output of wealth per head of population, in 2007 it ranked 37th for infant mortality and 36th for expectation of life at birth.

[3] Cochrane, A.L., 'The history of the measurement of ill health', *International Journal of Epidemiology* 1972; 1: 89–92.

[4] Typically, patients have more faith in technical measurements than in their own subjective experience, and therefore underestimate their own potential contribution to diagnosis. Subjectively reported breathlessness on exertion, particularly episodic breathlessness which may be absent during examination, is the most powerful independent predictor of early death from both lung and heart disease, even in men with no current evidence of pre-existing coronary disease (Carpenter, L., Beral, V., Strachan, D. et al, 'Respiratory symptoms as predictors of 27 year mortality in a representative sample of British adults', *British Medical Journal* 1989; 299: 357–61; Cook, D.G., Shaper, A.G., 'Breathlessness, lung function and the risk of a heart attack', *European Heart Journal* 1988; 9: 1215–22; Higgins, M.W., Keller, J.B., 'Predictors of mortality in the adult population of Tecumseh', *Archives of Environmental Health* 1970; 21: 418–24). Doctors who do not believe what their patients say about themselves are likely to make disastrous mistakes.

[5] Voters still assume that if a local hospital works badly, some NHS authority will somehow put it right; they assume a public service still exists, as every government has promised it will. Of course, this means there is no outright market failure, just a quasi-market. The most zealous marketeers, like Enthoven and Prof Julian le Grand, assure politicians that the only reason their reforms don't seem to work is that they have not been applied with sufficient ruthlessness. Meanwhile commercial providers take full advantage of the fact that once having responsibility to provide public service, they also are never allowed to fail, so their profits are assured.

[6] Effectiveness of treatment is harder to judge than most people imagine. Medical and popular definitions of whether a drug works are entirely different. For doctors, a drug is said to 'work' if in a formal trial there is a 5% or more difference between patients given a new drug, and control patients given either an established drug or a placebo. For patients, a drug is said to 'work' if it actually does so in most of them, at least more than half. For drugs regarded by doctors as effective, this is frequently not the case. For example, sildenafil

(Viagra): even at an individually optimised dose from 25mg to 200mg, only 48% of men find that it works for them at least 60% of the times they attempt intercourse, compared with 11% of men who find that a placebo 'works' on the same definition. If they use only a single 25mg tablet, success falls to 28% – in other words, the 25mg dose does not work 72% of the time (Christakis, N., 'Does this work for you?', *British Medical Journal* 2008; 337: 1025).

[7] The extent of potential error in decisions to operate is seldom appreciated, even by doctors. For example, judging from their prevalence at routine autopsy, from 9% to 21% of British adults have gallstones, with large and, so far as I know, still unexplained area differences (Barker, D.J.P., Gardner, M.J., Power, C., Hutt, M.S.R., *British Medical Journal* 1979; ii: 1389–92). Only about 18% of these people are likely to get pain or any other harmful consequence over 15 years' follow-up (Gracie, W.A., Ranschoff, D.F., *New England Journal of Medicine* 1982; 307: 794–800). Cholecystectomy (excision of the gallbladder) is now an almost completely safe procedure, with an intrinsic mortality risk of only 0.17% (*Annals of Surgery* 1993; 218: 129–37), and with rapid recovery if modern endoscopic methods are used. It has become so safe, and so undisturbing that since endoscopic methods largely replaced open surgery, the total NHS cholecystectomy rate has risen by 25%, and spending on cholecystectomies has risen by 11.4%, despite a 25% fall in cost per operation (Lam, C.-M., Cuschieri, A., Murray, F.E., *British Medical Journal* 1995; 311: 1092).

So upper abdominal pain is common, gallstones are common, and (excluding patients with acute cholecystitis, duct stones or obstructive jaundice, as all studies here quoted have done) their association is sometimes causal, but often fortuitous. Cholecystectomy therefore may or may not be a rational intervention, though it is safe, seldom painful and has a diminishing unit cost. Most follow-up studies show persistent pain in 20%–30% of patients after cholecystectomy for gallstones thought to be causal (Jess, P., Jess, T., Beck, H., Beck, P., *Scandinavian Journal of Gastroenterology* 1998; 33: 550–3). In a controlled prospective study, 233 consecutive patients seen by 75 Rotterdam GPs complaining of recurrent upper abdominal pain, and suspected of symptomatic gallstones, all had ultrasound scans. Of those with confirmed gallstones, 61% were in pain, compared with 45% of patients without gallstones. Those with confirmed gallstones were offered cholecystectomy. Of those who had the operation, 87% ceased to have pain, compared with 63% of those with confirmed gallstones who declined operation, and 83% of patients without gallstones who had no operation. These differences were not statistically significant (Berger, M.Y., Hartman, T.C.O., van der Velden, J.J.I.M., Bohnen, A.M., *British Journal of General Practice* 2004; 54: 574–9). In another study, case histories of 252 patients who had undergone cholecystectomy were shown to a panel of physicians and a panel of surgeons. The physicians agreed operations were appropriate in 41% of cases, inappropriate in 30%, and couldn't agree in 29%. The surgeons agreed operations were appropriate in 52%, inappropriate in 2%, and couldn't agree on 46% (Scott, E.A., Black, N., *Annals of the Royal College of Surgeons of England* 1992; 74: 97–101).

Despite this chaos, consensus criteria have been agreed by experts which are supposed to make rational choices possible. Using these, a one-year prospective study of all 960 patients on waiting lists of six Spanish hospitals for cholecystectomy concluded the operation was inappropriate in only 0.7% and uncertain in 7.9% (*European Journal of Public Health* 2004; 14: 252–7), a wonderful advance if it is true. We shall know that only after these patients have finished waiting, have had their cholecystectomies, and either lost or retained their pre-operative symptoms. Cholecystectomy rates for different populations in Britain still show huge variability without any rational explanation (Aylin, P., Williams, S., Jarman, B., Bottle, A., 'Dr Foster's case notes: variation in operation rates by Primary Care Trust, 1998–2004', *British Medical Journal* 2005; 331: 539).

[8] Wilkin, D., Hallam, L., Leavey, R., Metcalfe, D., *Anatomy of Urban General Practice*, London: Tavistock, 1987. NHS 'reform' has encouraged patients to access care directly through nurse-run direct telephone advice centres, often leading to referrals to Accident and Emergency departments in hospitals which GPs, who already know their patients and have wider diagnostic experience and training, might not have made. It is becoming increasingly difficult to measure what goes on in primary care, as it becomes fragmented by competing agencies, but the pattern has probably not changed much since the 1980s.

[9] Eisenberg, L., 'Science in medicine: too much, or too little and too limited in scope?', *American Journal of Medicine* 1988; 84: 483–91.

[10] Shaw, G.B., 'Preface' to *The Doctor's Dilemma*, London: John Constable, 1907.

[11] This was demonstrated dramatically by Stanley Milgram's experiments in 1961–62, showing that most ordinary citizens of New Haven, Connecticut, were willing to administer painful and even life-threatening electric shocks if instructed to do so by someone in apparently established authority (Blass, T., *The Man Who Shocked the World: The Life and Legacy of Stanley Milgram*, New York: Perseus Books, 2004; paperback: Basic Books, 2005).

[12] Participation in medical research has huge educational potential not only for health professionals but also for communities, particularly if they participate

repeatedly in different studies. In my own experience, this can provide first steps toward mass education in the nature of scientific reasoning and evidence (Hart, J.T., Smith, G.D., 'Response rates in south Wales 1950–1996: changing requirements for mass participation in human research', in Chalmers, I., Maynard, A. (eds), *Non Random Reflections on Health Services Research: On the 25th Anniversary of Archie Cochrane's Effectiveness and Efficiency*, London: BMJ Publishing Group, 1997, pp 31–57). This potential can be fully realised only in studies that stick to the same population through several generations, and so far as I know, nobody has ever measured the cumulative and collective effects of repeated community participation. Participants must be fully informed, and this should include discussion of trial design and its underlying logic. Randomisation of trial participants is particularly challenging and rewarding. In general, participants gain from scientific trials organised by bona fide independent agencies like the Medical Research Council (MRC) or university departments, in that caring professionals who undertake them are highly motivated and work to obsessionally high standards. However, there is now no evidence that participants in trials fare better than non-participants receiving the same care outside trials (Vist, G.E., Hagen, K.B., Devereaux, P.J., Bryant, D., Kristoffersen, D.T., Oxman, A.D., 'Systematic review to determine whether participation in a trial influences outcome', *British Medical Journal* 2005; 330: 1175–9), though this may have been true in the past, when systematic care of any kind was scarce.

[13] In the Glyncorrwg practice, in 1986 we reviewed 500 consecutive deaths from 1964 to 1985, all those occurring in a total population varying between 1,600 and 1,800, almost two-thirds of them at home. We had routine information about deaths in hospital, but enquiries about unexpected deaths in which errors seemed possible were generally treated with hostility, and access to hospital records was refused, so we were unable to estimate errors in hospital accurately. Of all these deaths 45% were preceded by avoidable causal factors of some kind, almost half of them (20%) attributable to my own errors (Hart, J.T., Humphreys, C., 'Be your own coroner: an audit of 500 consecutive deaths in a general practice', *British Medical Journal* 1987; 294: 871–4).

[14] Errors arising from not doing what you know may be more frequent than those arising from not knowing what you ought to do. In one study 40 years ago, in 55 audits of 37 topics relating to 5,499 patient records, 94% of errors were in performance, but only 6% were in knowledge (Ashbaugh, D.G., McKean, R.S., 'Continuing medical education: the philosophy and use of audit', *Journal of the American Medical Association* 1976; 236: 1485–8). Probably the most common reason for not doing what you know is that constrained circumstances and resources preclude optimal choices. Obviously

this study was done a long time ago. I don't know if anyone has looked into this important question in the same way more recently. If not, it obviously cries out for replication.

[15] That is, health gains exceed health losses. All medical interventions necessarily entail some possibility of health loss, so the outcome of care must always be a net product.

[16] Cambridge Group for the History of Population and Social Structure and Max Planck Institute for Demographic Research in Rostock, in *Science* 2002; 296: 1029–31.

[17] Boseley, S., 'Cubans tell NHS the secret of £7 a head health care', *Guardian*, 2 October 2000.

[18] MacDonald, T., *Hippocrates in Havana: Cuba's Health Care System*, Knebworth: Bolivar Books, 1997. The most powerful single contributor to health gain on a mass scale is maternal literacy. Mothers who can read and write, and therefore begin to understand and criticise and make their own decisions about child care and relationships with their partners, live longer and healthier lives, and so do their families (Briggs, N., 'Illiteracy and maternal health: educate or die', *Lancet* 1993; 341: 1063–4.)

[19] Ochoa, F.R., 'Situacion, sistema y recursos humanos en salud para el desarollo en Cuba', *Revista Cubana de Salud Pública* 2003; 29: 157–69.

[20] Cuban doctors currently earn an average $25 a month, but up to ten times as much if they work abroad in the Cuban overseas aid programmes (mainly in Venezuela and Bolivia) and their salaries are doubled after they return. Cuban medical workforce planning assumes a 2%–3% annual defection rate for doctors working abroad, an astonishingly low figure considering the hardships imposed by 50 years of strictly enforced blockade by the US (Feinsilver, J., 'Cuban health politics at home and abroad', in Panitch, L., Leys, C. (eds), *Morbid Symptoms: Health under Capitalism. Socialist Register 2010*, London: Merlin Press, 2009: 216–39).

[21] Agdestein, K., Roemer, M.I., 'Good health at a modest price: the fruit of primary care', *Journal of Public Health Policy* 1994; 15: 485–90.

[22] Wilkinson, R.G., Pickett, K.E., *The Spirit Level: Why More Equal Societies Almost Always Do Better*, London: Allen Lane, 2009; Wilkinson, R.G.,

Pickett, K.E., 'Income inequality and population health: a review and explanation, *Social Science & Medicine* 2006; 62: 1768–84.

[23] Idler, E.L., Angel, R.J., 'Self-rated health and mortality in the NHANES-I epidemiologic follow-up study', *American Journal of Public Health* 1990; 80: 446–52. See also Idler, E.L., 'Subjective assessments of health and mortality: a review of studies', *International Review of Health Psychology* 1992; 1: 33–54.

[24] For example, Garratt, A.M., Ruta, D.A., Abdalla, M.I. et al, 'The SF36 health survey questionnaire: an outcome measure suitable for routine use within the NHS?', *British Medical Journal* 1993; 306: 1440–4, and Paterson, C., 'Measuring outcomes in primary care: a patient-generated measure, MYMOP, compared with the SF-36 health survey', *British Medical Journal* 1996; 312: 1016–20 and 626–7).

[25] Measuring output by process is essential for putting NHS functions out to contract, and this, more than any inherent difficulty in measuring outcomes, has been a main reason for continued counting as a substitute for thought.

[26] Berwick, D.M., 'Measuring NHS productivity: how much health for the pound, not how many events for the pound', *British Medical Journal* 2005; 330: 975–6.

[27] Lakhani, A., Coles, J., Eayres, D., Spence, C., Rachet, B., 'Creative use of existing clinical and health outcomes data to assess NHS performance in England: Part 1 – performance indicators closely linked to clinical care', *British Medical Journal* 2005; 330: 1426–31, and Lakhani, A., Coles, J., Eayres, D., Spence, C., Sanderson, C., 'Creative use of existing clinical and health outcomes data to assess NHS performance in England: Part 2 – more challenging aspects of monitoring', *British Medical Journal* 2005; 330: 1486–92.

[28] For example, evaluation of cost-effectiveness of procedures should entail estimates of varying cascade effects on future risks of health loss from interventions at different points in time or on different pathological processes. The weights attached to these may profoundly affect funding and allocation of resources, even where some elements of planning have been retained, at the present state of quasi-privatisation reached by most West European health services (Brouwer, W.B.F., Niessen, L.W., Postma, M.J., Rutten, F.F.H., 'Need for differential discounting of costs and health effects in cost effectiveness analyses', *British Medical Journal* 2005; 551: 446–8).

[29] It is hard to believe that anyone still thinks the NHS has more to learn from industry than vice versa, but the advocates of total quality control, on the Japanese automotive model, are still saying this; see, for example, Marshall, M., 'Applying quality improvement approaches to health care: the health sector could learn much from industry', *British Medical Journal* 2009; 339: 819–20.

[30] McKeown, T., *The Role of Medicine*, Oxford: Blackwell, 1979.

[31] Illich, I., *Medical Nemesis: Limits to Medicine: The Expropriation of Health*, London: Marion Boyars, 1976.

[32] Smith, R., 'Review of new printing of Illich, I., *Limits to Medicine. Medical Nemesis: The Expropriation of Health*, London: Marion Boyars, 1974', *British Medical Journal* 2002; 324: 923.

[33] Johansson, S.R., 'Food for thought: rhetoric and reality in modern mortality history', *Historical Methods* 1994; 27: 101–25.

[34] Godber, G., 'An endangered thesis. Review of McKeown, T., *The Role of Medicine: Dream, Mirage or Nemesis?*, Oxford: Blackwell, 1979', *British Medical Journal* 1980; 280: 102.

[35] Cochrane, A.L., *Effectiveness and Efficiency: Random Reflections on Medical Care*, London: Nuffield Provincial Hospitals Trust, 1971.

[36] Hart, J.T., 'An assault on all custom: Cochrane's "Effectiveness and efficiency"', *International Journal of Health Services* 1973; 3: 101–4.

[37] Cochrane, A.L., St Leger, A.S., Moore, F., 'Health service "input" and mortality "output" in developed countries', *Journal of Epidemiology & Community Health* 1978; 32: 200–5.

[38] Bagehot, W., *The English Constitution*, London: 1867, republished Fontana 1963: 250–1. His own position was frankly stated: 'I can venture to say, what no elected member of parliament, Conservative or Liberal, can venture to say, that I am exceedingly afraid of the ignorant multitude of the new constituencies. I wish to have as great and as compact a power as possible to resist it' (p 281).

[39] We are repeatedly assured that the cultural difference between the UK and the US in public attitudes lies in priority for equity in Britain, but for consumer choice in America. This is certainly true of those who own, control and largely operate media sources of information and opinion, in both countries. But is

it really true of their common people? Health care reform was the biggest single issue in the 2008 presidential election, and Barack Obama was fully committed to it. Everyone understood this to mean that the 47 million US citizens without health insurance would be brought into a reformed system. Beyond doubt, Obama was elected, and elected on this platform, with a mandate to proceed with reform. By the middle of 2009 his opponents, both in the Republican Party and within the Democratic Party machine, and the insurance companies, which always fund both parties and organise opinion at all levels through lobbying and public relations companies, were able to create enough publicly displayed hysteria to put this democratic process into question, and all too easily convince apparently intelligent journalists that this mandate had somehow disappeared. According to a study published in the *American Journal of Medicine* (doi:10.1016/j.amjmed.2009.04.012), by 2007 nearly two-thirds of bankruptcies were linked to illness and medical bills, a rise of 50% over the figure in 2001. More than three-quarters of those thus bankrupted were medically insured at the start of their illness. All that was before the collapse of financial markets and rapid rise in unemployment. In the US, when you lose your job you lose your health care insurance. Maybe it's true that the 85% of US citizens who have access to more than crisis care can be frightened into forgetting about the 15% who have not, but the main difference between these two cultures is probably just that UK citizens have experience of inclusive free care.

[40] Hull, C.H. (ed), *The Economic Writings of Sir William Petty, together with the observations upon the Bills of Mortality, more probably by Capt. John Graunt*, New York: A.M. Kelley, 1963. The English revolution provides one of the first examples of innovative thinking and administrative action on public health. As Charles Webster has written, 'The collective evidence tends to support Bowden's view that the period 1620–1650 "witnessed extreme hardship in England, and were probably the most terrible years through which the country has ever passed." … The social planners of the Puritan Revolution proved to have a correct appraisal of the crisis of health facing the nation. Their first priorities – economic diversification and agricultural improvement – were measures particularly designed to insulate the lower classes against dearth and economic fluctuation. It was anticipated that improvements in diet and general well-being introduced by personal initiative would radically alleviate the problem of disease' ('The crisis of subsistence and health of the puritan revolution', *Bulletin of the Society for Social History of Medicine* 1976; 17: 8–10). This anticipated similar developments in France after 1789.

[41] Morabia, A., 'P.C.A. Louis and the birth of clinical epidemiology', *Journal of Clinical Epidemiology* 1996; 49: 1327–33; Lilienfeld, A.M., Lilienfeld, D.E.,

'Epidemiology and the public health movement: a historical perspective', *Journal of Public Health Policy* 1982; 3: 140–9; Foucault, M., *The Birth of the Clinic: An Archaeology of Medical Perception*, London: Tavistock Publications, 1973 (originally published as *Naissance de la Clinique*, Paris: Presses Universitaires de France, 1963).

[42] Codman, E.A., 'The product of a hospital', *Surgery, Gynaecology & Obstetrics* 1914; 18: 491–6. Reprinted in White, K.L., Frenk, J., Ordoñez, C. et al, *Health Services Research: An Anthology*, Washington DC: PAHO, 1992.

[43] Ferguson, T., McPhail, A.N., *Hospital and Community*, London: Oxford University Press, 1954.

[44] Roemer, M.I., Schwartz, J.L., 'Doctor slowdown: effects on the population of Los Angeles County', *Social Science & Medicine* 1979; 130: 213–18, and James, J., 'Impacts of the medical malpractice slowdown in Los Angeles County: January 1976', *American Journal of Public Health* 1979; 69: 437–43.

[45] For example, overall risk of deep vein thrombosis (DVT) in the legs is more than 20% after any major surgery, and more than 40% after orthopaedic surgery (National Institute for Health and Clinical Excellence, *Venous Thromboembolism. Reducing the Risk of Venous Thromboembolism (Deep Vein Thrombosis and Pulmonary Embolism) in Inpatients Undergoing Surgery*, Clinical Guideline 46, 2007). Few of these clots break off and spin off to impact in lung arteries, and even fewer are large enough to cause death from lung embolism, but many permanently reduce lung function, and even more predispose to leg ulcers later in life.

[46] Slater, P.E., Ever-Hadani, P., 'Mortality in Jerusalem during the 1983 doctors' strike', *Lancet* 1983; ii: 1306.

[47] In 1966, deaths attributed to appendicitis and appendectomies in Germany were two to three times higher than in any other country, and within Germany were one third higher in West Berlin than in the country as a whole. Appendectomy rates in Germany were twice as high as in the US or the UK, and were three times higher in white-collar workers than in manual workers. Though acute appendicitis occurs randomly and requires immediate surgery, appendectomies were performed almost five times as often on Thursdays as Sundays, and two to three times more often on weekdays than weekends. Though acute appendicitis mainly affects young people, most deaths attributed to it in Germany occurred over 50 years of age. In 959 cases where excised appendices had been examined under a microscope, only 25% showed evidence of acute appendicitis. Pflanz concluded that the high German death rate

attributed to appendicitis reflected not the incidence of acute appendicitis, but the frequency of appendectomy. German medical culture accepted diagnosis of 'chronic appendicitis' more commonly than other national cultures, and accepted a category of 'neurogenic appendicitis' unrecognised anywhere else. As few of these operations were reimbursed by private fees, he discounted greed as a motive for interference, but he found other, essentially cultural reasons why surgeons interpret doubt in ways that favour mechanistic interpretation of problems, and therefore mechanistic solutions (Lichtner, S., Pflanz, M., 'Appendectomy in the Federal Republic of Germany: epidemiology and medical care pattern', *Medical Care* 1971; 9: 311–30).

[48] Bunker, J.P., Barnes, B.A., Mosteller, F., *Costs, Risks and Benefits of Surgery*, New York: Oxford University Press, 1977.

[49] Bunker, J., *Medicine Matters after All: Measuring the Benefits of Medical Care, a Healthy Lifestyle, and a Just Social Environment*, Nuffield Trust series 15, London: The Stationery Office, 2001.

[50] Nolte, E., McKee, M., *Does Health Care Save Lives? Avoidable Mortality Revisited*, London: Nuffield Trust, 2004.

[51] Nolte, E., McKee, M., 'Measuring the health of nations: analysis of mortality amenable to health care', *British Medical Journal* 2003; 327: 1129–32.

[52] Hart, J.T., 'Rule of halves: implications of underdiagnosis and dropout for future workload and prescribing costs in primary care', *British Journal of General Practice* 1992; 42: 116–9.

[53] Wilber, J.A., Barrow, J.G., 'Hypertension – a community problem', *American Journal of Medicine* 1972; 52: 653–63.

[54] Kinmonth, A.L., Murphy, E., Marteau, T., 'Diabetes and its care – what do patients expect?', *Journal of the Royal College of General Practitioners* 1989; 39: 324–7.

[55] Stephens, D., 'Hearing aids – making the system work', *Soundbarrier*, December 1988; 4.

[56] Wormald, W.P.L., Wright, L.A., Courtney, P., Beaumont, B., Haines, A.P., 'Visual problems in the elderly population and implications for services', *British Medical Journal* 1992; 304: 1226–9.

[57] Prosser, S., Dobbs, F., 'Case-finding incontinence in the over-75s', *British Journal of General Practice* 1997; 47: 498–500.

[58] Fraser, S., Bunce, C., Wormald, R., Brunner, E., 'Deprivation and late presentation of glaucoma: case-control study', *British Medical Journal* 2001; 322: 639–43.

[59] Hin, H., Bird, G., Fisher, P. et al, 'Coeliac disease in primary care: case finding study', *British Medical Journal* 1999; 318: 164–7.

[60] Jones, A., 'Screening for asthma in children', *British Journal of General Practice* 1994; 44: 179–83.

[61] Jones, K., Lane, D., Holgate, S.T., Price, J., 'Asthma: a diagnostic and therapeutic challenge', *Family Practice* 1991; 8: 97–9.

[62] Chandna, S.M., Schultz, J., Lawrence, C. et al, 'Is there a rationale for rationing dialysis? A hospital based cohort study of factors affecting survival and morbidity', *British Medical Journal* 1999; 318: 217–23.

[63] Cooper, C., Melton, L.J., 'Vertebral fractures: how large is the silent epidemic?', *British Medical Journal* 1992; 304: 793–4.

[64] Isometsä, E., Henriksson, M., Heikkinen, M. et al, 'Suicide and the use of antidepressants: drug treatment of depression is inadequate', *British Medical Journal* 1994; 308: 915.

[65] Richardson, J., Feder, G., 'Domestic violence: a hidden problem for general practice', *British Journal of General Practice* 1996; 46: 239–42.

[66] Cunningham-Burley, S., Allbutt, H., Garraway, W.M., Lee, A., Russell, E.B.A.W., 'Perceptions of urinary symptoms and health care seeking behaviour amongst men aged 40–79 years', *British Journal of General Practice* 1996; 46: 349–52.

[67] Mair, F.S., Crowley, T.S., Bundred, P.E., 'Prevalence, aetiology and management of heart failure in general practice', *British Journal of General Practice* 1996; 46: 77–9.

[68] Sudlow, M., Thomson, R., Kenny, R.A., Rodgers, R., 'A community survey of patients with atrial fibrillation: associated disabilities and treatment preferences', *British Journal of General Practice* 1998; 48: 1775–8.

[69] King, M., Nazareth, I., 'Community care of patients with schizophrenia: the role of the primary care team', *British Journal of General Practice* 1996; 46: 231–7.

[70] Young, J.B., 'The primary care stroke gap', *British Journal of General Practice* 2001; 51: 787–8.

[71] Eagle, K.A., Goodman, S.G., Avezum, A., Budaj, A. et al, 'Practice variation and missed opportunities for reperfusion in ST-segment-elevation myocardial infarction: findings from the Global Registry of Acute Coronary Events (GRACE)', *Lancet* 2002; 359: 373–7.

[72] Bernal, P., Escroff, D.B., Aboudarham, J.F. et al, 'Psychosocial morbidity: the economic burden in a pediatric Health Maintenance Organisation sample', *Archives of Pediatric & Adolescent Medicine* 2000; 154: 261–6.

[73] Moore, S., Molyneux, D., 'Chronic disease in institutionalised patients', *British Medical Journal* 1997; 315: 1539.

[74] Hart, J.T., 'Semicontinuous screening of a whole community for hypertension', *Lancet* 1970; ii: 223–7.

[75] We soon realised that for blood pressure control, we needed to screen people over 65 as well as younger adults, and did so, though we never published these data. Using ultrasound sensors and following a strict research protocol, we also screened a 5-year cohort of newborn children and followed them up for 10 years, initially at 3-month intervals to age one, and annually thereafter. Even under apparently standard conditions and using research-quality measurements, we found these measurements so unstable that for clinical decisions they were clearly useless. In the light of this experience, the American Hypertension Society's encouragement of their paediatric specialoids to screen children for hypertension and treat those in the top 5% or so of the distribution with antihypertensive drugs seemed to us another unjustifiable example of a search for markets in a market-driven health care economy. Our other screening measures in childhood, most notably active search for childhood asthma and urinary tract infections, were very successful. In general, we found that effective anticipatory care for adults needed to start in childhood, and effective anticipatory care for the elderly needed to start in middle age. This meant that a large proportion of care needed to become proactive, initiated not by patients' symptoms but by objective assessment of avoidable risks.

[76] Hart, J.T., 'The marriage of primary care and epidemiology: continuous anticipatory care of whole populations in a state medical service' (Milroy lecture), *Journal of the Royal College of Physicians of London* 1974; 8: 299–314.

[77] When 'Well Men's Clinics' became fashionable in the 1980s, we didn't have enough well men to create one; we were too busy dealing with the problems turned up by proactive search. By UK standards this was an unusually sick population, but it was typical of those to be found wherever people were still employed in heavy industry, or had become unemployed by its collapse, or been transferred to lower-wage occupations. Poor people everywhere have poor health, so the potential added workload for their proactive primary care is colossal, a problem only beginning to be recognised in Scotland, and not yet recognised at all elsewhere in the UK.

[78] Battles raged in the 1970s between GP pioneers of whole-community screening for high blood pressure, and epidemiologists who opposed it. The issue was eventually resolved by calling continuous whole-population screening by primary care teams 'opportunist case-finding', and reserving the word 'screening' for the more formal procedures of epidemiologists and the burgeoning well-man and well-woman clinics of private health care.

[79] This approach to primary care was first introduced by the Dutch GP Cuys van den Dool (Van den Dool, C.W.A., 'Antizipierende Medizin', *Allgemeinmedizin international* 1974; 2: 56–61). Its origin is interesting. An epidemiology unit at the Hague medical school had done several cross-sectional surveys, screening for simple indicators of health such as blood haemoglobin concentration, weight for height, arterial pressure, glucose or protein in urine, and so on in his practice at Stolwejk. Newly detected abnormalities were surprisingly few, so the academic researchers lost interest. Van den Dool, on the other hand, found that if he applied the same routine screening techniques at routine encounters, to build up an evidence profile for all of his registered population over several years, this detected much more hitherto undetected illness. This was mainly because of higher response rates, particularly from people with symptoms (usually non-specific), who are less likely to attend for cross-sectional screening by staff they do not already know.

[80] Later work confirms that we had good reason to search for treatable but untreated chronic illness, with opportunities for prevention. Follow-up analysis of patients admitted to hospital in Australia found that 17% of admissions were prompted by acute events occurring within already established continuing disease. Roughly half of these events were judged readily preventable by

continuing anticipatory care in the community – preventable, but not prevented (*Medical Journal of Australia* 1999; 170: 411–15).

[81] Hart, J.T., Thomas, C., Gibbons, B., Edwards, C., Hart, M., Jones, J., Jones, M., Walton, P., 'Twenty five years of audited screening in a socially deprived community', *British Medical Journal* 1991; 302: 1509–13.

[82] Kaul, S., 'Twenty five years of case finding and audit', *British Medical Journal* 1991; 303: 524–5.

[83] The Glyncorrwg practice was adopted in 1974 as a research practice by the Medical Research Council's Epidemiology and Health Care Unit at Northwick Park Hospital, directed by Prof Tom Meade. The MRC paid for one additional doctor and additional office and nursing staff, to allow us to develop research studies of our own, mostly into sodium intake in relation to arterial pressure, and pilot studies for large multicentre research studies in primary care, from 1974 to 1992.

[84] Hart, J.T., Smith, G.D., 'Response rates in south Wales 1950–1996: changing requirements for mass participation in human research', in Chalmers, I., Maynard, A. (eds), *Non Random Reflections on Health Services Research: On the 25th Anniversary of Archie Cochrane's Effectiveness & Efficiency*, London: BMJ Publishing Group, 1997: 31–57.

[85] The importance of inclusive population denominators cannot be stressed too much. Countries such as the US whose care systems depend on consumer choice in a market can create such population denominators only in specially contrived situations such as university practices, usually sited in socially deprived areas otherwise lacking any good primary care provision. Though only a few British primary care units used the full potential of this facility for research, it certainly influenced thought at the leading edge of innovation, and dominated ideas from the 1970s onwards, not only among innovative GPs, but also at the British Department of Health. The present rush to consumerism and market choice has seriously impeded this trend, but is unlikely to reverse it.

[86] Hart, J.T., 'The Inverse Care Law', *Lancet* 1971; i: 405–12. Banal because one might as well cite the Inverse Shoe Law, stating that barefoot children are least likely to have shoes. The Inverse Care Law shocked people because, whereas they customarily regard shoes as a traded commodity (so that it seemed natural for Imelda Marcos to have 3,000 pairs while many Filipino children had none), health care they still regard as a human right, unsuited to

trade. This view of health care seems to be held more widely and tenaciously in British than in US culture.

[87] Hannay, D.R., 'Deprivation payments and workload', *British Journal of General Practice* 1997; 47: 663–4.

[88] Wilheim, D., Metcalfe, D.H.H., 'List size and patient contact in general medical practice', *British Medical Journal* 1984; 189: 1501–5.

[89] Stirling, A.M., Wilson, P., McConnachie, A., 'Deprivation, psychological distress, and consultation length in general practice', *British Journal of General Practice* 2001; 51: 456–60.

[90] Carlisle, R., Johnstone, S., 'Factors influencing the response to advertisements for general practice vacancies', *British Medical Journal* 1996; 313: 468–71.

[91] Doctors paid by capitation want to keep their patients as customers and therefore to please them. However, if doctors have established friendly relationships with their patients, as most still do, insulting these friends becomes a real problem. Dutch doctors, watching what happened to German doctors employed by Bismarck's *Krankenkassen*, had a large enough private market to defend their status as professional gentlemen, for whom sorting patients for entitlement to benefit would be demeaning. Though they accepted the beginnings of a much less inclusive insurance system for industrial workers in 1914, they refused to accept responsibility for certification of incapacity. This has been performed ever since by independent doctors salaried by the state. In 1990, the last time I looked at the figures, rates for short- and long-term sickness absence were 2.6% and 3.4% respectively in the UK, 5.0% and 3.3% in Germany, and 7.1% and 8.9% in the Netherlands. These relativities had been maintained over many years, so if the Dutch intention was to encourage sterner work discipline, it failed. Assessment may have been easier when men had to work hundreds of metres below ground, lying on puddled stone floors to hack as best they could, undercutting coal with a pick, with as little as 50cm between floor and roof so that even shoulder movement was hardly possible, and all this for coal cut and loaded for less than 2 shillings a ton, but sold at the pit head for 9 shillings and exported for over 12 shillings a ton. Judging from my own experience of certification of miners and steelworkers from 1961 to 1992, the most important factor in judging disability (apart from what patients themselves said) was knowledge of patients' previous work record, and their reputation among their workmates and wives. Mining communities were generally well informed about the many social and personal factors affecting attendance at work, including exhaustion, demoralisation, fear (absence always

rose after serious accidents or near-accidents), economic rewards of work and economic penalties for absence. In Glyncorrwg we had huge levels of short-term absence in the 1960s, when wages were disgracefully low. As soon as wages rose after the 1972 and 1974 strikes, morale rose and absence attributed to sickness or injury fell steeply. Though a few doctors always enjoyed acting for management, a large majority tended to give their patients the benefit of the huge doubts surrounding all such judgements. In my experience and in usual conditions (I exclude rugby international matches) true malingering was and still is a rare (but paradoxically disabling) disease (see Yelin, E., 'The myth of malingering: why individuals withdraw from work in the presence of illness', *Milbank Quarterly* 1986; 64: 622–49).

[92] Steinar Westin ('Challenges of changing political and socioeconomic structures', keynote speech at WONCA Conference, Hong Kong, 1995) cited referenced data on the following effects of unemployment found in controlled prospective studies:

Consultation rates with GPs	+22%
Referrals to specialists	+60%
Length of sickness absence	+50%
Death within 10 years	+50%–100%

From 1970, when the last mine in the Afan valley was closed, miners in Glyncorrwg travelled often long distances to mines elsewhere. In 1981, male unemployment in the Afan valley was officially estimated at 38%, based on claims for benefit in our travel-to-work catchment. Workers at two local factories had been working 12-hour shifts 7 days a week for the previous three months to complete urgent orders. A boy leaving our local school had written 55 job application letters without getting a reply. Three vacancies for apprentice electricians at the local steelworks attracted 7,000 applicants from all over Britain. In 1983, just before the year-long miners' strike, we measured unemployment in the Glyncorrwg practice population ourselves, based not on claims for benefit but on whether people had jobs (so that people claiming sickness benefit were included). Of all men aged 16–64, 48% had no work. Of young men aged 16–24, 60% had no work. After the strike, the British coal industry was virtually destroyed. Coal-mining communities entered two decades of appalling demoralisation, with very serious social and health consequences, particularly for young people, which are only beginning to diminish today. The UK economy still depends on coal, but virtually all of it is now imported.

[93] Independent contractor status ensures that GPs fund their practices at least partly from their own pockets; they can choose how much to spend on staff and equipment, and at what point they will take on a partner or salaried assistant to share case-load (but in the latter case, not the profits or power). In this, and the small-mindedness that so often follows from it, lies the most important reason to support the principle of state salaried service. Throughout my years in practice, my net income was never more than half the average net income for GPs, even though we were able to use our MRC-funded research staff to assist in some routine care. Much the same applied to other GPs who tried to provide optimal care in those years. I understand things are a bit better now.

[94] Of course, the improvements in health we secured in times of full employment would almost certainly not have withstood the later effects of defeat and return to pre-war levels of mass unemployment, especially effects such as drug dependence in teenagers, and I have no later data. Countries which, unlike the UK, sustained socialised health care systems with adequate funding, reduced or eliminated social class differences in mortality (Kunst, A.E., Geurts, J.J.M., van den Berg, J., 'International variation in socioeconomic inequalities in self reported health', *International Journal of Epidemiology & Community Health* 1995; 49: 117–23; Kunst, A.E., Mackenbach, J.P., 'The size of mortality differences associated with educational level. A comparison of 9 industrialized countries', *American Journal of Public Health* 1994; 84: 932–7; Kunst, A.E., Mackenbach, J.P., 'International variation in the size of mortality differences associated with occupational status', *International Journal of Epidemiology* 1994; 23: 742–50; Netherlands Central Bureau for Statistics, Erasmus University, Rotterdam, *International Variation in Socioeconomic Inequalities in Self Reported Health*, The Hague: SDU Publishers/CBS Publications, 1992). After they embarked on neoliberal 'reform' programmes, social class differences in mortality again increased. This pattern occurred in both Sweden and Finland (Whitehead, M., 'Health inequalities in Britain and Sweden', *Lancet* 1990; 335: 331; Whitehead, M., Evandrou, M., Haglund, B., Diderichsen, F., 'As the health divide widens in Sweden and Britain, what's happening to access to care?', *British Medical Journal* 1997; 315: 1006–9; Whitehead, M., Gustafsson, R.A., Diderichsen, F., 'Why is Sweden rethinking its NHS style reforms?', *British Medical Journal* 1997; 315: 935–9; Koskinen, S.V.P., Martelin, T.P., Valkonen, T., 'Socioeconomic differences in mortality among diabetic people in Finland: five year follow up', *British Medical Journal* 1996; 313: 975–8; Lynch, J.W., Kaplan, G.A., Cohen, R.D. et al, 'Childhood and adult socioeconomic status as predictors of mortality in Finland', *Lancet* 1994; 343: 524–7; Forssas, E., Keskimäki, I., Reunanen, A., Koskinen, S., 'Widening socioeconomic mortality disparity among diabetic people in Finland', *European Journal of Public Health* 2003; 13: 38–43).

[95] Hart, J.T., 'Two paths for medical practice', *Lancet* 1992; 340: 772–5.

[96] Even today, many members of the Labour Party and its MPs are reluctant to face the colossal gap between what spokespersons for New Labour say about their intentions for the NHS, and what they actually do, if they can get away with it. In the small print of the public services review launched in March 2007 by Prime Minister Blair was a proposal to discuss reducing free NHS treatment to a set of core services, with everything else provided and paid for by either direct charges or personal insurance (Timmins, N., 'NHS may be restricted to core services', *Financial Times*, 20 March 2007). The main obstacle to this has not been political resistance, but opposition from the Treasury, which still understands that insurance-based care and direct patient charges both inevitably entail huge increases in costs of administration. The point was made yet again by Wanless, on purely empirical grounds (Wanless, D., Appleby, J., Harrison, A., Patel, D., *Our Future Health Secured?*, London: King's Fund, September 2007). The appeal of insurance and direct charges lies partly in potential profit to insurance companies, but mainly in populist appeal to the tabloid press and the public ignorance it sustains – not at all in potential savings.

[97] Piece-rated income for GPs was introduced to NHS in 2003, rewarding general practices according to the proportions of patients with common chronic diseases for whom they achieved targets for quality of care (Quality and Outcomes Framework, QOF). It allowed GPs to exclude patients for whom treatment seemed impossible. Such exclusions seem to have been more frequent in poorer populations. A study of 7,637 practices in England now shows this scheme may nevertheless have reduced inequalities. They were categorised into five equal-sized groups according to deprivation scores. Over the first three years of the scheme, median achievement rose by 4.4% in the least deprived areas, compared with 7.6% for the most deprived areas. This reduced the original gap between these extremes from 4% in year 1 to 0.8% in year 3 (Doran, T., Fulwood, C., Kontopantelis, E,. Reeves, D., 'Effect of financial incentives on inequalities in the delivery of primary clinical care in England: analysis of clinical activity indicators for the quality and outcomes framework', *Lancet* 2008; 372: 728-36).

[98] With little public or parliamentary discussion, Margaret Thatcher moved the UK Department of Health from the classic model built around traditionally conservative civil servants, mistrustful of commerce and reluctant to change, towards leadership from NHS managers, sympathetic clinicians and recruits from the world of business. Starting with the Griffiths Report in 1983, and mightily stepped up by New Labour in 2000–05 (when Nigel Crisp was both

Permanent Secretary and Chief Executive of the NHS), the Department of Health became central manager of NHS England as a corporate enterprise, with a strong new professional management cadre thinking on business lines. They displaced civil servants from power in much the same way as they displaced medical and other professionals who dared to question the idea of public service as a business (Smith, R., 'The rise of Stalinism in the NHS: an unfree NHS and medical press in an unfree society', *British Medical Journal* 1994; 309: 1644–5). By 2006 the top leaders of this process, 30 people, included only one traditional Whitehall civil servant, the Permanent Secretary (Greer, S.L., Jarman, H., *The Department of Health and the Civil Service: From Whitehall to Department of Delivery to Where?*, Nuffield Trust, 2007). In the NHS commercial directorate, which handles all the many NHS contracts handed to commercial providers, only 8 out of 190 staff are civil servants. The rest are business executives paid at commercial rates, who in 2007 were estimated to cost between £20m and £30m annually (Timmins, N., 'Private sector role in pioneering healthcare scheme to be slashed', *Financial Times*, 13 November 2007). When political parties call for drastic reductions in civil service staff, these are the people a still-credulous public may imagine they have in mind. In fact, the ones who lose either their jobs, or the time to do their work in socially sensitive ways, will be those in daily contact with the poor and unemployed, granting or denying benefits.

[99] Doll, W.R.S., 'Monitoring the National Health Service', *Journal of the Royal Society of Medicine* 1973; 66: 729–40.

[100] Put at its simplest, per capita GDP in the US is 28% higher than in the UK and 41% higher than in France, so the US is said to be the world's wealthiest country. To produce this material wealth, US workers work 9% more hours than UK workers, and 16% more than French workers. Average annual holidays taken by US workers are 21% less than those taken by UK workers, and 34% less than those taken by French workers (de Wolff, A., *Bargaining for Work and Life,* Toronto: York University, 2003, Appendix: 62). UK men live an average of 0.87 years longer than in the US, and Frenchmen an average of 2.14 years longer (same figures for women are 0.94 years and 3.61 years respectively). (CIA, *World Fact Book,* accessed 2009). People in the US produce more wealth, but have less time and less life in which to enjoy it, so evidently per capita GDP is at best an inadequate, at worst a grossly misleading measure of success in human terms (Weale, M., 'Economic progress and health improvement: performance indicators should reflect both', *British Medical Journal* 2009; 339: 1097–8).

[101] Within Britain, inequality has reached extremes never before known. The UK is now a tax haven for the world's billionaires. Grant Thornton, tax accountants commissioned by *The Sunday Times* to provide data for their annual review of the wealthiest people in the UK, estimated the total assets of UK £billionaires at £126bn, on which they paid taxes totalling £14.7m. They estimated that about three in five of these £billionaires paid no personal income tax whatever (Maidment, P., 'The UK billionaires', *Forbes.com*, 7 December 2006).

[102] The proportion of all work now devoted to killing people, or credibly threatening to do so, is almost beyond comprehension. By 1990 the value of weapons, equipment and factories devoted to the US Department of Defense was 83% of the value of all plant and equipment in US manufacturing. Below is a table of the top 10 annual military budgets, rounded to the nearest billion dollars, as they have been officially admitted (actual sums are almost certainly much larger):

US 2008	$623bn
China 2004	$65bn
Russia	$50bn
France 2005	$45bn
UK	$43bn
Japan 2007	$42bn
Germany 2003	$35bn
Italy 2003	$28bn
South Korea 2003	$21bn
India 2005	$19bn

Estimated world total: $1,100bn (Johnson, C., 'Why the US has really gone broke', *Le Monde Diplomatique*, February 2008: 2–3).

If these dollars were transferred to health care, to save life rather than destroy it, the number of jobs created would be vastly greater than in weapons production, because health care is hugely more labour intensive. Would voters accept this? Evidence suggests that in the UK, public opinion is shifting as more people see the consequences of wars in the Middle East. In a public opinion poll in 2006, 51% of respondents supported renewal of Britain's Trident nuclear missiles, 39% opposed it. Today, 42% still support renewal, but 54% want Britain to abandon nuclear weapons altogether. Of Labour voters, a majority still supported possession of nuclear weapons in 2006, but today only 40% still believe the UK should retain nuclear weapons, and 59% are opposed. Even of Conservative voters, 41% now support abandoning nuclear weapons. The cost of renewing the Trident weapons system is estimated to be at least £20bn (Glover, J., 'Most voters want to scrap nuclear weapons – ICM poll', *Guardian*, 14 July 2009).

[103] Baumol, W.J., 'Social wants and dismal science: the curious case of the climbing costs of health and teaching', *Proceedings of the American Philosophical Society* 1993; 137: 612–37.

[104] Between 1978 and 2000, people employed in UK production, construction, transport and utilities fell from 40% to 24% of the total employed workforce, while those employed in education, health care, social work and other public services rose from 13% to 17%, broadly confirming Baumol's trends (MacGregor, D., 'Jobs in the public and private sectors', *Economic Trends*, June 2000 and June 2001, Table C). Between 2000 and 2004, UK manufacturing lost over 720,000 jobs, 18% of its total workforce. Successful competition requires larger investment in skills, research, development and innovation, for which well-funded universities, schools and health care are necessary foundations. In his paper *China, Europe and UK Manufacturing* (London: Trades Union Congress, 2005), TUC Chief Economist Ian Brinkley shows that though UK business and its government seem to think the only way to compete with China is to reduce labour costs and deregulate employment, companies in Germany, which they cite as having the highest labour costs and most burdensome regulation in the EU, have almost doubled the value of their exports to China over the past five years, growing five times faster than exports from the UK (*LRD Fact Service* 2005; 67: 105–6).

[105] Towse, R. (ed), *Baumol's Cost Disease: The Arts and Other Victims*, Cheltenham, UK/Northampton, MA: Edward Elgar, 1997.

[106] This issue has been excellently researched by John Appleby, Chief Economist at the King's Fund, an Establishment think-tank rarely far from government. Chancellor Gordon Brown accepted the 'fully engaged' option proposed by Derek Wanless in his review of UK spending on health care. Wanless comes from the world of business and has never been accused of socialist tendencies. On his estimates of projected spending, NHS spending as a percentage of GDP had risen from about 5.2% in 1977–78 to about 6.8% by 1997 (when New Labour took office) and nearly 8% in 2005 (at the end of New Labour's second term). Assuming 'full engagement', he forecasts this will rise to 9% in 2007–08, 11% in 2012–13, 12% in 2017–18, and 12.5% by 2022–23. Though NHS spending today is seven times higher in real terms than in its infancy in 1950, spending on all other goods and services has also risen threefold, without any disastrous effects on our economy or culture. If

the British economy grows at 2% a year, this allows NHS spending to reach 30% of GDP by 2055, by which time present spending on all other goods and services will have doubled (Appleby, J., 'Economic growth and NHS spending', *Health Service Journal*, 6 January 2005: 22). It would not be difficult to present these figures in ways that would terrify voters, rather than help them to understand the real meaning of rising material productivity. Judging from Conservative and New Labour campaigning in the 2005 general election, we shall soon see this occur, particularly if, as now seems likely, 2% annual growth rates cannot be sustained in market economies led only by search for profit.

[107] Baumol's hope that those owning the means of production of wealth and influence over popular beliefs would voluntarily invest their growing surplus in higher culture, more thoughtful education, or more humane and effective health care for the whole of society as human rights and an expanding social wage, rather than pocket it for themselves, is not credible. His economic ideas were imaginative, but his politics were Quixotic. Nothing shows this better than his own choice of a name for his discovery: he called the increasingly unaffordable cost of personal labour throughout the arts, education, and health care 'Baumol's disease', and most economists who developed this topic seem to have accepted this term. In fact, what he had found was not a disease, but an anomalous and threatened fragment of health, somehow surviving within profit-driven societies.

[108] From March 2008, competing NHS Hospital Trusts in England have been permitted to spend on advertising their services, explicitly including celebrity endorsements.

[109] Woolhandler, S., Himmelstein, D.U., 'Costs of care and administration at for-profit and other hospitals in the United States', *New England Journal of Medicine* 1997; 336: 769–74.

[110] People who already use private agencies for health care or to educate their children (among them, a growing proportion of Labour MPs) can't see this. Most of these agencies disguise themselves so far as possible as charities, truly devoted to that subset of the population either born to rule, or who have through their own hard work fought their way up the ladder, and thus proved their superiority, at least to themselves. Private sector schools, and perhaps to some extent private health care facilities, have a unifying effect on those who use them, against the rest of society: sectional solidarity, or collective selfishness.

Chapter Three

[1] For example: '… the failure of the market to insure against uncertainties has created many social institutions in which the usual assumptions of the market are to some extent contradicted. The medical profession is only one example, though in many respects an extreme one. All professions share some of the same properties. The economic importance of personal and especially family relationships, though declining, is by no means trivial in most advanced economies; it is based on non-market relations that create guarantees of behavior which would otherwise be afflicted with excessive uncertainty. Many other examples can be given. The logic and limitations of ideal competitive behavior under uncertainty force us to recognize the incomplete description of reality supplied by the impersonal price system' (Arrow, K.J., 'Uncertainty and the welfare economics of medical care', *American Economic Review* 1963; 53: 941–73).

[2] Lee-Potter, J., *A Damn Bad Business: The NHS Deformed*, London: Victor Gollancz, 1997.

[3] The word 'free' has many contradictory meanings. Here I mean free for entrepreneurs to buy, sell and invest, not that patients don't have to pay.

[4] Woolhandler, S., Himmelstein, D., 'Paying for national health insurance – and not getting it', *Health Care Costs*, July/August 2002: 88–98. Their precise estimate was that 59.8% of US health care spending was funded from taxes, 15% more than government estimates because those did not include public employees' health care benefits, or tax subsidies related to health care.

[5] Trisha Greenhalgh has provided a beautifully simple example of this. Commenting on a worthy but orthodox paper on factors relating to obesity in childhood, she found that though the authors rightly remembered to control for differences in education in mothers, which like other effects of social class are closely and causally associated with obesity, they completely omitted this from their list of potential interventions to prevent or treat obesity. As she rightly remarks, 'interventions aimed at increasing the health literacy of the primary care giver have far greater potential [than clinical interventions] for achieving a slimmer cohort of primary school children' (Greenhalgh, T., 'Early life risk factors for obesity in childhood: the hand that rocks the cradle rules the world', *British Medical Journal* 2005; 331: 453). The omission is typical.

[6] Spence, J., 'The need for understanding the individual as part of the training and function of doctors and nurses', in *The Purpose and Practice of Medicine*, London: Oxford University Press, 1960, pp 271–80.

[7] Hoffman, C., Rice, D., Sung, H.Y., 'Persons with chronic conditions: their prevalence and costs', *Journal of the American Medical Association* 1997; 277: 1473–9.

[8] Even before the 1980s, when NHS responsibility for long-term care of the elderly chronic sick was quietly dropped by a Conservative government, without serious opposition from either the Labour Party or the Liberal Democrats, care rose above the level of Poor Law warehousing in only a minority of pioneering geriatric units (Rodgers, J.S., Gray, J.A.M., 'Long stay care for elderly people: its continuing evolution', *British Medical Journal* 1982; 285: 707–9). Most remained little better than in Charles Dickens' time (Townsend, P., *The Last Refuge*, London: Routledge & Kegan Paul, 1962, and Townsend, P., 'The structured dependency of the elderly: a creation of social policy in the 20th century', *Ageing & Society* 1981; 1: 5–28). A huge new investment was needed to meet the needs of an ageing society (Acheson, E.D., 'The impending crisis of old age: a challenge to ingenuity', *Lancet* 1982; ii: 592–4). Without any public consultation or electoral mandate, the ruling consensus solved this problem first by declaring it insoluble (Jeffreys, M., 'The over-eighties in Britain: the social construction of a panic', *Journal of Public Health Policy* 1983; 4: 367–72), then by turning its back on it, and handing responsibility to private nursing homes run for profit. Whereas healthy growth of geriatric medicine for all of the people in Britain was betrayed, in the US it never even existed (Carboni, D.K., *Geriatric Medicine in the United States and Great Britain*, Contributions to the Study of Ageing 1, Westport, CN/London: Greenwood Press, 1982, pp 1–97).

[9] Dowrick, C., May, C., Richardson, M., Bundred, P., 'The biopsychosocial model of general practice: rhetoric or reality?', *British Journal of General Practice* 1996; 46: 105–7.

[10] A total of 776 male outpatients aged 55 or more who were attending a US Veterans' Administration hospital clinic were randomised to continuity of providers, or to discontinuity. Over 18 months' follow-up, men randomised to continuity had almost half as many hospital admissions (20% versus 39%) and shorter average length of stay (15.5 days versus 25.5 days). They also thought their providers were more thorough, knew more and were more interested in patient education (Bunker, J., Wasson, J.H., Sauvigne, A.E., Mogielnicki, R.P.,

Frey, W.G., Sox, C.H., Gaudette, C., Rockwell, A., 'Continuity of outpatients medical care in elderly men: a randomized trial', *JAMA* 1984; 252: 2413–17).

[11] Oye, R.K., Bellamy, P.E., 'Patterns of resource consumption in medical intensive care', *Chest* 1991; 99: 685–9.

[12] For example, incidence of childhood diabetes has risen throughout Europe since the 1950s, at annual rates of increase varying from 3% to 6%. Most ominously, this rate of increase is highest in the youngest age group, children under four. Identical twin studies show that this is probably caused by a major environmental change of some sort, but far more investment is going to new methods of treatment than into the nature of this change, or how to tackle it ('EURODIAB ACE Study Group', *Lancet* 2000; 355: 873–6).

[13] Cook, R.I., Render, M., Woods, D.D., 'Gaps in the continuity of care and progress on patient safety', *British Medical Journal* 2000; 320: 791–4.

[14] A characteristic example of what happens when care is fragmented between specialists, with no one person responsible for overall coordination of care and everyone minding only their own business, was reported in 2005. Care of an elderly woman with toxic effects from lithium treatment for depression was spread across three sites delivered by six teams. She died from treatable kidney failure (Gannon, C., 'Will the lead clinician please stand up?', *British Medical Journal* 2005; 330: 737). This was a common professional experience, attracting much subsequent correspondence.

[15] About one quarter of new entrants to British public health now have substantial prior experience in primary care as trainee GPs, many of them mature students who have shifted their careers. These form an entirely new and refreshing force in what had become a dangerously stagnant and complacent specialty.

[16] This can be done through what's known as critical event audit, or critical event analysis (Greenhalgh, T., 'Critical event audit', *British Medical Journal* 2001; 323: 1195). A critical event includes not only disasters that actually occurred, but near misses that almost occurred, but fortunately not quite, which are far more numerous, and where it may be easier to get truthful accounts from participants. The principle was established long ago for study of coal-mining accidents.

[17] A contemporary local colleague always treated all acute childhood illness with broad-spectrum antibiotics, with or without any precise diagnosis. Such

an indiscriminate policy might have prevented this death. On the other hand, community prevalence of antibiotic-resistant bacteria, including MRSA, is closely and causally related to rates of prescribing antibiotics in primary care. Prevalence in hospitals is much higher, mainly because antibiotics are far more heavily prescribed there. Blunderbuss clinical medicine is no solution.

[18] BC 41(3), from DIPEx website, now www.healthtalkonline.org, quoted by Herxheimer, A., 'Gathering and assessing narrative evidence', paper read at Conference on Integration of Narrative with Science in Medicine, London, 3 December 2003.

[19] Almost three-quarters of UK patients have been registered with their GP for five years or more, which should mean that GPs usually have some idea of their patients' stories already, and don't have to start from zero. In these circumstances 10 minutes is probably right as an average, with a few consultations needing up to 25 minutes. Consultations longer than this often go round in circles and may then be counterproductive. Better to come again in a day or two, when the whole problem may appear quite different. US experience suggests that a consultation with a new patient takes 22.6 minutes compared with 17.7 minutes for an established patient (Mechanic, D., 'How should hamsters run? Some observations about sufficient patient time in primary care', *British Medical Journal* 2001; 323: 266–8). Kaplan suggested at least 20 minutes was needed for patients to participate in decisions, but in my experience this was usually attainable within 10 minutes, given continuity and good records.

[20] Time to sit down is a recent assumption, confined to developed economies. Before the NHS, employed workers below administrative grades could consult a GP either through the Lloyd George panel (through the Insurance Act of 1911), or by paying a private fee. For GPs to maximise income, there had to be a difference between what they gave as a legal entitlement and what they sold for a fee. In some practices in industrial areas, this difference included the right to sit down. Panel patients were offered no chair to sit on. They had to stand up to say their piece. This was still happening in the early 1980s when I visited Spanish practices based on a similar national insurance scheme, though I'm sure it is now long gone. For different reasons, the same barbaric conditions existed in some working-class practices in the US around the same time, organised so that patients could be examined on a couch, but had no opportunity to sit and talk; otherwise, as such physicians would explain, they might never stop talking (Turner, J., 'The American dream', *GP Magazine*, 14 October 1977).

[21] Department of Health, *The National Survey of NHS Patients: General practice: 1998*, www.doh.gov.uk/public/nhssurvey.htm.

[22] Freeman, G.K., Horder, J.P., Howie, J.G.R., Hungin, A.P., Hill, A.P., Shah, N.C., Wilson, A., 'Evolving general practice consultation in Britain: issues of length and context', *British Medical Journal* 2002; 324: 880–2.

[23] Ridsdale, L., Carruthers, M., Morris, R., Ridsdale, J., 'Study of the effect of time availability on the consultation', *Journal of the Royal College of General Practitioners* 1989; 39: 488–91.

[24] Verby, J.E., Holden, P., Davis, R.H., 'Peer review of consultations in primary care: the use of audio-visual recordings', *British Medical Journal* 1979; 1: 1686–8.

[25] Mechanic, D., 'How long should hamsters run?' Some observations about sufficient patient time in primary care', *British Medical Journal* 2001; 323: 266–8.

[26] Beckman, H.B., Frankel, R.M., 'The effect of physician behavior on the collection of data', *Annals of Internal Medicine* 1984; 101: 692–6. When a similar study was repeated in 1998, average time before interruption had risen to 22 seconds (Marvel, M.K., Epstein, R.M., Flowers, K., Beckman, H.B., 'Soliciting the patient's agenda: have we improved?', *Journal of the American Medical Association* 1999; 281: 283–7).

[27] Hart, J.T., 'Innovative consultation time as a common European currency', *European Journal of General Practice* 1995; 1: 34–7.

[28] Grol, R., Wensing, M., Mainz, J., Ferreira, P., Hearnshaw, H., Hjortdahl, P., Oleson, F., Ribacke, M., Spenser, T., Szécsényi, J., 'Patients' priorities with respect to general practice care: an international comparison', *Family Practice* 1999; 16: 4–11.

[29] Squires, B., Learmonth, I., 'Empowerment of patients: fact or fiction', *British Medical Journal* 2003; 326: 710.

[30] Andersson, S.-O., Mattsson, B., 'Length of consultations in general practice in Sweden: views of doctors and patients', *Family Practice* 1989; 6: 130–4.

[31] Švab, I., Katic, M., 'Let the patients speak', *Family Practice* 1991; 8: 182–3. This study was so simple, and its evidence so counter-intuitive for most older health professionals, that it deserves to be used regularly as a learning

experience for undergraduates, illustrating most of the main qualities needed for original research in unexpected settings.

[32] Cromarty, I., 'What do patients think about during their consultations? A qualitative study', *British Journal of General Practice* 1996; 46: 525–8; and Pollock, K., Grime, J., 'Patients' perceptions of entitlement to time in general practice consultations for depression: qualitative study', *British Medical Journal* 2002; 325: 687–90.

[33] Gottlieb, B., 'Non-organic disease in medical outpatients', *Update* 1969; 5: 917–22.

[34] Speckens, A.E.M., van Hemert, A.M., Spinhoven, P. et al, 'Cognitive behavioural therapy for medically unexplained physical symptoms: a randomised controlled trial', *British Medical Journal* 1995; 311: 1328–32.

[35] Bridges, K.W., Goldberg, D.P., 'Somatic presentation of DSM III psychiatric disorders in primary care', *Journal of Psychosomatic Research* 1985; 29: 563–9; and Weich, S., Lewis, G., Donmall, R., Mann, A., 'Somatic presentation of psychiatric morbidity in general practice', *British Journal of General Practice* 1995; 45: 143–7.

[36] Slater, E., 'Diagnosis of "hysteria"', *British Medical Journal* 1965; 1: 1395–9.

[37] Crimlisk, H.L., Bhatia, K., Cope, H., David, A., Marsden, C.D., Ron, M.A., 'Slater revisited: six year follow up study of patients with medically unexplained motor symptoms', *British Medical Journal* 1998; 316: 582–6.

[38] A review of 27 publications concerning 1,466 patients whose symptoms had initially been considered to have no organic cause, and then followed for a mean five years since 1965, showed a decline in misdiagnosis from 23%–36% in the 1950s to 2%–6% by the 1990s (Stone, J., Smyth, R., Carson, A., Lewis, S., Prescott, R., Warlow, C., Sharpe, M., 'Systematic review of conversion symptoms and "hysteria"', *British Medical Journal* 2005; 331: 989–91).

[39] Lloyd, K.R., Jenkins, R., Mann, A., 'Long term outcome of patients with neurotic illness in general practice', *British Medical Journal* 1996; 313: 26–8; Moncrieff, J., Kirsch, I., 'Efficacy of antidepressants in adults', *British Medical Journal* 2005; 331: 155–9; Sims, A., Prior, P., 'The pattern of mortality in severe neuroses', *British Journal of Psychiatry* 1978; 133: 299–305; Sims, A., 'Mortality in neurosis', *Lancet* 1973; ii: 1072–5; Maricle, R.A., Hoffman, W.F., Bloom,

J.D. et al, 'The prevalence and significance of medical illness among chronic mentally ill outpatients', *Community Mental Health Journal* 1987; 23: 81–90.

[40] Stewart-Brown, S., Layte, R., 'Emotional health problems are the most important cause of disability in adults of working age: a study in the four counties of the old Oxford Region', *Journal of Epidemiology & Community Health* 1997; 51: 672–5.

[41] Schulz, R., Beach, S.R., Ives, D.G., Martire, L.M., Ariyo, A.A., Kop, W.J., 'Association between depression and mortality in older adults: the Cardiovascular Health Study', *Archives of Internal Medicine* 2000; 160: 1761–8. Despite this convincing evidence of the lethal consequences of depression, meta-analyses of randomised controlled trials show little evidence of clinically (rather than statistically) significant net benefit from antidepressant drugs (Moncrieff, J., Kirsch, I., 'Efficacy of antidepressants in adults', *British Medical Journal* 2005; 331: 155–9). Despite this poor evidence, they remain a gigantic international pharmaceutical market.

[42] This should not be misinterpreted to mean that people can make all parts of their bodies do anything they want simply by thinking and wishing hard enough, any more than the world can be changed by thinking and wishing about it.

[43] Kroenke, K., Mangelsdorff, D., 'Common symptoms in ambulatory care: incidence, evaluation, therapy and outcome', *American Journal of Medicine* 1989; 86: 262–6.

[44] Katon, W.J., Walker, E.A., 'Medically unexplained symptoms in primary care', *Journal of Clinical Psychiatry* 1998; 59 (suppl 20): 15–21.

[45] Bosanquet, N., Pollard, S., *Ready for Treatment: Popular Expectations and the Future of Health Care*, London: Social Market Foundation, 1997, pp 98–103.

[46] Hannay, D.R., Maddox, E.J., 'Incongruous referrals', *Lancet* 1975; ii: 1195–7. Of 1,344 people registered at a health centre, 23% had at least one severe or apparently serious medical symptom during the previous two weeks for which they had not consulted a doctor, compared with 9% who had consulted a doctor for a medical symptom causing insignificant pain or disability, and not apparently serious.

[47] Fijten, G.H., Muris, J.W.M., Starmans, R. et al, 'The incidence and outcome of rectal bleeding in general practice', *Family Practice* 1993; 10: 283–7.

[48] A poll of GP readers of *Pulse* newspaper in 2008 showed only one third of 500 respondents believed the NHS would be free at point of contact in 10 years' time. Eighty per cent of GPs said they would not support any further private sector involvement in the NHS, but 84% said they did not believe the NHS would exist in its present form in 10 years' time (Guardian Unlimited blogs, 10 April 2008). Nick Bosanquet and Stephen Pollard undertook their own survey of public opinion, from which they drew the following conclusions:

> The most striking general finding … is the gap between expectations and wants. Broadly, the public wants the NHS to offer everything, and to offer it free; 65% say, for instance, that NHS services should always be free. But, crucially, a mere 13% expect that they *will* be free in ten years' time. Some 67% think that the NHS will provide fewer services and those no longer covered will only be available privately, even though 80% do not like such a prospect. It is on this expectations gap that modernisers should focus. With expectations so clearly dampened, the battle is already half won … ideas for reform based on a wholesale switch to non-state insurance schemes are politically fanciful. Even when presented with today's reality of often long waits for non-emergency treatments … 74% still cling to the NHS rather than paying for private speed. The message is clear. Modernisers need to approach the task of reform not through grand plans involving large lump sum payments or a sudden and widespread switch to private provision, but through sums of money that are easy to contemplate, and that chime with other services.… This survey simply shows what the public will stomach today. It is now up to the politicians and opinion formers to move the argument on. (*Ready for Treatment: Popular Expectations and the Future of Health Care*, London: Social Market Foundation, 1997: 98–103)

[49] For a balanced assessment favourable to surgical intervention, see Crawford, E.D., 'PSA testing: what is the use?', *Lancet* 2005; 365: 1447–9.

[50] Ciatto, S., 'Reliability of PSA testing remains unclear', *British Medical Journal* 2003; 327: 750.

[51] Punglia, R.S., D'Amico, A.V., Catalona, W.J., Roehl, K.A., Kuntz, K.M., 'Effect of verification bias on screening for prostate cancer by measurement of prostate-specific antigen', *New England Journal of Medicine* 2003; 349: 335–42.

[52] Lenzer, J., 'FDA's counsel accused of being too close to drug industry', *British Medical Journal* 2004; 329: 189.

[53] On 18 March 2009 the *New England Journal of Medicine* released two pre-publication interim reports of two large controlled trials of PSA screening for prostate cancer, one in Europe, the other in the US. The European trial found 20% more deaths in unscreened controls than in men screened, but also that for each death delayed, 47 other lives were substantially impaired by treatment (by impotence, incontinence or other side effects). The US trial found a statistically insignificant trend for more deaths in the screened group. The *Daily Mail, The Daily Mirror, The Independent, Guardian* and *The Scotsman* all reported the European trial as a potential reduction of prostate cancer deaths by one fifth, none mentioned the US trial and none reported the data on side effects, or that 1,410 men had to be screened to postpone one death (Ben Goldacre, *Guardian*, 21 March 2009). PSA is an extremely useful measure of activity in prostate cancer cells, once a firm clinical diagnosis has been made, confirmed by biopsy. As a diagnostic tool for screening, it is simply confusing.

[54] By 2005, direct payments from patients accounted for over 20% of total health care spending in Belgium, Spain, Portugal, Italy, Hungary and Poland (Jemiai, N., Thomson, S., Mossialos, E., 'An overview of cost sharing for health services in the European Union', *Euro Observer* 3, Autumn 2004). By 2010, even Sweden had introduced substantial direct charges: Kr140 (£12) for a GP consultation, Kr300 (£25.70) for a specialist consultation or visit to a hospital A&E department, Kr80 (£6.85) for each night spent in a hospital bed, and the full cost of prescriptions up to Kr900 (£77) a year, then reduced rates to a maximum of Kr1,800 (£154) a year. The Wales Labour Party, supported by its coalition partner Plaid Cymru, has stayed faithful to the principles of 1948. The Welsh Assembly took a decision, opposed only by the Conservative Party, to abolish prescription charges in 2007. Since then there have been no step changes in prescribing rates to suggest that either professional or patient behaviour has changed. A steady 4%–6% annual rise in prescriptions has continued, mainly for cardiovascular disease, as it has also in England, where high charges have been maintained by central government. Wales has always had a high per capita prescription rate, but its ranking has not changed compared with England. Wales has the lowest net ingredient cost per prescription in the UK, and 84% of prescribing is generic (Jewell, T., 'Have dispensed items really risen with free prescriptions?', *British Medical Journal* 2008; 337: 591).

[55] Creese, A., 'User fees', *British Medical Journal* 1997; 315: 202–3.

[56] Evans, R.G., Barer, M.L., 'The American predicament', OECD Policy Studies 7, *Health Care Systems in Transition*, Paris: OECD, 1990, pp 80–5.

[57] Moses, S., Manji, F., Bradley, J.E., 'Impact of user fees on attendance at a referral centre for sexually transmitted diseases in Kenya', *Lancet* 1992; 340: 463–6, and Editorial, 'Charging for health services in the third world', *Lancet* 1992; 340: 458–9.

[58] de Sardan, J.P.O., 'Africa: no money, no treatment', *Le Monde Diplomatique*, June 2004: 15.

[59] Williams, P., Tarnspolsky, A., Hand, D., Shepherd, M., 'Minor psychiatric morbidity and general practice consultation', *Psychological Medicine*, Monograph Supplement 9, 1986.

[60] Corney, R.H., 'A survey of professional help sought by patients for psychosocial problems', *British Journal of General Practice* 1990; 40: 365–8.

[61] Goldberg, D., Williams, P., *A Users' Guide to the General Health Questionnaire (GHQ)*, Windsor: NFER-Nelson Publishing, 1988.

[62] Barsky, A.J., 'Amplification, somatization, and the somatiform disorders', *Psychosomatics* 1992; 33: 28–34.

[63] Starfield, B., Wray, C., Hess, K. et al, 'The influence of patient-practitioner agreement on outcome of care', *American Journal of Public Health* 1981; 71: 127–31. Though doctors like to imagine that they can predict their patients' decisions about their care, we have excellent evidence that this is not so. Joel Ménard ran a hypertension follow-up clinic at a Paris teaching hospital, where staff knew patients well and maintained continuity of care. Objective measures of how assiduously patients adhered to their treatment plans showed no correlation between predicted and actual behaviour, nor any association of behaviour with education or social class, though doctors thought these would be powerful predictors (de Goulet, P., Ménard, J., Vu, H.-A. et al, 'Factors predictive of attendance at clinic and blood pressure control in hypertensive patients', *British Medical Journal* 1983; 287: 88–93). Similar results were found in the Netherlands when predicted and actual behaviour were compared for patients' capacity to change diet, smoking or exercise habits (Verheijden, M.W., Bakx, J.C., Delemarre, I.C.G., Wanders, A.J., van Woudenbergh, N.M., Bottema B.J.A.M., van Weel, C., van Staveren, W.A., 'GPs' assessment of patients' readiness to change diet, activity and smoking', *British Journal of General Practice* 2005; 55: 452–7). In both cases, researchers reached a simple conclusion: nobody knows what patients can do until they are allowed to try, which means that they all have to be asked, and all their answers have to be listened to.

[64] Burack, R.C., Carpenter, R.R., 'The predictive value of the presenting complaint', *Journal of Family Practice* 1983; 16: 749–54.

[65] In a classic experiment, eight sane researchers presented at 12 psychiatric hospitals in five states of the US, falsely claiming they had heard voices. They otherwise behaved normally. Persuading staff that they were sane, and could leave hospital, took from 7 to 19 days. All but one was diagnosed as schizophrenic on admission. Out of 118 real patients these researchers met on the admissions ward, 35 recognised that these impostors were sane, and were probably doing an experiment, but none of them was detected by staff. The researchers then warned staff at a teaching and research hospital, which had denied this could have happened there, that over the next three months one or more pseudopatients would present for admission in the same way. Though none was in fact offered for admission, 41 out of 193 patients presenting for admission were diagnosed confidently as pseudopatients by at least one member of staff (Rosenhan, D.L., 'On being sane in insane places', *Science* 1973; 179: 250–8).

[66] Pringle, J., *Living with Schizophrenia – by the Relatives*, London: National Schizophrenia Fellowship, 1974.

[67] Editorial, 'Dying with their rights on', *Lancet* 1989; ii: 1492.

[68] Wing, J.K., 'Epidemiology of schizophrenia', *Journal of the Royal Society of Medicine* 1987; 80: 134–5.

[69] The lifetime risk of schizophrenia is 1% for all social classes, with true prevalence unrelated to social class, but average age at first hospital admission for schizophrenia at 28 years for most affluent patients is more than 8 years earlier than for poor patients. Others rank appropriately between these two extremes. In other words, the Inverse Care Law applies.

[70] Followed up 15 years after a first episode of schizophrenic disorder, about 25% have recovered completely and no longer need treatment (Wiersma, D. et al, 'Natural course of schizophrenic disorders: a 15-year follow-up of a Dutch incidence cohort', *Schizophrenia Bulletin* 1998; 24: 75–85). See also Turner, T.H., 'Long term outcome of treating schizophrenia: antipsychotics probably help – but we badly need more long term studies', *British Medical Journal* 2004; 329: 1058–9.

[71] This was established by the important MRC studies at Northwick Park (Johnstone, E.C., Crow, T.J., Johnson, A.L., MacMillan, J.F., 'The Northwick

Park study of first episodes of schizophrenia. I. Presentation of the illness and problems relating to admission', *British Journal of Psychiatry* 1986; 148: 115–20; Crow, T.J., MacMillan, J.F., Johnson, A.L., Johnstone, E.C., 'The Northwick Park study of first episodes of schizophrenia. II. A randomised controlled trial of prophylactic neuroleptic treatment', *British Journal of Psychiatry* 1986; 148: 120–7; MacMillan, J.F., Crow, T.J., Johnson, A.L., Johnstone, E.C., 'The Northwick Park study of first episodes of schizophrenia. III. Short-term outcome in trial entrants and trial eligible patients', *British Journal of Psychiatry* 1986; 148: 128–33; and MacMillan, J.F., Gold, A., Crow, T.J., Johnson, A.L., Johnstone, E.C., 'The Northwick Park study of first episodes of schizophrenia. IV. Expressed emotion and relapse', *British Journal of Psychiatry* 1986; 148: 133–43).

[72] 'Psychosocial interventions for schizophrenia', *Effective Health Care*, August 2000.

[73] Rollin, H., 'In my own time: schizophrenia', *British Medical Journal* 1979; 1: 1773–5.

[74] Bagley, C., 'There is nothing postmodern in what people with schizophrenia want', *British Medical Journal* 2001; 323: 449–50.

[75] Timimi, S., *Pathological Child Psychiatry and the Medicalisation of Childhood*, Hove: Brunner-Routledge, 2002.

[76] Medawar, C., *Power and Dependence: Social Audit on the Safety of Medicines*, London: Social Audit, 1992.

[77] Taylor, E., Sandberg, S., Thorley, C., Giles, S., *The Epidemiology of Childhood Hyperactivity*, Oxford: Oxford University Press, 1991, pp 93–113.

[78] Consensus criteria for diagnosis of ADHD in the US are as follows: six or more out of nine frequently observed inattentive behaviours, and six or more out of nine frequently observed hyperactive or impulsive behaviours. Some of these must have been present before age 7, and some must cause impairment in two or more settings (for example at home, at school or at work). They must provide clear evidence of clinically significantly impaired social, academic or occupational functioning, and they must not be more readily attributable to some other mental disorder (American Psychiatric Association's *Diagnostic and Statistical Manual of Mental Disorders*, 4th edn, Washington, DC: American Psychiatric Association, 1994). On these generous criteria even US prevalence rates seem surprisingly modest.

[79] Jick, H., Kaye, J.A., Black, C., 'Incidence and prevalence of drug-treated attention deficit disorder among boys in the UK', *British Journal of General Practice* 2004; 54: 345–7.

[80] 'Stimulant drugs for severe hyperactivity in childhood', *Drug & Therapeutics Bulletin* 2001; 39: 52–4.

[81] Kewley, G.D., 'Personal paper: attention deficit hyperactivity disorder is underdiagnosed and undertreated in Britain', *British Medical Journal* 1998; 316: 1594–6.

[82] Roberts, J., 'Behavioural disorders are overdiagnosed in the US', *British Medical Journal* 1996; 312: 657.

[83] Levine, M.D., Oberklaid, F., 'Hyperactivity: symptom complex or complex symptom?', *American Journal of Diseases in Childhood* 1980; 134: 409–14.

[84] Guevara, J.P., Stein, M.T., 'Evidence based management of attention deficit hyperactivity disorder', *British Medical Journal* 2001; 323: 1232–5. Arguments for and against were presented by David Coghill and Harvey Markovitch respectively in *British Medical Journal* 2004; 329: 907–9.

[85] Mayor, S., 'Warning against overuse of drugs for inattentive children', *British Medical Journal* 1996; 313: 770.

[86] 'Drug company breaks 30 year agreement on patient advertising', *British Medical Journal* 2001; 323: 470.

[87] Marwick, C., 'US doctor warns of misuse of prescribed stimulants', *British Medical Journal* 2003; 326: 67.

[88] Timimi, S., 'Effect of globalisation on children's mental health', *British Medical Journal* 2005; 331: 37–9.

[89] Hampton, J.R., Harrison, M.J.G., Mitchell, J.R.A., Prichard, J.S., Seymour, C., 'Relative contributions of history-taking, physical examination, and laboratory investigation to diagnosis and management of medical outpatients', *British Medical Journal* 1975; ii: 486–9, and Peterson, M.C., Holbrook, J.H., Hales, D.V. et al, 'Contributions of the history, of physical examination, and of laboratory investigation in making medical diagnosis', *Western Journal of Medicine* 1992; 156: 163–5.

[90] Peppiatt, R., 'Eliciting patients' views of the cause of their problem: a practical strategy for GPs', *Family Practice* 1992; 9: 295–8. Of 1,000 consecutive consultations with a single GP, 150 patients volunteered causal ideas, and another 266 gave causal ideas when asked. Of these ideas, 30% proved useful for diagnosis. The most useful were ideas about cancer, anxiety, age, occupation and heart disease.

[91] A recent paper noted that '… with the rapid growth in new diagnostic technologies there is now a suggestion that it is more efficient and cost-effective to employ a technician to undertake a battery of investigations rather than have an expensive clinician spending time listening to patients' (Summerton, N., 'The medical history as a diagnostic technology', *British Journal of General Practice* 2008; 58: 273–6). That suggestion may not get far with experienced clinicians, but will be of intense interest to their managers.

[92] For practice to follow scientific method, diagnosis should follow a hypothetico-deductive pathway, forming successive hypotheses which further evidence is designed either to validate or refute. We have good evidence that this pattern is rarely followed in practice. Most clinicians, most of the time, rely on empiricism, recognising common patterns familiar from experience. We also have good evidence that most serious errors occur in this pattern recognition mode rather than hypothetico-deductive mode. Progress in part depends on a general shift to more scientific modes of thought, by both professionals and patients (Hopayian, K., 'Why medicine needs a scientific foundation retaining the hypotheticodeductive model', *British Journal of General Practice* 2004; 54: 400–4).

[93] A classic example is investigation of headache, the commonest of all symptoms presented in primary care. Brain tumours account for less than 0.1% of the lifetime prevalence of headache. (Goadsby, P.J., 'To scan or not to scan in headache', *British Medical Journal* 2004; 329: 469–70). The threshold suggested by NICE as reasonable for referral for brain scans in headache is a 1% risk of tumour, estimated by clinical judgement of symptoms. The alternative is watchful waiting. For headache, low imaging threshold may be cost-effective because patients who have been scanned, with a negative result, use substantially less resources in the following year than those unscanned. However, imaging threshold at 1% risk leads to false positive rates around 6% (Hamilton, W., 'The price of diagnosis', *British Journal of General Practice* 2008; 58: 837–8). We need also to remember that most brain tumours either are inoperable, or are metastases from cancer elsewhere – either of these is essentially incurable.

[94] Studies in the US show that the most-wanted item in consultation is explanation of patients' problems. Even in that culture, which sets such a high value on technical investigations, diagnostic tests and other sorts of support were all rated lower than explanation (Williams, S., Weinman, J., Dale, J., Newman, S., 'Patient expectations: what do primary care patients want from the GP and how far does meeting expectations affect patient satisfaction?', *Family Practice* 1995; 12: 193–201).

[95] Frank, J.D., 'The placebo is psychotherapy', *The Behavioral & Brain Sciences* 1983; 6: 291–2. Placebo is usually a misnomer, because it implies intention to deceive (Latin *placebo* = I please). A better term would be 'caring effects', because the main operator seems to be the patient's belief that at last she has found someone competent and willing to help (Hart, J.T., Dieppe, P., 'Caring effects', *Lancet* 1996; 347: 1606–8). To assess their real effects, placebo or caring effects need to be measured not against active treatments, but three ways: against an active drug, against placebo, and against no treatment at all. This has been done, showing virtually no independent effect of placebo pills; the important ingredient is not the pill, but the person who gives it (Hrobjartsson, A., Gotzsche, P.C., 'Is the placebo powerless? An analysis of clinical trials comparing placebo with no treatment', *New England Journal of Medicine* 2001; 344: 1594–602). More or less supportive environments in which treatments are given influence their effectiveness. For example, having a view of trees through a window seemed to speed recovery from surgery (Ulrich, R.S., 'View through a window may influence recovery from surgery', *Science* 1984; 224: 420–1). Such environmental effects seem to be general (Di Blasi, Z., Harkness, E., Ernst, E., Georgiou, A., Kleijnen, J., 'Influence of context effects on health outcomes: a systematic review', *Lancet* 2001; 357: 757–62). This may not be surprising, but should be taken into account in design of NHS buildings. Most primary care health centres in Britain still look like our schools – cheap and soon dilapidated.

[96] De Gruy, F., Columbia, L., Dickinson, P., 'Somatisation disorder in a family practice', *Journal of Family Practice* 1987; 25: 45–51.

[97] Fink, P., 'Surgery and medical treatment in persistent somatising patients', *Journal of Psychosomatic Research* 1992; 36: 439–47, and Escobar, J.L., Golding, J.M., Hough, R.L. et al, 'Somatisation in the community: relationship to disability and use of services', *American Journal of Public Health* 1987; 77: 837–40.

[98] Davies, N., 'The most secret crime', *Guardian*, 2 June 1998.

[99] Portegijs, P.J.M., Jeuken, F.M.H., van der Horst, F., Kraan, H.F., Knottnerus, J.A., 'A troubled youth: relations with somatization, depression and anxiety in adulthood', *Family Practice* 1996; 13: 1–11.

[100] Hooper, P.D., 'Psychological sequelae of sexual abuse in childhood', *British Journal of General Practice* 1990; 40: 29–31.

[101] Richardson, J., Feder, G., 'Domestic violence against women', *British Medical Journal* 1995; 311: 964–5.

[102] Katon, W., Kleinman, A., Rosen, G., 'Depression and somatization: a review. Part 1', *American Journal of Medicine* 1982; 72: 127–35.

[103] Dunea, G., 'Nonsenserine', *British Medical Journal* 1991; 303: 253.

[104] Howe, A., '"I know what to do, but it's not possible to do it" – general practitioners' perceptions of their ability to detect psychological distress', *Family Practice* 1996; 13: 127–32.

[105] Angela Coulter and colleagues tracked the full sequence from self-selection by patients through referral by GPs to final selection for hysterectomy for excessive menstrual bleeding (Coulter, A., Klassen, A., McPherson, K., 'How many hysterectomies should purchasers buy?', *European Journal of Public Health* 1995; 5: 123–9). They found that most critical decisions were made not by specialists, but at primary care level. Once people got referred into the hospital pipeline, few escaped surgery. Most significant choices were made by GPs, shared sometimes with patients, more often unshared, particularly with working-class women. The quality of primary care thus became the main determinant of surgical efficiency, chiefly depending on the extent to which patients' full health agendas were considered, without hasty resort to referral for surgery as a way both to save consultation time, and to ensure that patients were satisfied that something substantial was being done. Hysterectomy rates for this indication are now rapidly falling, to about two-thirds less than a decade ago (Reid, P.C., Mukri, F., 'Trends in number of hysterectomies performed in England for menorrhagia: examination of health episode statistics, 1989 to 2002–3', *British Medical Journal* 2005; 330: 938–9). They now show little variability between different NHS areas. This contrasts with cholecystectomy rates, which still show huge unexplained variation between areas, and have not been subjected to similar intelligent scrutiny (Aylin, P., Williams, S., Jarman, B., Bottle, A., 'Dr Foster's case notes: variation in operation rates by Primary Care Trust, 1998–2004', *British Medical Journal* 2005; 331: 539).

[106] Mulley, A.G., 'The need to confront variation in practice', *British Medical Journal* 2009; 339: 1007–9.

[107] Diagnostic errors are inevitably more frequent in older patients with multiple disorders. They occur first, because clinicians tend to look for single, large and static explanations for clinical events, and second, because the errors inherent in each step of diagnosis are compounded when they follow multiple pathways. Old people also present difficulties for interpretation of measurements, where normal values are based on evidence from younger people. Mathematical analysis of these factors suggests that failing to make a diagnosis when a disease is present, or making a diagnosis when a disease is not present, are both likely to occur about twice as often in old as in younger patients (Fairweather, D.S., Campbell, A.J., 'Diagnostic accuracy: the effects of multiple aetiology and the degradation of information in old age', *Journal of the Royal College of Physicians of London* 1991; 25: 105–10).

[108] Chris Gunstone gives a good account of five recent cases illustrating this point, with which most experienced clinicians or surviving relatives are likely to sympathise (Gunstone, C., 'Cancer in the elderly – a case for informed pessimism?', *British Journal of General Practice* 2005; 55: 648).

[109] Coulter, A., McPherson, K., Vessey, M.P., 'Do British women undergo too many or too few hysterectomies?', *Social Science & Medicine* 1988; 27: 987–94. Since then, British rates have continued to rise.

[110] Lilford, R.J., 'Hysterectomy: will it pay the bills in 2007?', *British Medical Journal* 1997; 314: 160–1.

[111] It seems strange that nobody has yet developed a simple technique for measuring menstrual loss objectively, but perhaps there is not much demand for this. At the Oxford John Radcliffe Hospital, Margaret Rees used accurate research measurements of menstrual flow to see whether treatment could address patients' real concerns more accurately and rationally, with less resort to surgery (Rees, M.C.P., 'Role of menstrual blood loss in management of complaints of excessive menstrual bleeding', *British Journal of Obstetrics & Gynaecology* 1991; 98: 327–8.). She studied 17 patients aged 30–45 referred for treatment of heavy menstruation, but with measured menstrual blood loss between 15ml and 60ml, way below the consensus threshold. She gave them a clear explanation of how they compared with other women, and then explored related problems constituting their own personal patterns of illness, rather than the standard disorder defined as menorrhagia. Three years after being told their blood loss was normal and did not need treatment, she

found 14 had accepted this, a huge gain in efficiency. However, two were still taking medication for menorrhagia, and one had managed to get herself a hysterectomy.

This suggests that more rational discussion and better communication has a more than 80% success rate, but there is other evidence that the other 20% may feel happier after a hysterectomy, and this includes a lot of people. Coulter and her colleagues found that, of patients who had complained of mild to moderate menorrhagia, 83% who had had hysterectomies were satisfied with their treatment, compared with only 45% of patients treated by medication, though objectively these treatments were equally successful in controlling bleeding (Coulter, A., Peto, V., Jenkinson, C., 'Quality of life and patient satisfaction following treatment for menorrhagia', *Family Practice* 1994; 11: 394–401). Results were only marginally different for women complaining of severe bleeding. Her study of consultations about heavy menstrual bleeding between 483 patients and 129 GPs showed that, when given an opportunity to choose between treatment options (medication, hysterectomy or other operative techniques such as endometrial ablation), about one third of patients wanted to participate in this decision and had a strong treatment preference. Strongest predictors for this wish were higher education and previous consultations for gynaecological disorders – patients who were more confident, knowledgeable and assertive. This must partly account for the astonishing fact that UK women who left school without any educational qualification are 15 times more likely to have a hysterectomy than women with a university degree. Despite much greater cost barriers, there are similar social differences in the US.

[112] Ligation of internal mammary arteries in hope of improving perfusion of heart muscle in coronary heart disease became popular in the US and Italy in the late 1940s, with convincingly high early success rates. By 1954 initial enthusiasm had waned sufficiently for a search for scientific evidence to be possible. Using random allocation to sham and real operations on internal mammary arteries for treatment of angina caused by coronary heart disease, Beecher showed that both were equally effective for about one third of patients in terms of consumer satisfaction at short-term follow-up, though obviously sham operations had no objective effect on coronary bloodflow (Beecher, H.K., 'Surgery as placebo: a quantitative study of bias', *Journal of the American Medical Association* 1961; 176: 1102–7, and Benson, H., McCallie, D.P., 'Angina pectoris and the placebo effect', *New England Journal of Medicine* 1979; 300: 1424–9). Such experiments are no longer possible, but I see no reason why more recent procedures should not have similar transient subjective effects in the same proportion of patients.

[113] Sackett, D.L., Rosenberg, W.M.C., Gray, J.A.M. et al, 'Evidence based medicine: what it is and what it isn't', *British Medical Journal* 1996; 312: 71–2.

[114] To compare one treatment with another (including no treatment at all) in as nearly as possible identical groups of people seems a very simple idea, self-evidently useful even to the most primitive healers. This was not so, revealing that what now seems self-evident was an idea unthinkable for earlier generations. So far as I know, the earliest example of any such comparison was a trial of blood-letting in the Peninsular War, reported in 1816 (Hamilton, A.L., *Dissertatio medica inauguralis de synocho castrensi*, Edinburgh: J. Ballantyne, 1816). Sixty-six sick soldiers were alternately bled or not bled. Of those bled, 35 died. Of those not bled, two died (quoted from Chalmers, I., 'Comparing like with like: the evolution of prospective control of selection biases', paper read at conference on beating biases in therapeutic research: historical perspectives, at Osler-McGovern Centre, Green College, Oxford, 2002: 9–10). This dramatic result seems to have had no lasting effect on practice. Forms of blood letting for non-specific illness were still in use in France and in Russia until well after the Second World War. The first modern trial published in English with strictly randomised controls was the MRC trial of streptomycin for tuberculous meningitis, designed by Philip D'Arcy Hart and Marc Daniels (D'Arcy Hart, P., 'Randomised controlled clinical trials', *British Medical Journal* 1991; 302: 1271–2).

[115] For political and cultural reasons that deserve more study than they have received, this happened much earlier in Britain and the British Commonwealth, Ireland, the US, Netherlands and Scandinavia – broadly, the English-reading medical sphere – than elsewhere in Europe. With the outstanding exception of Cuba, it was ignored or suppressed by states trying to build socialist economies.

[116] Sullivan, F., Mitchell, E., 'Has general practice computing made a difference to patient care? A systematic review of published reports', *British Medical Journal* 1995; 311: 848–52. Ominously, this study found that doctor-initiated and medical content increased with computerisation of records, but patient-initiated social content fell.

[117] We found checklists essential for complete performance of necessary tasks, in the systems of anticipatory care we developed in Glyncorrwg for detection and management of common chronic forms of ill health. However, we had also to recognise their potentially stultifying effect on imagination, and their tendency to replace health outcome by data recording as the aim of care. They easily degenerate into rituals, eventually disconnected from clinical judgement of any kind, an old story repeated again and again in the history of

medicine. I met a striking example in the 1950s, when I worked occasionally as a locum school medical officer. At a large secondary modern school the school nurse explained that in that two-hour session I had to examine about 100 children. When I said there was no way I could do this within the time available, she explained that these were 'just cursories'. All I had to do, she said, was to look at their tonsils, examine their hearts (by which she meant, to apply a stethoscope to the left side of their chest) and look at the soles of their feet. At some time in the remote past, some doctor in the schools medical administration had decided that the three most important conditions to search for were large tonsils (ripe for ritual tonsillectomy), rheumatic heart disease (common until the 1950s, but then rapidly nearing extinction) and plantar warts (known to, and apparently dreaded by, all teachers as verrucas; they are self-limiting and need no treatment other than washing more often). Checklists and guidelines start from good intentions and best contemporary evidence, but they tend to fossilise sooner than their pioneers anticipate. The value of surgical checklists was recently rediscovered and confirmed. A study of 3,733 patients before and 3,955 patients after introduction of a 19-item checklist at every operation showed a 47% fall in post-operative deaths, from 1.5% to 0.8%, and a 36% fall in in-hospital complications, from 11% to 7% (Soar, J., Peyton, J., Leonard, M., Pullyblank, A.M., 'Surgical safety check lists: improve collaborative teamwork, minimise surprises, and reduce harm to patients', *British Medical Journal* 2009; 338: 186–7). However, surgical checklists have existed as far back as anyone can remember. Without them, swabs, artery forceps, even the occasional rubber glove get left in the peritoneal cavity from time to time, by even the finest surgeons. The problem is that the less often errors occur, the easier it becomes to tick all the boxes without really looking to see whether an error is in fact present.

[118] Spenser, T., 'Guidelines as an integral stage in quality development', *Family Physician (Israel)* 1993; 21: 37–9.

[119] Fairfield, G., Hunter, D.J., Mechanic, D., Rosleff, F., 'Managed care: origins, principles and evolution', *British Medical Journal* 1997; 314: 1823–6.

[120] Feder, G., Griffiths, C., Highton, C. et al, 'Do clinical guidelines introduced with practice based education improve care of asthmatic and diabetic patients? A randomised controlled trial in general practice in East London', *British Medical Journal* 1995; 311: 1473–8.

[121] The NHS hospital equivalent of QOF is called Payment By Results (PBR). The 'results' in question are, of course, results for management, not for health gain; in other words, both QOF and PBR are forms of piecework as used in

industrial manufacture, which tends to raise productivity but reduce quality, unless tightly supervised and regulated. Introduction of PBR in NHS England was associated with a reduction in average hospital stay of only 0.08 of a day more than in NHS Scotland, where, like in Wales, it has not been introduced. This contrasts with the US, where it was associated with a reduction in average stay of more than one whole day, an effect soon summarised as 'discharge quicker and sicker' (Anderson, G.A., 'The effects of payment by results', *British Medical Journal* 2009; 339: 523–4). Perhaps US doctors are simply more accustomed to such incentives, and therefore more responsive to them.

[122] Hart, J.T., Hart, M., *Present State and Future Needs of Primary Care in Kazakhstan and Kirghizstan: Report of a Visit March 18–April 8, 1995*, London: Royal Free Hospital Department of Primary Health Care, 1995.

[123] Choudhry, N.K., Stelfox, H.T., Detsky, A.S., 'Relationships between authors of clinical practice guidelines and the pharmaceutical industry', *Journal of the American Medical Association* 2002; 287: 612–17.

[124] Hawkes, N., 'NICE goes global: NICE decisions on NHS drug funding have attracted attention abroad, but can the international interest be turned into profit?', *British Medical Journal* 2009; 338: 266–7.

[125] 'NICE told to break its close links with pharmaceutical industry by WHO adviser Kees de Joncheere', *British Medical Journal* 2003; 327: 637.

[126] Hart, J.T., 'What evidence do we need for evidence based medicine?', Cochrane lecture 1997, *Journal of Epidemiology & Community Health* 1997; 51: 623–9.

[127] Williamson, C., 'Ensuring that guidelines are effective: give them to the patient', *British Medical Journal* 1995; 311: 1023.

[128] Eaton, L., 'Website of experiences hopes to reach more patients', *British Medical Journal* 2008; 337: 896–7. After relaunch, DIPEx provided 30 to 50 separate patient's experiences for each of about 50 topics.

[129] *The Expert Patient*, London: Department of Health, August 2001.

[130] Several professional bodies have very successfully developed expert patients, including children, to teach trainee medical specialists and GPs. All note that this depends on a profound change in professional culture (Donaghy, F.,

Boylan, O., Loughrey, C., 'Using expert patients to deliver teaching in general practice', *British Journal of General Practice* 2010; 60: 136–9.

[131] Association of the British Pharmaceutical Industry, *The Expert Patient Survey*, October 1999, London: ABPI, 1999.

[132] Market & Opinion Research International, for Developing Patient Partnerships, formerly the Doctor Patient Partnership (DPP), *Medicines and the British*, London: MORI, 2003.

[133] Barlow, J.H., Turner, A.P., Wright, C.A., 'A randomised controlled study of the arthritis self-management programme in the UK', *Health Education Research* 2000; 15: 665–80, and Lorig, K.R., Sobel, D.S., Stewart, A.L., Brown, B.W., Bandura, A., Ritter, P. et al, 'Evidence suggesting that a chronic disease self-management programme can improve health status while reducing hospitalisation. A randomised trial', *Medical Care* 1999; 37: 5–14.

[134] Shaw, J., Baker, M., '"Expert patient" – dream or nightmare?', *British Medical Journal* 2004; 328: 723–4.

[135] Greenhalgh, T., 'Research methods 2: whose evidence is it anyway?', *British Journal of General Practice* 1998; 48: 1448–9.

[136] Many factors have converged to produce the present global crisis of capitalism, but possibly the most important has been the rapid growth of fictional capital during the past decade, above all trading in future expectations and debts, with no measurable basis in reality. In this period national wealth has appeared to become completely detached from the real economy of production of goods and services. As this provided the material base for gentrification (*embourgeoisement*) on a mass scale, we may anticipate a retreat towards renewed proletarianisation – or whatever popular word replaces that fossilised term.

[137] From cautious critic of a marketised NHS during Conservative administrations, Julian Le Grand, Richard Titmuss Professor at the London School of Economics and Political Science, has become a zealous advocate of what he and Titmuss, the pioneer of gift relationships, once opposed. At a recent conference he suggested that patients with chronic health problems be given their own NHS budgets to spend at whatever points of retail sale they might choose, public or private. When she became Health Minister, Patricia Hewitt promised to consider this proposal carefully, before she returned to the back benches and a directorship with Boots, a major new applicant for

NHS contracts (Harding, M.-L., 'Patients could get their own budgets, Number 10 says', *Health Services Journal*, 19 May 2005: 5). Since then the proposal seems to have been at least temporarily shelved. Its most effective opponent has probably been the Treasury, which knows that such a US-style market would be unaffordable in the UK, and just as extravagant and inefficient as in the US. Ordinary members of the Labour Party have never been asked for their opinion.

[138] Quality-Adjusted Life Years (QALYs) were designed by health economists at the University of York as a sort of universal currency for policy decisions, a measure of effectiveness for all treatments (Rosser, R.H., 'From health indicators to quality adjusted life years: technical and ethical issues', in Hopkins, A., Costain, D. (eds), *Measuring the Outcomes of Medical Care*, London: Royal College of Physicians of London 1990, pp 1–16). It has been useful for a few rather limited interventions, like joint replacements or bypass grafts, but can never keep pace with the rate of innovation, real or imagined, because the evidence needed to calculate them is still not available for most treatments, and takes many years to accumulate – by which time new treatments have been introduced.

[139] Hawkes, N., 'Why is the press so nasty to NICE?', *British Medical Journal* 2008; 337: 788.

[140] By international standards, broadcast news in the UK, including stations funded by advertising, is relatively impartial. But how does the BBC define impartiality? By giving a fair hearing to spokespersons for all three main political parties. The leaders of all these parties agree on the nature of 'reform' of the NHS. They differ only on the pace and extent of 'reforms', not the principle. Virtually all broadcasters exclude or marginalise anyone defending the principle of a gift economy in the NHS, with its plans and transactions open to scrutiny, and fully accountable to MPs in Parliament. This set of principles still has implicit mass support among the electorate, though it is seldom set out explicitly. We still have occasional documentary broadcasts, wherein a few brave professionals dare to limit their career prospects by telling the truth as they see it.

[141] This has helped to ensure that NHS prices for virtually all health care-related processes are much lower than in the US, even for products actually produced in the US. For example, heart pacemakers, selling in the US for $35,000 each, are available to the NHS for $5,000 – and, of course, free to NHS patients (BBC Radio 4 news broadcast, 24 August 2009).

[142] In US terminology, charts.

[143] Do you remember a game called Chinese whispers? When one junior doctor hands over responsibility for a patient to another doctor on the next shift, he or she is supposed to undertake a handover – a brief account of the main problems which that patient currently presents. Using fictional patient scenarios, with junior doctors giving verbal handovers to colleagues, 67% of data were lost in the first handover. By the fifth handover, 97% was lost. When this was repeated using written notes, loss by the fifth handover fell to 13%, which was further reduced to 3% when written notes were structured (Bhabra, G., Mackeith, S., Monteiro, P., Pothier, D., 'An experimental comparison of handover methods', *Annals of the Royal College of Surgeons of England* 2007; 89: 298–300). Structured records are a major advance, but constant vigilance is needed to keep even these alive, active and free from ritual observance.

[144] This function depends on continued existence of stable, registered populations in primary care, and defined population catchments for hospitals. Both of these are threatened by present policies promoting consumer choice, self-referral to a variety of competing sources of primary care, and multiple competing pathways both for entry to care and for referral to specialist advice. Fortunately new patterns of staff and patient behaviour take time to get established, particularly when change is imposed from above, has little support from public opinion, and still less from professional opinion. Despite more than 25 years of encouragement first from Conservative and then from New Labour governments, patients remain overwhelmingly loyal to their GPs and rarely move from one practice to another unless they move to a new home; competition between GPs is probably less now than it has ever been. What little competition exists between specialists or between hospitals still depends almost entirely on experience and opinions of primary care staff, hardly at all on the experience and opinions of patients as consumers. Any government decision to retreat from consumerism would almost certainly be greeted with relief by staff, and all but a small (though probably influential) proportion of patients.

[145] They actually came into use in 1916, but rarely contained useful information until after the Second World War.

[146] Interviewed about his recollections of practice when he started in the 1950s, soon after the NHS began, a Paisley GP described the then customary attitude to medical records in Scottish industrial practice:

> We had Lloyd George [records] and we kept them in cabinets ... these were our receptionist's pride and joy and not taken out at any time. They were stored, everything was stored there, but we never used the

files. The files were not brought out for us to use. So [as an incoming partner] I didn't have any knowledge of the patient coming to see me. The patients would come with all their bottles, with all the medication, and say: 'Doctor, that's what I'm getting', and I would just write out what the medication was. But we never got the files out. The partners' attitude at that time was 'Well, we know the patients, we don't need files – I've known them all their life ... why would I want to write anything down?' We kept the letters from the hospital in a pile, which just got bigger and bigger.' (Michell, E., Smith, G., 'An oral history of general practice 9: record keepers', *British Journal of General Practice* 2003; 53: 166–7).

As a locum in the 1950s and 1960s, that was exactly my experience.

[147] Ward, L., Innes, M., 'Electronic summaries in general practice: considering the patient's contribution', *British Journal of General Practice* 2003; 53: 293–7.

[148] Pyper, C., Amery, J., Watson, M., Crook, C., 'Patients' experiences when accessing their on-line electronic patient records in primary care', *British Journal of General Practice* 2004; 54: 38–43.

[149] My nearest city, Swansea, is served by two large NHS hospitals, Morriston and Singleton, both now quasi-independent Trusts. In the pre-'reform' NHS they had similar paper records, and exchanged information freely, though inefficiently. About 12% of records were missing at any particular time. 'Reform' introduced competition between these hospitals, so each Trust developed its own IT system, each incompatible with the other. Fortunately, competition did not develop very far, the Trusts soon agreed to specialise in different, complementary fields, so outpatients still moved frequently from one to the other. Whereas paper records could follow them on loan, there was, and still is, no way to transmit computer-held data between them.

[150] Benson, T., 'Why general practitioners use computers and hospital doctors do not – Part 1: incentives', *British Medical Journal* 2002; 325: 1086–9, and Benson, T., 'Why general practitioners use computers and hospital doctors do not – Part 2: scalability', *British Medical Journal* 2002; 325: 1090–3.

[151] Langton, A., 'Sharing patient information electronically throughout the NHS: change of culture is needed', *British Medical Journal* 2003; 327: 622–3.

[152] deKare-Silver, N., 'Choose and book: whose choice is it anyway?', *British Medical Journal* 2005; 330: 1093.

[153] There are still no official figures for the cost so far of the proposed central IT system for NHS England. Informed estimates vary from £6.2bn to £20bn (Kmietowicz, Z., 'Tories promise to scrap "top-down, bureaucratic" NHS IT programme', *British Medical Journal* 2009; 339: 361).

[154] Williams, J., 'National programme for IT: the £30 billion question', *British Journal of General Practice* 2005; 55: 340–2.

[155] Cross, M., 'Electronic records may not be available in hospitals until 2015', *British Medical Journal* 2008; 336: 1153.

[156] Williams, J., 'National programme for IT: the £30 billion question', *British Journal of General Practice* 2005; 55: 340–2.

[157] Dove, G.A.W., Wigg, P., Clarke, J.H.C. et al, 'The therapeutic effect of taking a patient's history by computer', *Journal of the Royal College of General Practitioners* 1977; 27: 477–81.

[158] Brownbridge, G., Evans, A., Wall, T., 'Effect of computer use in the consultation on the delivery of care', *British Medical Journal* 1985; 291: 639–41; Ridsdale, L., Hudd, S., 'Computers in the consultation: the patients' view', *British Journal of General Practice* 1994; 44: 367–9; Sullivan, F., Mitchell, E., 'Has general practice computing made a difference to patient care? A systematic review of published reports', *British Medical Journal* 1995; 311: 848–52. On average, consultations using a computer-held rather than written record add almost one minute to consultation time. In the British NHS situation, where average time available is seldom more than 10 minutes, though doctor-initiated clinical content tends to increase, patient-initiated social content tends to fall.

[159] Progressive teaching of this sort depends on having sufficient staff for teaching in small groups, close to real patients. According to the Report of the Academic Careers Sub-committee of Modernising Medical Careers and the UK Clinical Research Collaboration (2005), the number of UK clinical academics had declined from 4,000 in 2001 to 3,500 by 2005, with the number of clinical lecturers falling by 30% over the same period, while medical schools were trying to double their intake of medical students and output of doctors because of serious staff shortages at all levels. The decline in teaching staff was attributed to lack of career structure, inflexible patterns of clinical and academic training, shortage of supported posts, and income differentials favouring clinical rather than academic work. Government pledged an initial £2.5m for 2005–06 to establish a new integrated training programme for clinical academics. Even

this drop in the ocean could disappear through impending cuts in all higher education, to reduce public debts incurred to save UK banks.

[160] Spokespersons for the Department of Health have assured the press that data of these sorts will be excluded from the future shared NHS patient records now being developed in its National Programme for Information Technology (NPfIT: www.connectingforhealth.nhs.uk). This assurance is a typically glib conclusion from people whose model of NHS activity is episodic surgery, as though illness could ever be wholly separated from the people that have it. Data will certainly have to be partitioned in various subsets, with different levels of access, an extremely difficult task which can succeed only if patients are supported by professional carers with sustained and intimate experience of their family circumstances.

[161] In US usage, EKG.

[162] In the US, by 2008, 60% of prostatectomies were being performed by 400 robots. In UK there were only nine, doing around 10% of operations. The surgeon sits at a console viewing a three-dimensional televised image, pushing buttons, while robot machinery operates through a keyhole incision. UK robotic operations now total over 20,000 a year, but this is said only to be the beginning (Mayor, S., 'Robotic prostatectomy transmitted live to engineers', *British Medical Journal* 2008; 336: 687).

[163] Bagge, E., Bjelle, A., Eden, S., Svanborg, A., 'Osteoarthritis in the elderly: clinical and radiological findings in 79 and 85 year olds', *Annals of the Rheumatic Diseases* 1991; 50: 535–9.

[164] Naylor, C.D., Williams, J.I., 'The Ontario panel on Hip and Knee Arthroplasty. Primary hip and knee replacement surgery: Ontario criteria for case selection and surgical priority', *Quality in Health Care* 1996; 5: 20–30.

[165] Frankel, S., Eachus, J., Pearson, N. et al, 'Population requirement for primary hip-replacement surgery: a cross-sectional study', *Lancet* 1999; 353: 1304–9. This paper was first submitted for publication in the *British Medical Journal*, but was turned down by its editorial committee on policy rather than scientific grounds – an interesting example of unconscious censorship (Frankel, S., Ebrahim, S., Smith, G.D., 'Limits to demand for health care: authors' reply', *British Medical Journal* 2001; 322: 735).

[166] To show the potential profit from hip replacement as a transnationally traded commodity, see the following data on different EU costs of hip replacement:

Country	Total cost	Medical staff	Other staff	Other costs
England	€3,628	€535	€123	€2,970
Netherlands	€4,779	€669	€378	€3,732
Denmark	€5,155	€202	€179	€4,774
France	€5,233	€728	€216	€4,279
Germany	€4,080	€596	€417	€3,067
Italy	€6,482	€229	€111	€6,142
Spain	€3,016	€400	€109	€2,507
Hungary	€968	€93	€191	€684
Poland	€1,561	€52	€10	€1,509

These costs are not adjusted for purchasing power parity, because this would conceal differences in staff pay which largely account for price differences (Health Benefits & Services Costs in Europe studies published as supplement to *Health Economics* 2008; 17: S8–S103). Members of the European Parliament are currently being pressed by EU administration to agree to free trade in surgical procedures between all member states, so that patients can be referred wherever they choose, with costs met by the health service in their own country. The financial consequences for competing English NHS hospital trusts, if workload becomes redistributed by price, are obvious.

Chapter Four

[1] In the more remote areas of developing economies, for example former Soviet Central Asia and many parts of Africa, real general practitioners existed at least up to the 1970s, tackling surgical and obstetric emergencies as well as the entire range of medical care at that time. To meet such doctors and listen to their stories is a chastening experience. In fully industrialised economies, we don't make doctors like that any more, but unless our economies completely fall apart, we no longer need them. The term 'general practitioner' has long been as obsolete as the British habit of describing what Americans call a doctor's office as a 'surgery'. It would be much better to call us community generalists.

[2] These patricians were an extremely small minority of a profession only precariously accepted as either learned or gentlemanly. As late as 1859, a surgeon major in the British Army who had won the Victoria Cross was excluded from a ball staged by Queen Victoria for holders of the VC, on the grounds that medical officers were not gentlemen. They were first accepted as royal guests only in 1891 (Cantlie, N., *A History of the Army Medical Department*, Vol 1, Edinburgh: Churchill Livingstone, 1974). In the US, social standing of doctors was even lower. When Charles W. Elliot became president of Harvard in 1869, anyone who chose could come off the street and enter

the Harvard School of Medicine. He proposed a number of reforms, among them lengthening the school year from four to nine months, and insisting that all candidates pass a written examination to get a degree. The dean of the medical school thought these 'improvements' would destroy the school. 'I had to tell him', the dean is reported to have said, 'that he knew nothing about the quality of Harvard medical students. More than half of them can barely write' (Brown, E.L., *Physicians and Medical Care*, New York: Russell Sage Foundation, 1937, pp 16–17). Doctors today rarely appreciate how recently they acquired the standing they now regard as natural.

[3] Two of these bone-setters from North Wales, Hugh Owen Thomas (1834–91) and his nephew Robert Jones (1858–1933), essentially founded orthopaedic surgery in the English-speaking world. By their clinical success they compelled the Royal College of Surgeons to accept them into the profession.

[4] There seem to have been such people in virtually all coal-mining communities, at least until the NHS started in 1948, dealing mainly with abscesses, soft-tissue injuries and back pain. They were usually repaid for their work in kind, together with the social recognition associated with effective care without pomposity. They were well remembered, particularly for occasions when their advice seemed wiser than that offered by doctors.

[5] When I entered practice in London in 1952, relations between GPs and midwives (state registered, well trained, and employed by London County Council) were often strained, sometimes openly hostile. Midwives were still seen as competing for trade. Cooperative relationships developed fairly fast once fees dropped out of the equation. Not so in the US, where in many states the medical profession managed to get midwifery made illegal. The consequence was more medical interventions in essentially normal deliveries, and therefore much higher maternal mortality rates (Loudon, I., 'On maternal and infant mortality 1900–1960', *Social History of Medicine* 1991; 4: 29–73).

[6] Reiser, S.J., *Medicine and the Reign of Technology*, London/New York: Cambridge University Press, 1978.

[7] These middle-class patients 'abusing' a facility intended for the poor seem to have gained very little. As a casualty officer at St Bartholomew's Hospital, London in 1879, Dr (later the poet) Robert Bridges saw 120 outpatients personally over a period of one hour and ten minutes – a rate of one patient every 35 seconds. At the same time, in another London hospital, three casualty officers dealt with 500 patients each morning (Rivington, W., *The Medical Profession*, Dublin, 1879).

[8] All this was much less true outside the cities and industrial areas of Britain, until GP-surgeons were expelled from cottage hospitals in 1948 and replaced by consultant specialists. In smaller market towns, GPs in the carriage trade usually had appointments at local cottage hospitals, funded by local charities and subscription, and did most of the routine surgery. They maintained a 'specialoid' role, similar to that long characteristic in the US, where the division between specialists and generalists has only recently approached the completeness reached long ago in Britain. For example, a report in 1974 from the American College of Cardiology found that though in Boston, Miami and New York there were more than 10 cardiologists per 100,000 population, 70% of these had office-based rather than hospital-based practices, and half were not specialist Board-certified (*Lancet* 1974; i: 617). These 'specialoids', pretenders to specialism without continuing hospital responsibility or higher qualifications, were gradually squeezed out by development of US medical care as a corporate business in the last third of the 20th century. The process was well described by Paul Starr (Starr, P., *The Social Transformation of American Medicine*, New York: Basic Books, 1983).

[9] Stevens, R., *Medical Practice in Modern England*, New Haven: Yale University Press, 1966.

[10] This was powerfully reinforced by the *Loi Debré*, which consigned the top 20% of achievers in final undergraduate examinations to become specialists, and left the rest to find whatever place they could in the hierarchy. Primary care is still thus classified by law as the lowest rung of responsibility and public respect.

[11] This view was embraced uncritically by Frank Honigsbaum in a book whose conclusions seem still widely accepted by historians (Honigsbaum, F., *The Division in British Medicine: A History of the Separation of General Practice from Hospital Care 1911–1968*, New York: St. Martin's Press, 1979). At a CIBA Foundation meeting where Honigsbaum presented his work, Sir George Godber was in the chair. After hearing the presentation, his first words were: 'I have never heard such rubbish before in all my life.' Sir George, by common consent probably the most innovative and powerful Chief Medical Officer the UK has ever had, was very aware of the rapid development of UK general practice as a new, population-based specialty, then well under way. Honigsbaum never understood this.

[12] This definition was provided in the *Red Book* setting out the terms of the GP contract. Apart from one major revision in 1967 to encourage group practice, better buildings and employment of office and nursing staff, the *Red Book* stood virtually unchanged from 1948 to 1988.

[13] Campbell, E.J.M., Scadding, J.G., Roberts, R.S., 'The concept of disease', *British Medical Journal* 1979; ii: 757–62.

[14] In recognisably modern form, this reification began in the 18th century, along with the Linnaean classification of animals and plants. It peaked towards the end of the 19th century, when rapid advances in bacteriology provided a model for diseases as predatory parasites, occupying their human hosts and thriving at their expense. This was reinforced and vulgarised by medical practice, and above all by medical trade. Merchants of health care needed ways to simplify the otherwise unmanageably complex health problems of real patients. They needed simplified language in which to explain and think about problems, and intelligible ways in which to justify their work and fees. This had negative as well as positive consequences. Medical students and nurses learned bestiaries of disease, as if they were independent species, stalking the jungle of life in search of prey, in which patients as people could be studied with veterinary objectivity, mundane vehicles of interesting diseases. Pharmacologists looked for magic bullets with which to shoot them, designed to hit the diseases but not the patients. They assumed that though each disease was different, each patient was more or less the same. Both sets of ideas worked better than any previous philosophy. Arsphenamine targeted syphilis in 1910, sulphonamides targeted streptococcal infections in 1935, penicillin targeted staphylococci and many other infections in 1943, and for the next couple of decades new breakthroughs in treatment of infectious disease became almost annual events. These were real breakthroughs, not media hyperbole. If you look at graphs of maternal mortality for the 1930s, with introduction of sulphonamide antibiotics in 1935 it falls off a cliff. Penicillin did the same for lobar pneumonia and syphilis, immediately after the Second World War.

[15] Marinker, M., 'On the boundary', *Journal of the Royal College of General Practitioners* 1973; 23: 83–94.

[16] Hart, J.T., 'Hidden agendas of earlier diagnosis', in Zander, L. (ed), *Change: The Challenge for the Future*, Royal College of General Practitioners Annual Symposium 1983, London: RCGP, 1984, pp 54–63.

[17] Riddle, M.C., 'A strategy for chronic disease', *Lancet* 1980; ii: 734–6.

[18] Greenfield, S., Kaplan, S.H., Ware, J.E., Yano, E.M., Frank, J.H., 'Patients' participation in medical care', *Journal of General Internal Medicine* 1988; 3: 448–57.

[19] Some of this expanding co-morbidity is an artefact of nomenclature. An increasing proportion of disorders still recognised and labelled as diseases are in fact particular forms of more general senescence. How many of these are found depends mainly on how hard they are looked for. Professional perceptions of patients' problems as single and simple, or multiple and complex, depends on how they think, the diagnostic labels in current use, and on available resources for diagnosis – above all, consultation time. In a review of the literature on co-morbidity in 1995, the proportion of consultations perceived as involving two or more different conditions varied from less than 1% to over 50% in different studies of different populations (van den Bos, G.A.M.,'The burden of chronic diseases in terms of disability, use of health care and healthy life expectancies', *European Journal of Public Health* 1995; 5: 29–34). Obviously these differences were mainly in perception, rather than in what was there to perceive. Typically, in a practice of 12,000 patients studied for six months, patients introduced at least one other problem in 43% of consultations for follow-up of chronic disease. Of these other problems 23% required new medication and 7% required referral to a specialist (Beale, N., Searle, M., Woodman, J.,'Use made by patients of chronic disease surveillance consultations in general practice', *British Journal of General Practice* 1992; 42: 51–3).

[20] One study of elderly US patients hospitalised for heart failure found 38% also had diabetes, 33% had chronic lung disease, 30% had atrial fibrillation and 18% had prior stroke. Such people are rarely included in clinical trials of new medications, but are in fact typical of those most likely to receive them (Heiat, A., Gross, C.P., Krumholz, A.M.,'Representation of the elderly, women and minorities in heart failure clinical trials', *Archives of Internal Medicine* 2002; 162: 1682–8).

[21] A study of women in Glasgow with breast cancer showed no social differences in quality of care or access, but much higher proportions with other major health problems, and also worse outcomes, for patients with the lowest incomes (Macleod, U., Ross, S., Twelves, C., George, W.D., Gillis, C., Watt, G.C.M.,'Primary and secondary care management of women with early breast cancer from affluent and deprived areas: retrospective review of hospital and general practice records', *British Medical Journal* 2000; 320: 1442–5).

[22] Smith, G.D., Hart, C., Blane, D., Hole, D.,'Adverse socioeconomic conditions in childhood and cause specific adult mortality: prospective observational study', *British Medical Journal* 1998; 316: 1631–5.

[23] Mold, J.W., Stein, J.F., 'The cascade effect in the clinical care of patients', *New England Journal of Medicine* 1986; 314: 512–4.

[24] Foucault, M., *The Birth of the Clinic: An Archaeology of Medical Perception*, London: Tavistock Publications, 1973.

[25] Most news reports of newly found risks of drinking alcohol or coffee, eating meat or fish, gaining or losing weight and so on, concern evidence of association, not evidence of causation. For example, we aim at 100% immunisation of children, starting around three months of age, but most cases of cerebral palsy are undetectable until later than this (because even anatomically, the central nervous system is not fully developed until after the first year of life). There is therefore a close association between immunisation and appearance of cerebral palsy soon after. Many parents understandably assume that this association is causal. Fears of this sort largely account for about 20% of parents failing to protect their children from infections such as measles, which is itself a known occasional cause of permanent brain damage. Almost every week we have reports of this sort, with no discussion either of the difference between associations and causes, or the difference between suggested causes supported or unsupported by any biologically plausible hypothesis. The problem arises partly from sensationalist editorial policies, but also from researchers desperate to attract funding by drawing public attention to their work.

[26] Kenneth Calman (Calman, K.C., 'Cancer: science and society and the communication of risk', *British Medical Journal* 1996; 313: 799–802) gave a vivid example of the difference between absolute and relative risks of death attributable to taking the low-dose oral contraceptive pill, or not taking it, or just being pregnant:

	Attributable deaths per million woman/years	
	Absolute risk	*Relative risk*
Non users	0.5	1.0
Low dose pill users	3.0	6.0
Pregnancy	6.0	12.0

Just going through a pregnancy raised the actual number of deaths attributable to pregnancy from one to 12 in two million non-pregnant, non-pill taking women over a period of one year, compared with women not pregnant, and not taking the pill. Using a low-dose oral contraceptive pill raised the actual number of deaths from one to three, compared with non-takers. Both pregnancy and pill-taking raised relative risk, but in both cases absolute risks were extremely small. As oral contraception was very efficient in preventing pregnancies, and pregnancies raised risks four times more than the pill, oral contraception seems to be a usually safer choice than either no contraception at all, or barrier methods such as condoms or diaphragms, with a much higher failure rate.

[27] McConnachie, A., Hunt, K., Emslie, K., Hart, C., Watt, G., '"Unwarranted survivals" and "anomalous deaths" from coronary heart disease: prospective study of general population', *British Medical Journal* 2001; 323: 1487–91.

[28] Richards, H.M., Reid, M.E., Watt, G.C.M., 'Socioeconomic variations in responses to chest pain: qualitative study', *British Medical Journal* 2002; 324: 1308–10.

[29] At 10kg or more over normal weight (optimal for health, not average: Body Mass Index 20–25), mortality from all causes is 46% above average at ages 15–34, 30% at 35–49, 18% at 50–65, but hardly at all above average over 65. There are many good reasons why older people should try to control their weight, but early mortality is not one of them. Body Mass Index (BMI) is metric weight, divided by the square of metric height.

[30] Whatever other factors may modify this process, obesity necessarily entails excess of energy intake over energy expenditure. Adult bodies need around 1,600 calories a day simply to sit down or lie in bed, rising to around 3,800 for a tall man doing really heavy work, like a coal miner or a lumberjack. In all fully industrialised countries, energy expenditures through physical work have fallen dramatically. This has happened obviously for working men, less obviously but probably equally for women still confined to domestic work, as both industrial and domestic work have shifted to machines. At the same time, actual hunger, as excess of energy expenditure over intake, has been virtually abolished, because of the much higher productivity of industrialised labour. In fully industrialised countries, poor people still have poor diets, but their deficiencies are in quality and variety, not calorie intakes. In both Britain and North America, obesity has become the most visible outward sign of social class. So far, at least, social class differences in obesity in Britain seem less than in the US. The Scottish Public Health Observatory reports obesity (BMI = 30+) in 19.6% of adult men in the richest fifth of all men, compared with 25.5% of the poorest fifth. The social gradient is much steeper for women: 21% of the richest fifth, compared with 32.1% of the poorest (www.scotpho.org. uk/home/Clinicalriskfactors/Obesity/obesitydata/obesity_deprivation.asp, accessed 13 February 2009).

[31] A simple concept, still underused: people with central obesity have a belly circumference greater than their hip circumference. This simple measurement has greater predictive power than BMI.

[32] Reaven, G.M.,'Role of insulin resistance in human disease', Banting lecture 1988, *Diabetes* 1988; 37: 1595–1607, and Eckel, R.H., Grundy, S.M., Mer, P.Z., 'The metabolic syndrome', *Lancet* 2005; 365: 1415–28.

[33] Cochrane, A.L.,'Science and syndromes', *Postgraduate Medical Journal* 1965; 41: 440–2.

[34] The phrase comes from an influential letter by Sir Clifford Albutt to *The Times* (Albutt, T.C., 'The Act and the future of medicine', *The Times*, 3 January 1912), predicting the end of good clinical medicine among general practitioners if Lloyd George's Insurance Act was applied. In fact, good clinical medicine in industrial practice had scarcely begun, and the Act was an important step towards making it possible to achieve 36 years later. However, Albutt's pessimistic assessment seemed fully confirmed 40 years later by Joseph Collings' survey of the state of general practice into which the NHS was born in 1948 (Collings, J.S., 'General practice in England today', *Lancet* 1950; i: 555–85). Interestingly, similar studies around the same time showed similar results in the US (Peterson, O.L., Andrews, L.P., Spain, R.S., Greenberg, B.G., 'An analytical study of North Carolina general practice, 1953–1954', *Journal of Medical Education* 1956; 31(12): part 2, p 1) and in Canada (Clute, K.F., *The General Practitioner*, Toronto: University of Toronto Press, 1963).

[35] Even today, long after the necessity of skilled generalists to lead primary care was recognised by all orthodox rhetoric, only 10% of US medical graduates enter primary care residency programmes. The other 90% train as specialists. Only about 30% of US doctors now in practice are in any kind of primary care, even on the loosest possible definition, compared with about 50% in the UK (on a similar definition) and most other EU countries.

[36] One of the first British GPs to collect data systematically from his practice, John Fry, coined a useful term for doctors in the US who claimed to have specialist skills, but had no substantial base in any hospital department. He called them 'specialoids' (Fry, J., *Medicine in Three Societies: A Comparison of Medical Care in the USSR, the US and UK*, Aylesbury: MTP, 1969). They were not eliminated from operative surgery until the 1980s. Before then US operative mortality was higher in the US as a whole than in the NHS, though not in centres of excellence for those who could afford to reach them.

[37] British Medical Association, *Charter for the Family Doctor Service*, London: BMA, 1965.

[38] This was developed in a classic paper by John Horder, well worth reading today: Horder, J.P., 'Physicians and family doctors: a new relationship', *Journal of the Royal College of General Practitioners* 1977; 27: 391–7 (published simultaneously in *Journal of the Royal College of Physicians of London*).

[39] The Charter reimbursed 70% of staff wages up to a maximum of two whole-time-equivalent staff per GP, with the GPs paying for the other 30%. It reimbursed 100% of the cost of premises, and allowed GPs to retain the full value of any consequent capital appreciation. Until the business crash of 2007–08, huge sums consequently accrued to GPs on retirement, in areas where property values were rising. Where they were falling, as in most industrial and all post-industrial areas, there was no such incentive for investment in buildings. Bosanquet and Leese (Leese, B., Bosanquet, N., 'Family doctors: their choice of practice strategy', *British Medical Journal* 1986; 293: 667–70) found that on five indicators of improvement (employment of practice nurse, improved or purpose-built premises, participation in training, possession of ECG, follow-up clinics), 32% of practices (high investors) accounted for 71% of positive scores. Nearly all the high-investing practices were in affluent areas. Looking at a northern coal-mining area between 1986 and 1992, the same authors found more practices in affluent expanding districts than in poorer declining districts had invested in premises and staff, and provided more services. Their costs were higher, and so were their incomes. However, practices in poorer districts had made a larger mean absolute increase in investment, resulting in an overall reduction in polarisation of standards (Leese, B., Bosanquet, N., 'Family doctors and change in practice strategy since 1986', *British Medical Journal* 1995; 310: 705–8). It was a mixed picture, but suggested that public investment through the pockets of GPs as independent contractors was less efficient than direct investment by the state in what people need, though that is my conclusion, not that of these authors.

[40] According to Dr Gerard Vaughan, Conservative Minister for Health in 1985, costs to taxpayers per consultation were then as follows:

At hospital outpatient departments	£50.00
At GP medical centres	£5.00

At first sight, a patient consulting a GP seemed to cost ten times less than a patient seeing any hospital specialist, however junior. A consultation with a retail pharmacist cost government nothing at all.

[41] Rivett, G., *From Cradle to Grave: Fifty Years of the NHS*, London: King's Fund, 1998, p 411. A much more influential model was developed by Dr Geoff Marsh, working in Teesside, referred to later in this chapter.

[42] Clarke, K., 'Working for patients: medical education, research and health', Speech by Secretary of State to medical profession, 10 July 1989, official press release.

[43] A second, back-up clutch system was provided by hospital accident and emergency (A&E) departments, providing episodic patch-up care for patients either unable to access primary care or without confidence in it. In decaying urban centres this was a major gap in the NHS care system, causing serious concern in the 1980s, when it was rightly regarded as a sensitive indicator of primary care performance. Self-referrals to A&E departments are now expanding relentlessly, along with an increasing diversity of walk-in clinics and phone-in advice centres, in line with the consumerist policies favoured by both Conservative and New Labour governments, regardless of the damage this does to continuity, or of the inefficiencies inherent in caring for people you do not already know. When I worked in the South Wales valleys, most GPs still did most of their own suturing for minor injuries. As in other areas far from the nearest hospital, direct self-referral to A&E was negligible in the Glyncorrwg practice, so our workload data were a dependable measure of the volume of primary care in our locality.

[44] As far back as hospitals have existed, their A&E departments (or equivalent casualty and outpatient departments) have always been used more by poor people. Socio-economic factors are strongly associated with emergency admission rates, but not with elective admission rates through GP referral (Reid, F.D.A., Cook, D.G., Majeed, A., 'Explaining variation in hospital admission rates between general practices: cross sectional study', *British Medical Journal* 1999; 319: 98–103). Countries with poorly developed or socially less accessible primary care systems have consequently inflated A&E departments. For example, in 2004, 30% of the Los Angeles population was uninsured, and depended on what remained of its public hospital care system to provide emergency care. This system was itself in fiscal crisis, facing a projected loss of over $700m between 2003 and 2005. Owing to rapid expansion of for-profit private hospitals, West Coast public hospitals had shrunk to only 6% of total hospital facilities, but provided 55% of care for the uninsured, who accounted for 35% of their admissions and 55% of their outpatient visits (Berliner, H.S., 'The crisis of the Los Angeles County Public Hospital system: a harbinger for the nation', *International Journal of Health Services* 2004; 34: 313–22).

[45] Though the NHS presents no legal or economic barriers to access, there can be many administrative barriers in areas of social deprivation and high primary care workload. About half the people sent to prison in Britain are not registered with a GP, often reflecting drug dependence, psychotic mental illness, or both. Homeless people, now a rapidly rising group, are a similar case, so are people with learning difficulties, street sex workers, asylum seekers and refugees, people with chronic psychotic mental illness, and Romany travellers. Providing they have access to friendly care, most of these patients are high users with complex needs, so, as self-employed contractors, many GPs do their best to avoid them. Less businesslike GPs, who believe that these people need and benefit from care more than any other social group, end up with a disproportionate number of such patients, in many cases enough to make ordinary practice impossible. The current solution is to create specialised practices in urban areas with a high concentration of such people, and more recently to exclude asylum seekers and illegal immigrants from NHS care (Taylor, K., 'Asylum seekers, refugees, and the politics of access to health care: a UK perspective', *British Journal of General Practice* 2009; 59: 765–72). Specialised practices have been provided, at least for homeless people, in about two-thirds of Primary Care Trust districts in England, but these services remain very incomplete. Patient registration is essential for effective forward planning and assessment of results, but many of these special schemes still deliberately exclude registration, because of perverse disincentives related to funding either by the NHS or by local government.

[46] Loudon, I., 'The principle of referral: the gatekeeping role of the GP', *British Journal of General Practice* 2008; 58: 128–30.

[47] Impressed by the effect of NHS gatekeeping on costs, many other European countries later adopted this policy. A study comparing those with and without a gatekeeping referral system showed that GPs with a gatekeeper responsibility tended to function more effectively in all dimensions (Boerma, W.G., van der Zee, J., Fleming, D.M., 'Service profiles of general practitioners in Europe', *British Journal of General Practice* 1997; 47: 481–6).

[48] For definition and origin of the term 'specialoid', see notes 8 and 36 above. Taylor, T.R., 'Pity the poor gatekeeper: a transatlantic perspective on cost containment in clinical practice', *British Medical Journal* 1989; 299: 1323–5.

[49] That such investment was justified is supported by US experience. Across the US mortality fell by 14.4 deaths per 100,000 people during an 11-year period in areas where the number of primary care doctors rose by one per 10,000 people. The effect was greatest on black mortality – that is, on those with highest health care needs (Shi, L., Macinko, J., Starfield, B., Politzer, R.,

Xu, J., 'Primary care, race and mortality in US states', *Social Science & Medicine* 2005; 61: 65–75).

[50] Gillam, S., 'Rising hospital admissions: can the tide be stemmed?', *British Medical Journal* 2010; 340: 275–6. Health care consultants Caspe Healthcare Knowledge Systems found that NHS hospital admissions rose by 6% annually from 2007 to 2009, compared with 4.6% in the preceding three years, 'threatening bankruptcy' for the service. Steve Gillam, at the Cambridge Institute of Public Health, points out that despite an expected shortfall of £8.4bn in NHS funding since the banking crisis, 'A multitude of new access routes ... have eroded the gatekeeping function of GPs', and that development of polyclinics 'in process if not in structure – is compromising continuity of care and reducing access to just those practitioners who may be able to contain and manage comorbidities in the community'.

[51] Fry, J., *Medicine in Three Societies: A Comparison of Medical Care in the USSR, USA and UK*, Aylesbury: MTP, 1969.

[52] Hayes, T.M., Harries, J., 'Randomized controlled trial of routine hospital clinic care versus routine general practice care for type II diabetes', *British Medical Journal* 1984; 289: 728–30.

[53] Darzi, A., *High Quality Care for All: NHS Next Stage Review Final Report*, London: Department of Health, 2008. The polyclinic idea seemed to appeal to specialists, and was endorsed with uncritical enthusiasm by the editor of the *Lancet*, despite the journal's long-standing hostility to both New Labour and Conservative policies for the NHS: 'For doctors, it feels that at long last, their call for clinical leadership in policy making has been heeded. It is now up to the profession to take this exceptional opportunity and make it work for patients' (Horton, R., 'The Darzi vision: quality, engagement and professionalism', *Lancet* 2008; 372: 1–2). After several polyclinics had been built in London and a few other cities, mostly organised and staffed by corporate for-profit providers but sometimes by consortia of GPs trying to keep corporate competitors off their turf, Lord Darzi resigned in 2009, returning to his clinical interests as a colorectal surgeon and oncologist. When his venture first began, he seems to have believed that all patients needed was to have direct access to specialists by self-referral, as in France and several other EU countries, and as many journalists and politicians already do, bypassing the NHS whenever they can afford it. In an interview with the *Guardian*, 29 December 2007, Lord Darzi explained that the essential problem with the NHS was not a lack of funding or expertise, but the way different parts connect. Patients in search of

treatment must navigate a maze – and may not end up at the door of those best equipped to treat them:

> Take the example of a patient in London who develops abdominal pain in the evening; they tolerate the pain overnight, then they go to see their GP, who says they need to see a consultant … What follows is a time-consuming and costly back-and-forth: to the consultant, to the hospital for an ultrasound scan, to the consultant to discuss the results, to the hospital for a surgery pre-assessment, to the hospital again for an operation, back to their GP with a wound problem … if you did your shopping this way … If Tesco provided you with that service, you wouldn't go there. If you booked your flights that way you'd be all over the place.

By the time Darzi resigned, he seems to have recognised the logistic consequences of sending everyone with acute abdominal pain straight to a specialist abdominal surgeon. Dr Ian Gibson, an MP, gave Parliament an excellent example of where direct self-referral to specialists may lead, on 8 June 2009. A patient presented with abdominal pain and asked for a scan. His father had just died from stomach cancer. He probably had nothing wrong with his stomach, but had previously undetected severe hypertension 224/124, diabetes, probable angina and early kidney failure. He was smoking 40 cigarettes a day, was depressed, and was drinking excess alcohol. What he wanted was a scan, but what he needed was generalist care – to be looked after.

[54] By September 2008, strongly encouraged by government, over 3,600 NHS patients per month were choosing to have planned surgery in a private rather than NHS hospital, but paid for by the NHS. This was still less than 1% of the total NHS elective case-load in England (Kmietowicz, Z., 'Patients take £7.6m a month out of NHS as they choose and book private sector treatment', *British Medical Journal* 2008; 337: 1372–3). Responding to public disquiet, then Health Minister Alan Johnson announced a planned reduction of private sector involvement in the NHS by two-thirds. What under Prime Minister Tony Blair was first meant to entail about £6bn of NHS business over five years was to be reduced to around £2.5bn. The Minister admitted that almost £93m had already been spent on procurement, and there were potentially tens of millions of pounds still to be paid out for cancellation of contracts (Timmins, N., 'Return to the true path?', *British Medical Journal* 2007; 335: 1066–7). After more public disquiet, and with many commercial providers disappointed by their profits, in October 2009 another Health Minister, Andy Burnham, announced a return to New Labour's initial promise to make existing NHS institutions the preferred providers for all care, and as I write in March 2010,

that remains government policy – until the next change. This step back from *de facto* preference for commercial providers was instantly denounced by NHS Partners Network, their trade body, as 'completely irresponsible' (Timmins, N., 'NHS will now be "preferred provider" of care, says Burnham', *British Medical Journal* 2009; 339: 827). Whatever ministers may say, probably any UK government, New Labour or Conservative, will still try to shift responsibility from the state to private providers, but so long as NHS hospitals still exist, people will probably continue to vote with their feet. The most serious and lasting damage to the NHS, and to staff morale and therefore to productivity, has not been the percentage of NHS work shifted to private providers, but the business culture pervading NHS management and imposed on all activities, irrelevant to and impeding rational clinical decisions.

[55] Some expert observers seem to think primary generalists may continue to develop care, but outside the NHS. 'If … [conflicts between professionals and politicians, within unchanged public health services, are resolved only partially and piecemeal, then] … privatisation of primary care would appear to be a solution, to retain maximal free practice for those who can pay directly, whilst allowing maximal industrialisation for others who cannot' (Iliffe, S., 'From general practice to primary care: the industrialisation of family medicine in Britain', *Journal of Public Health Policy* 2002; 23: 33–43).

[56] Marsh, G.N., Kaim-Caudle, P., *Team Care in General Practice*, London: Croom Helm, 1976. He showed good evidence that the team care he organised had favourable selective effects on the health of a poor Teesside community (Marsh, G., 'Clinical medicine and the health divide', *Journal of the Royal College of General Practitioners* 1988; 38: 5–9, and Marsh, G.N., Channing, D.M., 'Comparison in use of health services between a deprived and an endowed community', *Archives of Disease in Childhood* 1987; 62: 392–6).

[57] At least as a mode of thought among managers and policy-formers, standardisation of care has already reached alarming proportions, apparently remote from mundane experience of either patients or staff in UK primary care. For example, in San Francisco, workers at the University of California carried out a randomised trial of an automated telephone for people wanting advice on managing their diabetes (Handley, M.A., Shumway, M., Schillinger, D., 'Cost-effectiveness of automated telephone self-management support with nurse care management among patients with diabetes', *Annals of Family Medicine* 2008; 6: 512–8). As I write in March 2010, automated telephone responses, on every subject from buying a railway ticket to how to unfreeze your computer screen, evoke intense irritation or hostility from most people most of the time. Most people still feel elated when they at last hear a human

voice that listens to them, speaks to them in their own language, from somebody who sounds as though they share some of their own experience. However, where the only human voices still accessible have no time to waste on simple frailties, people may be grateful for any help they can get, from machines which have more time than human beings, may even speak many languages, and transmit a message devised by consensus experts. This study showed marginal benefits, in a society which has apparently given up trying not to become a machine. According to received wisdom, if cost-benefit is proved, this has to be the way forward. Reviews of this subject in the UK, though more cautious, offer no substantial resistance to this trend (Croft, P., Porcheret, M., 'Standardised consultations in primary care: are beneficial for some conditions, but should their extent be limited?', *British Medical Journal* 2009; 338: 668–9). To break out of the machine and restore a human face requires courage and imagination.

[58] Prof Chris Ham, an influential health policy expert who led the marketisation of the NHS but retained a reputation for some scepticism, suggested in 1996 that GPs could work more cost-effectively with larger patient lists (Ham, C., 'The NHS could benefit from fewer GPs and more nurses', *General Practitioner*, 9 August 1996). At that time, virtually everyone else still believed that most GPs had to look after too many patients. The average list size was then about 1,800 people of all ages, and the BMA's optimal recommended size was about 1,500. 'One model for the future', Ham wrote, could be the 'GP as specialist in family medicine. Triage would be carried out by qualified nurses and doctors would be called on only when needed.' He thought the NHS could then be run with half as many GPs. He, and thousands of others like him who think of NHS patients as a group that never includes themselves, seems oblivious of the judgements described in Chapter Three, which have to be made by whoever has responsibility for first encounters.

[59] More than 30 years ago, Marshall Marinker dared to admit that most urban families were served by different GPs, that most GPs knew little about many of the families they served, and that many patients benefited by seeing a GP they did not know, or actually sought care from someone to whom they were virtually anonymous (Marinker, M., 'The myth of family medicine', *World Medicine* 16 June 1976: 17–19). Family medicine, in the practical sense that, for example, written records for the whole household were filed together so that the problems of one family member could be easily considered in their full family context, was a reality, but scarce. Primary care is a much larger and more objective category, which makes no claims or assumptions about leadership, motivation, or how it is organised.

[60] Until 1966, these nurses worked almost completely independently from GPs. Before the NHS, relations between urban GPs and community nurses were often poor and sometimes hostile, because fee-earning GPs saw them as potential competitors. This was especially true of midwives, seen as competitors for trade, and health visitors, seen as competitors for authority. In the countryside relations were more human and very much better. Potentially serious divisions persist today, between GPs as employers of practice nurses and care assistants, and nursing staff employed by their own NHS authorities. As before, these divisions tend to be overlooked or ignored by administrators, but they can lead to serious inefficiency and unhappiness. With a single public employer they could probably be eliminated.

[61] Like every other progressive development in primary care, this was opposed by the New Labour government's policies (Heath, I., 'The perversion of choice', *British Medical Journal* 2009; 339: 1005). Health Minister Andy Burnham denounced GPs who tried to set boundaries for recruitment of patients, so that they served a geographically defined community. In a policy speech he announced government's intention to promote patient choice in primary care, as it had already done for specialist referral, so that patients may register with any GP willing to accept them, no matter how remote from where they live, opening the prospect of some GPs promoting themselves nationally, employing assistants to cope with whatever additional workload (and income) this may generate. The Conservative shadow minister said that, though welcome, this step was coming too late, so it seems this policy is set to continue.

[62] Drennan, V., Davis, K., *Trends over Ten Years in the Primary Care and Community Nurse Workforce in England*, London: University of London, St Georges, 2008.

[63] According to a Department of Health review published in July 2006 (*Regulation of the Non-Medical Healthcare Professions*), health care assistants (HCAs) were still unregulated and unregistered, and had no national minimum entry requirements, and so far as I can make out, this has not changed. According to the Royal College of Nursing, though numbers were growing rapidly, the Department of Health did not know how many were working in the NHS. According to data from Manchester University in 2002, HCAs in primary care in that region were doing 33% of all measurement interventions, and 28% of preventive or treatment interventions.

[64] US medical students, through their Pharmfree campaign, and New York doctors through No Free Lunch ('Just say no to drug reps') have led the way to greater professional self-respect (Moynihan, R., 'Who pays

for the pizza? Redefining the relationships between doctors and drug companies. 1: Entanglement', *British Medical Journal* 2003; 326: 1189–92; '2: Disentanglement', *British Medical Journal* 2003; 326: 1193–6). GPs can keep themselves better informed by reading their professional journals than by giving scarce time to professional brain washers, but, in the UK at least, their professional organisations set no example.Virtually all postgraduate educational activities still get as much support as they can from commercial sponsors, and all pay the price. In 2009 the State of Vermont made it illegal for companies dealing in pharmaceuticals or treatment devices to make gifts to doctors or any other health care professionals or institutions (*New England Journal of Medicine* 2009; 361: 8–9). The world did not come to an end.

[65] In 2002, 10 US pharmaceutical companies listed by *Fortune* had total combined international sales of $217bn (£106.6bn). Of this sum, 14% was spent on research and development, and 31% on marketing and administration. Roughly half of all pharmaceuticals are now 'me too' variants (Goldacre, B., 'Bad science: evil ways of drug companies', *Guardian*, 8 August 2007). I have no comparable figures for the UK industry. All pharmaceutical companies are extremely conscious of their poor public image, and do their best to conceal essentially marketing developments (consumer research, packaging, presentation and design of products that are irrelevant to their efficacy) in their research budgets.

[66] MORI poll reported in *bmaNews*, 12 March 2005.

[67] Chest clinics and venereal disease clinics were left with local government from 1948 until 1974, and so were not then a part of the NHS. By the time public health functions were removed from local government and absorbed into the NHS, tuberculosis seemed largely overcome and syphilis seemed close to extinction. This whole experience now seems almost forgotten.

[68] Control of HIV through sexually transmitted disease clinics obviously provides a more recent example of all this, but as HIV and AIDS had not arrived in my community before I retired, I have no experience of how it was coped with.

[69] In the Glyncorrwg centre, by the 1980s we were running weekly evening follow-up clinics for high blood pressure and diabetes, and monthly clinics for schizophrenia. These were a considerable burden on staff, all of whom needed to get back to their families, so it was no small thing to add to this another 10 minutes or so to discuss why people had not come, what should be done about them, and who should have responsibility for doing it. Proactive

follow-up of this kind is the most visible difference between demand-led care and anticipatory care. It was extremely effective, particularly for people with schizophrenia treated with monthly depot injections of antipsychotic drugs. When these patients did not attend, they were visited at home by a doctor who knew them well enough to restore trust and persuade them to resume treatment. In our area, psychiatrists in those days were unfortunately not willing to allow any of their community nursing staff to help us, or even to discuss policies for shared care.

[70] The conventional way to refer to more comprehensive and inclusive judgements is to describe such approaches as holistic. It has become extremely popular among liberally inclined healthcare workers of all kinds, but I have not found it useful. The central idea of holism is that any evolved whole is greater than the sum of its parts, and that no single thing can be fully understood in isolation from its extended context. Though this is obviously true, it does nothing to get us beyond banal observation. Holism originated as a quasi-philosophy advanced by Jan Smuts in 1926, in his book *Holism and Evolution*. Known in South Africa as Janni the fox, Smuts managed in a single life to combine three large reputations – as a leader of the Boers' guerilla resistance to the English, as senior statesman and recurrent Prime Minister of the Union of South Africa and champion of the British Empire, and as a philosopher. To achieve this on the basis of white supremacy in a country where people of European descent were outnumbered eight to one by people of African descent, a supremacy he never questioned, required a philosophy fitted for contemplation of reality rather than struggle to change it. So it has been for holism, a soapy term which evades necessary conflict.

[71] Starfield, B., 'Primary and specialty care interfaces: the imperative of disease continuity', *British Journal of General Practice* 2003; 53: 723–9.

[72] The story of the Quality and Outcomes Framework (QOF) shows the extent to which highly placed experts have always underestimated the work of lowly placed workers in primary care. Projected costings assumed that few practices would reach more than 80% of targets for recorded data, and most would fall far short of this. In fact, even in the first year (2004–05), most practices were reaching over 90% of their targets, so they had to be paid for this, though such sums had not been anticipated or budgeted. Neither government nor news media have ever acknowledged this gross underestimation both of what GPs and their staffs were already doing, and how quickly they adapted this to the new shape of demands. The QOF is an immense achievement, codifying virtually every aspect of the necessary work of primary care in all fields, not just clinical activities, but all aspects of practice organisation,

recording, relationships with patients and populations, educational work, and so on, even including arrangements for patients and their organisations to suggest additional features in future. Its weaknesses lie in the extent to which it may encourage bureaucracy, gaming and over-management, and deter imagination and innovation beyond its defined curriculum.

[73] Davidoff, F., Haynes, R.B., Sackett, D., Smith, R., 'Evidence Based Medicine. A new journal to help doctors identify the information they need', *British Medical Journal* 1995; 310: 1085–6.

[74] Guthrie, C., 'Prevention and cure of type 2 diabetes. Let's move upstream from obesogenic environments please', *British Medical Journal* 2002; 325: 965.

[75] Guthrie, C., Letter to *British Medical Journal* 2001; 323: 63–4.

[76] *Road Traffic and Health*, London: BMA, 1997.

[77] This includes the New Labour government brought to power in 1997 on a pledge, among other things, to reverse this policy. Since 1997, at least 187 more school and local playing fields have been sold (James Chapman, *Daily Mail* website, 30 March 2008).

[78] Welsh Assembly policy may have had a surprisingly large impact in a relatively short time. Surveys of 4,000 11- to 18-year-olds by the British Market Research Bureau every six months over the past 15 years show a rapid decline in weekly swimming in England, from 25% in 1993 to 12% in 2008. There was a decline with age, from 14% of 11- to 15-year-olds to 9% of 16- to 18-year-olds. The highest levels of swimming were in Wales, where 25% of 11- to 15-year-olds still swim every week, compared with 10% in London, Yorkshire, Humberside and the North of England.

[79] It took several decades for the pioneering work of Jerry Morris on the relation of physical inactivity on coronary heart disease even to begin to influence medical practice (Morris, J.N., Chave, S.P.W., Adam, C., Sirey, C., Epstein, L., Sheehan, D.J., 'Vigorous exercise in leisure time and the incidence of coronary heart disease', *Lancet* 1973; i: 333–9). This was partly because how people actually live their real lives, outside an experimental setting, was an extremely difficult research subject, from which it was almost impossible to produce data so undeniably conclusive as dieting studies.

[80] In Glyncorrwg, local initiatives of this sort, which our staff helped to lead, eventually got us three miles of cycle track, three fishing ponds, and a mountain

biking centre now listed as world ninth for popularity with aficionados. Our community still has its own football and rugby teams, playing on their own public fields, even though we have only about 500 families in the community, and almost all the shops and many houses are boarded up.

[81] In my experience in a developed democracy, it is necessary only once to organise a busload of patients to lobby local authorities for an obviously necessary and urgent material change, for every subsequent threat to be taken seriously. From then on, the threat rarely needs to be implemented.

Chapter Five

[1] An estimated 40% of the world population has no access to a toilet or latrine. Ninety per cent of the world's sewage is discharged to soil, sea or fresh water (George, R., *The Big Necessity: The Unmentionable World of Human Waste and Why it Matters*, New York: Holt Paperbacks, 2009).

[2] Petty was the founding father of modern economics and public health, a genius who deserves to be better known. There is an adequate account of his work in George Rosen's *History of Public Health* (New York: MD Publications, 1958; expanded edition: Baltimore, MD: Johns Hopkins University Press, 1993), but the best of all short accounts is in A.V. Anikin's *A Science in its Youth: Pre-Marxian Political Economy* (Moscow: Progress Publishers, 1975).

[3] Ringen, K., 'Edwin Chadwick, the market ideology, and sanitary reform: on the nature of the 19th century public health movement', *International Journal of Health Services* 1979; 9: 107–20.

[4] The Elizabethan Poor Law established Boards of Guardians, whose members were appointed from local landowners and gentry. In one form or another, they were responsible for the care of the indigent right up to 1948.

[5] The most outstanding example was Middlesex County Council, which developed many excellent hospitals on the outskirts of London. Most people expected these to become the model for the NHS, but Bevan was aware of extreme differences in political maturity between different areas of the UK. Local government control would have precluded a truly national NHS. He was also aware of the price he paid: local democratic control of hospital administration was postponed – he thought for only a few years; in fact, indefinitely.

[6] A notable example of this has been consistent campaigning by the Royal College of Physicians and the BMA, far in advance of government, for legislative action against the promotion of nicotine and alcohol, against powerful resistance from commercial interests.

[7] In Manchester, Britain's first centre of mass industrialisation, by the middle of the 19th century roughly two-thirds of all deaths had received prior medical attention of some kind, a rough indicator of the extent to which this had become regarded as important either for survival, or at least for a dignified death (Evidence of Dr John Leigh, physician to the Manchester Union and Registrar of Births and Deaths, *Parliamentary Papers, Report from the Select Committee on Medical Relief*, Shannon: Irish University Press, 1854. Quoted by Bloor, D.U., 'The union doctor', *Journal of the Royal College of General Practitioners* 1980; 30: 358–64).

[8] Doctors with least training were glad to serve poor areas in any paid capacity, but had virtually no time or other resources to apply medical science as it was beginning to be understood in the most progressive teaching hospitals. George Bernard Shaw, who knew better than most the realities of care for the poor from experience as an elected member of the St Pancras Board of Guardians, provided a classic description in his preface to *The Doctor's Dilemma* (London: John Constable, 1907):

> The only way [the GP serving the poor] can preserve his self respect is by forgetting all he ever learnt of science, and clinging to such help as he can give without cost merely by being less ignorant and more accustomed to sick beds than his patients. Finally he acquires a certain skill at nursing cases under poverty-stricken domestic conditions, just as women who have been trained as domestic servants in some huge institution with lifts, vacuum cleaners, electric lighting, steam heating and machinery that turns the kitchen into a laboratory and engine-house combined, manage, when they are sent out into the world to drudge as general servants, to pick up their business in a new way, learning the slatternly habits and wretched makeshifts of homes where even bundles of kindling wood are luxuries to be anxiously economised.

[9] Sale or purchase of goodwill in general medical practice was made illegal throughout the UK by the NHS Act in 1948, with compensation to GPs already in practice. It was hoped that new doctors would be selected as partners by old doctors according to their skills, rather than their capital. The law was strictly enforced; retiring doctors who inflated the price of their house as a way of making incoming doctors pay for goodwill in attractive areas were

liable to get caught by the Medical Practices Committee. The GPs' Charter of 1966 provided state funding for primary care buildings, but left ownership in the hands of GPs. In most cities, this led to huge capital appreciation, so that old doctors gained large additions to their already generous pensions, and new doctors found they might have to pay hundreds of thousands of pounds to enter a partnership. In 2004, the UK New Labour government completed destruction of this part of the 1948 Act by abolishing the Medical Practices Committee (which had controlled distribution of GPs to encourage them to go to areas with a shortage of doctors, and prevent them going to areas of surplus). Blair's government made sale of goodwill legal again. An obvious consequence was to make it easier for transnational corporate providers to take over the care of large populations, with minimal local opposition from established GPs. A less obvious, but probably intended, effect was to strengthen established GPs' status as independent contractors, quasi-private owners of a public service.

[10] Because other European countries were not yet fully industrialised, none of them developed so simple a system. Germany in particular, generally regarded as the pioneer of socially organised primary care, developed a system owing much more to the traditions of the GP carriage trade, with fees for items of service and co-payments from patients within a personal insurance system, rather than wholly free access in a tax-based system. Both British and German GPs had a fierce sense of personal ownership of their fiefdoms in primary care, but flat-rate capitation on the one hand and fees-for-service on the other led to profoundly different medical cultures. For this and many other reasons, France and Germany have remained bastions of liberal free trade in primary care, while Holland, Scandinavia and the Mediterranean countries came closer to the British model.

[11] In late 19th- and early 20th-century society, minimum professional income meant enough to wear a suit, collar and tie, keep a bicycle or horse and trap (or after the First World War, a car), a wife, one or possibly two live-in servants, a varying but usually large number of children, and private education for them, usually with priority for boys. Doctors had relatively low social status until science began to give them some credibility. When a colleague who worked in the most prestigious practice in Port Talbot was called in the 1930s to the local mansion, he was only allowed to enter through the tradesmen's entrance. When the Royal Physician, Lord Horder, arrived by train from London to confirm the diagnosis made by this mere GP, he was allowed in through the front door. The NHS virtually eliminated poor doctors, but many of them still liked to imagine better days when they had been more respected and appreciated.

[12] In 1896 the *Lancet* sent a correspondent around Britain to report on the terms and conditions of service of doctors serving industrial workers and their families, resulting in publication of a classic, 'The Battle of the Clubs'. In Southampton the *Lancet* correspondent found about a quarter of the population registered in Club schemes, from which doctors earned 4 shillings a head annually for unlimited access to medical advice and medicines. The Southampton Board of Guardians contracted medical care for its 2,000 indigent poor for an annual fee of £5 a head. In 1893 these 2,000 had 500 medical visits at 2½ pence (contemporary coinage) per visit. In Portsmouth, the Medical Benefit Society contracted for unlimited access to advice and medicine for dockyard workers and their families for a weekly fee of ½ pence a head. One GP contracted to this scheme kept a ledger showing 1,958 home visits and 4,650 office consultations for fees totalling £38 11s 1d, an average of 1.4 pence per consultation. For larger specific items of service there were higher scales.

To understand these sums one needs to know something of contemporary prices and earnings. From 1883 to 1913 the value of money stayed almost unchanged. The purchasing power of £1 in 1883 fell over the next 100 years to 3½ (new decimal) pence by 1983, 3.5% of its original value. It may be more meaningful to look at a few prices around 1905. A new brick-built terrace house cost about £150, or £100 if built in stone. Adult miners' earnings by 1914 averaged around £145 a year, with large differences between younger, fitter men able to hew high tonnage from the coalface, and less fit or older men working on transport, timbering, repairing and the many other skills needed to keep a mine in production. Hewers worked underground for an eight-hour day, six days a week, cutting and loading coal entirely by hand. Boys of 14 started at 60 old pence a week, £31 a year. All this compared well with £15 a year for a six-and-a-half-day week for girls forced by absence of local paid work into exile in London as live-in housemaids. It compared badly with economist Alfred Marshall's estimate of £500 a year as a reasonable income for a university professor, or the £1,000 a year inherited by Beatrice Webb on her marriage to Sydney, to support their lifelong enterprise as theorists for mainstream English social democracy (Harrison, R.J., *The Life and Times of Sidney and Beatrice Webb: 1858–1905, the Formative Years*, London: Macmillan Press, 2000). Coal miners were never rich, but they were not too poor to afford subscriptions of around 6 old pence (£0.025) each week for their Medical Aid Schemes.

[13] Williams, C., *Democratic Rhondda: Politics and Society 1885–1951*, Cardiff: University of Wales Press, 1996. The best way I know to understand these ideas in contemporary terms is to read Robert Blatchford's *Merrie England*, first published in 1893, but reprinted in facsimile, with an excellent new foreword,

by Journeyman Press in 1976. The first edition sold 25,000 copies, leading to a reprint which sold over 700,000 copies within a few months, later reaching nearly a million. The Independent Labour Party, precursor of the Labour Party and the first British socialist party with a mass base, was formed in the same year. Before publication of *Merrie England*, there were fewer than 500 socialists in the whole county of Lancashire, an area of concentrated industry; 12 months later there were 50,000. It was translated into Welsh, Dutch, German, Swedish, Italian and Spanish, and a US edition is said to have sold roughly as many copies as the original in Britain. Blatchford knew how to write for people only beginning to read newspapers. He was inspired mainly by William Morris, the first Englishman to develop Marxism imaginatively and try to apply it to his own field of work. Blatchford was a vulgariser, whose popularity partly depended on trimming socialist ideas to fit existing common sense; whatever didn't fit, he amputated. Like others with such an eclectic approach, as soon as the 1914 war broke out, he became an equally successful propagandist for the slaughter of man by man.

[14] In 1911, the total annual income of all 32,000 British doctors was estimated by the *British Medical Journal* at £8 million, resulting in an average annual income of £250, and a median income somewhat less than £200. Compared with care for the rest of Britain's labouring poor in the early 20th century, the Welsh miners' medical schemes were well funded and their doctors well paid. This depended on the poundage system, unique to Wales. Everywhere else, friendly societies took fixed subscriptions unrelated to income, but in Wales the schemes took 3 or 4 pence for every £1 earned, deducted at the colliery office, so that funding for health care rose and fell with earnings. These were linked in turn to the pithead price of coal and the prosperity of the entire industry. Coal prices fluctuated, often wildly, but tended to move upwards throughout the first two decades of the 20th century, when coal was the main source of energy and had an apparently unlimited domestic and export market. In some schemes poundage was paid straight to the contracted doctors, in which case any investment in care was a deduction from their personal income. This guaranteed that little investment was made even in premises, equipment or clerical staff, let alone specialist doctors or nurses. But in the larger, more politically and socially conscious schemes which are of much greater interest, poundage was paid not to the doctors, but to a miners' medical aid fund from which doctors' salaries were paid, leaving the rest for investment in better buildings, equipment, staff, training, and whatever other measures the Scheme committees thought conducive to the health of subscribers and their families.

[15] Until early in the 20th century, the South Wales coal owners were mostly small entrepreneurs, themselves either miners or descended from miners, who

therefore lived close to their labour force. The miners' medical aid schemes were already well established before large companies, like Powell Duffryn and Insoles, whose major decisions could be taken remote from the workforce, came to dominate the mining economy.

[16] Until well into the 20th century, most operations were done in patients' homes on the kitchen table. In my own practice in Glyncorrwg, my GP predecessors held a minor operating session every Sunday morning until 1948, when patients first gained access to free care at Neath and Swansea hospitals by fully trained surgeons. Obstetric care was usually excluded. If it was required, because a birth seemed too difficult for a midwife to manage, GPs still charged a fee, unless obstetric care was included in their contract.

[17] Marx and Engels' influence in the South Wales coalfield is excellently documented in Hywel Francis and Dai Smith's *The Fed: A History of the South Wales Miners in the 20th Century* (London: Lawrence & Wishart, 1980). Their influence in the UK Labour movement as a whole, and the often strange forms that it took, are excellently described and objectively assessed in Caroline Benn's superb biography of Keir Hardie, still generally agreed to be the father of the Labour Party (Benn, C., *Keir Hardie*, London: Random House, 1992). Possibly her best summary is on pp 69–70, describing Hardie's considerable correspondence with Engels after Marx's death, during the socialist revival toward the end of the 19th century:

> All [Hardie's] negative references are clearly to the SDF [Hyndman's Social Democratic Federation] and not to Marxism, and to the SDF revolution-around-the-corner, upon which Hyndman – and many gurus of the left since – sought to hook hearers. Hardie deplored this, and so did the 'Marx family'. Nor can Hardie's words be interpreted to mean he deplored ideology, when he had written to Engels specifically that, 'We are not opposed to ideals and recognizing ... their power in inspiring men, we are more concerned in the realisation of an ideal than the dreaming of it.'

Before his death Engels joined the Independent Labour Party, precursor of the Labour Party itself, as an ordinary member (Benn, C., *Keir Hardie*, London: Random House, 1992, p 100). There is no evidence that he or anyone else thought this indicated a departure from Marx's ideas.

[18] Dr Alastair Wilson of Aberdare told me how his father, a GP sympathetic to workmen and a rare medical supporter of the Lloyd George Insurance Act, would attend operations for hernia at the cottage hospital, alongside a GP

colleague equally notorious for his unswerving support for Guest, Keen & Baldwin, the local coal and steel employers. Each would stoutly assert that the cause of the hernia – from exceptional work strain (for the Miners' Federation) or from a congenital weakness (for GKB) – was plain to see. There could in fact have been no visible evidence either way.

[19] Speaking of cottage hospitals in the mining valleys in the run-up to the NHS, Bevan claimed that though government described them as voluntary hospitals, many got 97.5% of their revenue from miners' subscriptions (Bevan, A., *Hansard*, 30 April 1946, vol 422, col 47. Quoted in Powell, M., 'Wales and the National Health Service', *Llafur* 2000; 8(1): 34).

[20] Earwicker, R., 'Miners' Medical Services before the First World War: The South Wales Coalfield', *Llafur* 1981; 3(2): 39–52, and Falk, L.J., 'Coal miners' Prepaid Medical Care in the United States, and some British Relationships 1792–1964', *Medical Care* 1966; 4: 37–42.

[21] Coal was mined where it was found, resulting in many relatively isolated settlements where every aspect of life became organised around this single industry. In South Wales isolation was reinforced by mountains dividing each valley from its neighbours, resulting in a characteristically mixed, often contradictory culture, common to all mining communities: independent self-reliance but also divisive parochialism, combined with disciplined solidarity against external enemies. Compared with England's ancient north-eastern and Midland coalfields, deep mining was a late development in Wales except around the iron and steel industries in Merthyr Tydfil. Welsh coal mining became a major economic and social force only from about 1860, but from then onwards development was extremely rapid, leading to an international in-migration to the South Wales valleys at roughly the same rate as to the Klondike in the US over the same period.

[22] Day-to-day decisions about the schemes were taken by elected committees, initially dominated by colliery officials but from around 1900 by the South Wales section of the Miners' Federation of Great Britain, locally known as 'the Fed' (Francis, H., Smith, D., *The Fed: A History of the South Wales Miners in the 20th Century*, London: Lawrence & Wishart, 1980). Meetings of the kind where major decisions were taken concerning the medical aid societies and their disputes with the BMA have been well described by Steve Thompson (Thompson, S., 'A proletarian public sphere: working class provision of medical services and care in south Wales, c.1900–1948', chapter 5 in Borsay, A. (ed), *Public Service or Private Commodity? Medicine in Wales, c.1800–2000*, Cardiff: University of Wales Press, 2003):

In any mass meeting of colliers or other workmen in South Wales, the usual practice was for anybody who had something to say to stand up and make their comment. Debate was open to anyone with anything to express on a particular matter regardless of position or status. Furthermore, oratory at these public meetings involved an interactive relationship between speaker and audience that ensured that the opinions and feelings of society members were clearly expressed. Newspaper reports of meetings show that speakers were constantly being interrupted with cries of approval or objection from those present, so that even usually inarticulate groups and individuals could make their feelings felt in a very direct way and play some part in determining actions and policies.

Such scenes are sometimes described as 'Athenian democracy', forgetting that two-thirds of the population of Attica were then slaves, with no rights whatever. Miners are among the founders of true participative democracy. The nature of coal mining is entirely different from factory production, leading to few national disputes but many local disputes with employers. At least until the 1930s, production of coal depended almost entirely on men working in extremely variable and often unpredictable conditions, assisted very little by machines. Miners were paid according to the amount of large coal they produced, and the workforce rose or fell according to world market demand, leading alternately to mass overwork and mass unemployment. This gave every trade unionist personal experience of wage negotiations at the point of production, a keen interest in the work of the union and a deep appreciation of the value of solidarity in all its aspects. Whenever local lodges of the Fed had to take important decisions affecting a whole colliery, or a whole village dependent upon it, mass meetings were held, well attended by everyone affected. For the concept of democracy to have any real meaning, it must in some way be measurable. Its most suitable yardstick could be the extent to which decisions are taken by people who will themselves suffer their consequences. Using this measure, the rise and eventual decline of the miners' medical aid societies was a rise and eventual decline of participative democracy. Even as late as the 1970s, long after every trace of local democratic control of the NHS had vanished, meetings of this kind were still possible where Welsh mining communities needed to discuss any major issue of common concern. Archie Cochrane, the pioneer of epidemiology in South Wales after the Second World War, got the miners' union to organise such meetings for him in the Rhondda Fach, through which he gained informed cooperation from around 90% of his target population for a demanding programme of research into tuberculosis and pneumoconiosis, setting a new world standard for population response. Our research studies in Glyncorrwg for the Medical

Research Council all began with whole-community meetings of this kind, with exactly the sort of informal participation Thompson describes.

[23] The first hospital in the Rhondda Valleys opened in 1896, with only four beds serving almost 100,000 people. Even by 1914 provision had risen only to 88 hospital beds serving 180,000 people (Egan, D., *Coal Society: A History of the South Wales Mining Valleys*, Llandyssul: Gomer Press, 1987, p 90).

[24] Thompson, S., 'A proletarian public sphere' (see note 22 above for full reference details).

[25] At a national level this opportunity was first recognised by Beatrice Webb in her Minority Report to the Royal Commission on Poor Law reform in 1909, though her proposals were ignored in the Majority Report. Far less known are proposals for a nationalised public medical care system oriented to public health aims made in 1911 by Dr Benjamin Moore (1867–1922), founder of British medical biochemistry and a pioneer of 20th-century health economics. He estimated that about 250,000 UK deaths annually could have been prevented by a medical care system organised to apply current knowledge fully to the whole population. His ideas were presented in his book *Dawn of the Health Age* (London: J. & A. Churchill, 1911), and through the State Medical Service Association (SMSA) formed by him and a small but authoritative group of like-minded medical intellectuals in 1912. This attracted much attention in the medical press for two years, until all progressive thought was drowned by war hysteria. It never seems to have reached doctors in the front line of care in industrial areas. Though discussion revived briefly in 1918, the SMSA lapsed into passivity after Moore's premature death in the post-war pandemic of influenza. The SMSA wound up in 1929, but some of its remaining members resurfaced in 1931 with the birth of the Socialist Medical Association (SMA, renamed Socialist Health Association [SHA] in the 1970s). The SMA was affiliated to the Labour Party, and it introduced plans for a free, universal and comprehensive state medical service into Labour's national policy in 1934. The SHA is now divided. Its Welsh and Scottish regions still promote the NHS as a gift economy, through the Welsh Assembly and the Scottish Parliament. The SHA in England remains ambiguously tied to whatever New Labour does next.

[26] Collings, J.S., 'General practice in England today', *Lancet* 1950; i: 555–85.

[27] Irvine, D., Jeffreys, M., 'BMA Planning Unit survey of general practice 1969', *British Medical Journal* 1971; 4: 535–43.

[28] Leese and Bosanquet studied GP investment strategies from 1966 to the early 1980s, when government began to support such investment with large subsidies (Bosanquet, N., Leese, B., 'Family doctors: their choice of practice strategy', *British Medical Journal* 1986; 293: 667–70). On five indicators of improvement (employment of practice nurse, improved or purpose-built premises, participation in training, possession of ECG, follow-up clinics) 32% of practices (high investors) accounted for 71% of positive scores. Nearly all the high-investing practices were in affluent areas. Even with large subsidies, investment in areas of continued industrial decline with falling populations made no business sense.

[29] In the words of coalfield historian Ray Earwicker ('Miners' medical services before the First World War: the South Wales coalfield', *Llafur* 1981; 3(2): 39–52) it was:

> the system of pay-as-you-earn deductions that gave the miners' medical clubs their strength. But it was the acquisition of financial control of the clubs through a Workmen's Fund and initiation of a salaried medical service that gave the South Wales clubs their distinctive character. Dispute over the issue of control was settled between the employers and workmen. Employer resistance was minimal. ... The colliery doctors petitioned the employers against this change but it was promptly rejected. The doctors, poorly organised, were forced to acquiesce ...

This soon changed once the big disputes between miners and their doctors began in the early 20th century, when the BMA became as fierce a union as any other.

[30] I have dealt with this in greater detail in *A New Kind of Doctor: The General Practitioner's Part in the Health of the Community* (London: Merlin Press, 1988).

[31] Though the miners had potential allies in Benjamin Moore and his eminent medical colleagues, these medical intellectuals were socially and geographically too distant from both miners and miners' doctors to form any effective political alliance. British doctors at the bottom of the professional pile rarely saw themselves as intelligentsia in the European and Latin American traditions exemplified by Chekhov, Semashko, Štampar, Evang, Guevara and Barghouti.

[32] The Ebbw Vale dispute was almost exactly repeated in 1934, when my father, Dr Alex Tudor-Hart, together with several other doctors, was recruited by the South Wales Miners' Federation to work for the Llanelli Workmen's Medical Aid Scheme after the local doctors, supported by the BMA, withdrew from

their previous contracts. The miners, tinplate and foundry workers of Llanelli were trying to develop a larger scheme similar to that in Tredegar, with major surgery performed by specialists rather than their GPs. They proposed to pay for these by reducing the proportion of poundage paid to their contracted GPs, who would also have lost fees previously paid to them for surgery. After a bitter and divisive dispute lasting 18 months, the old doctors still retained most of the patients, though the new scheme was generally recognised as a more rational system. The BMA's chief negotiator was Dr Charles Hill, who later led BMA resistance to the NHS. The dispute was finally settled by arbitration, giving the BMA most of what it wanted, but allowing recruitment of enough salaried specialist staff for the influential Political and Economic Planning Report of 1936 to propose it as a model for the future NHS (Davies, R., 'Workers and medical services', in Edwards, J. (ed), *Tinopolis: Aspects of Llanelli's Tinplate Trade*, Llanelli Borough Council, 1995, pp 162–9).

[33] As Rhodri Morgan (who became leader of the Labour Party in Wales against sustained opposition from Blair) is fond of recalling, the Conservative Party in Wales has never succeeded in winning an elected majority, in the whole time since common people began to get a vote. This is in contrast to Scotland, where the Conservatives still remain powerful in many rural areas.

[34] The imperialist wings of the Liberals, Conservatives, Fabians and reforming civil servants like Sir Robert Morant led a vigorous pre-emptive reform movement on the eve of the First World War, which laid the foundations for 20th-century education and welfare services completed after the Second World War. This was a conscious effort to assimilate vulgarised socialist ideas to an imperialist programme, assuring British citizens privileged status as servants of a dominant imperial power. In this way the progressive perceptions of Charles Darwin, which had destroyed the hold of the Anglican Church over the minds of industrial workers, were easily adapted to social Darwinism and the ranking of races. Social Darwinism provided the seeds for fascism. The close association between eugenic concepts of racial purity and the birth of modern state welfare is a necessary and useful embarrassment for socialists, deserving more thought than it has so far received. The depth and extent of change needed in state services to make them into services of, by and for the people, rather than means for social control, has always been underestimated.

[35] This policy had some success. Though the German Social Democrats became the world's largest and leading socialist party, developing an internally inclusive independent culture which before 1914 seemed on course eventually to provide the world's first socialist state, Bismarck's insurance schemes shifted the Social-Democratic agenda from revolution to reform, and helped to ensure

that by the end of the 19th century the revolutionary legacy of Karl Marx seemed safely castrated.

[36] Lloyd George knew from his actuaries that male life expectancy in 1911 averaged only about 12 months of life after retirement at 65. Proposals today to raise retirement age to 70 would mean that in many unhealthy inner-city areas, pensions might again become 'affordable' to the top of society, in much the same way. At present death rates, if retirement age were raised to 70, 30.6% of men would never collect their pension because they had already died. Biggest losers would be in the poorest London boroughs, of which Hackney is the worst, where 48.3% never reach their 70th birthday (TUC report, *Work Till You Drop*, London: TUC, 2004).

[37] The Poor Law was intended not only to drive the poor into factories, but to strengthen the existing social hierarchy by heading off revolution. William Farr, founder of Britain's uniquely excellent health statistics (which provided important evidence used in Marx's *Capital*), wrote in the 1870s that the new Poor Law was 'an insurance of life against death by starvation, and of property against communistic agitations'.

[38] Grigg, J., *Lloyd George: The People's Champion, 1902–1911*, London: Eyre Methuen, 1978, p 325.

[39] Wall, A., 'Reforming the reforms', in Iliffe, S., Mostyn, J., Ross, R. (eds), *From Market Chaos to Common Sense: Papers on Future Policies for Health*, London: Medical World/Socialist Health Association, 1993.

[40] Wall, A., 'So what would YOU do then, Andrew Wall?', *British Journal of Health Care Management* 2002; 8: 151–3.

[41] Hari, J., 'This corruption in Washington is smothering America's future: how do you regulate banks effectively, if the Senate is owned by Wall Street?', *Independent*, 29 January 2010.

[42] Labour Party general election manifesto, 1997.

[43] A major step in commercialisation of all public services was the New Labour government's decision, soon after it was elected in 1997, to adopt the Conservative Party's plans to replace funding for public service projects by the Treasury, by funding from private investors through the Private Finance Initiative (PFI). These were contracts, usually for 30 years, for commercial companies to build schools, hospitals and other public service facilities, and

in some cases to staff them, and then rent them back to education authorities, the NHS, or whatever public agency had accepted this sleight of hand. When PFI was introduced by a Conservative government it was derided by the Labour Party in opposition as covert privatisation, as indeed it was. It was extremely costly, because governments can borrow at much lower rates of interest than any commercial agency (because they carry the risk that their contractors may fail). For example, the only hospital in Wales built through PFI, Baglan Moors hospital serving Neath and Port Talbot, cost £54m to build, but the NHS will have to pay Baglan Moor Healthcare just under £270m over the next 28 years. Like all PFI projects, the entire transaction is covered by commercial secrecy. The government has claimed that 88% of PFI projects were delivered on time and within budget, compared with 70% of public service projects delivered late, and 73% over budget. Allyson Pollock's research team at the Centre for International Public Health at the University of Edinburgh looked at the five studies cited by the Treasury to support these claims. Two were by the National Audit Office (NAO), which concluded that as they were based entirely on interviews with PFI project managers, they offered no basis for proof of efficacy of any method of procurement. A third study by a private company contained no comparative data on either method of procurement. The fourth study cited by the Treasury was still covered by commercial secrecy and therefore not accessible for analysis, despite original assurances that it would be published. The fifth and final study was the only one containing any comparative data. This was commissioned by the Treasury from a PFI consultancy and engineering company. Even this compared cost and time overruns in 39 public schemes with just three out of 451 operational PFI schemes, it excluded any PFI schemes already considered failed or problematic, and used different baselines for public and PFI schemes from which to calculate escalations in cost. Throughout the 30 years or so of PFI contracts, all remain secret from the public and unaccountable to MPs in Parliament. The contracts can be traded as commodities on the stock exchange, so there is never an assurance that the contractor originally approved by NHS negotiators will retain responsibility for implementation. Multi-million-pound shareholdings in education, NHS and transport projects are changing hands in secret deals between contractors and financiers, releasing immense cash windfalls for business, at taxpayers' expense. To its credit, the devolved Welsh Assembly government got out of this rush to corruption as soon as it could.

[44] Consequences for NHS funding are as yet uncertain. Ominously, the UK government has hired the US management consultancy McKinsey Corporation to advise on how to reduce the NHS annual budget by around £20bn. A report exists, as yet unpublished, but leaked to the *Health Service Journal* (Vize, R., 'McKinsey have plotted a course, NHS managers must

lead through it', *HSJ*, 2 September 2009). This proposed a nearly 10% cut in overall staffing (137,000 jobs), reduced entry to medical schools in anticipation of impending medical unemployment, a 40% cut in hospital inpatients by reducing both numbers ('nearly 40% don't need to be there') and length of stay, and selling £8.3bn-worth of hospital estates. The following day, McKinsey neither confirmed nor denied accuracy of these leaked proposals. A government minister implied that the entire report had been rejected, but said nothing about any alternative ways either to reduce costs or to maintain funding. Traditionally, we generally believed that politicians were elected and paid to develop policies, and senior civil servants were appointed and paid to apply them. To avoid conflicts of interest, both were then supposed to work widely separated from the world of commerce. When and where did any elected representatives of the people decide to merge commerce with public service?

[45] Himmelstein, D.U., Woolhandler, S., 'The corporate compromise: a Marxist view of health maintenance organizations and prospective payment', *Annals of Internal Medicine* 1988; 109: 494–501.

[46] Kmietowicz, Z., 'Contract for GPs in England "failed to live up to expectations"', *British Medical Journal* 2008; 337: 833. There is now one enterprising GP in the Midlands with a very large practice who has no partners. He employs 19 salaried GP assistants. Under the new laws introduced by Tony Blair and agreed by a large majority of Labour MPs, when he chooses to retire he will be able to sell this practice to whoever offers the highest bid. Of practices in the East End of London borough of Newham employing salaried GPs, and surveyed by Dr Osman Bhatti, more than three-quarters failed to pass on the 1.5% rise in GP pay recommended in 2009 by the Doctors and Dentists Review Body. More than half of these salaried GPs, who were responsible for reaching QOF targets, received no extra pay, though these are supposed to be incentive payments. Few practice partnerships gave their salaried assistants contracts conforming to BMA guidelines, excusing this by saying they couldn't afford them. Back to the 1930s.

[47] Data on recent GPs' annual net earnings from NHS work, after deduction of practice expenses, from the NHS Information Centre were reported in *bmaNews*, 30 January 2010:

Net NHS earnings	n	2007–08 %	2006–07 %	2005–06 %	2004–05 %
>£250,000	260	0.8	0.8	0.9	0.5
£200,000–£250,000	650	1.9	2.2	2.4	1.4
£150,000–£200,000	3,560	10.6	10.7	11.4	7.4
£100,000–£150,000	13,220	39.3	40.8	42.9	36.2
£50,000–£100,000	13,610	40.5	39.5	36.4	45.6
<£50,000	2,320	6.9	6.0	5.9	9.0

These data confirm median earnings well below figures generally quoted in news media.

[48] Personal communication from Dr Bess Barrett, NE Derbyshire Primary Care Trust, 6 February 2006. Subsequent published references include: Robinson, F., 'No private matter: taking the fight against commerce to the courts', *The New Generalist* 2006; 4: 58–61; Barrett, E.D., 'Can general practitioners compete with big business? Changing drivers in the NHS', *British Medical Journal* 2006; 332: 1335–6; Arie, S., 'Can GPs compete with big business?', *British Medical Journal* 2006; 332: 1172–3.

[49] Timmins, N., Masters, B., Knight, R., 'US health executive offered top NHS role', *Financial Times,* 30 April 2007.

[50] Here is what Richard thought in 1996 about transnational investments in publicly provided, non-profit health services:

> In September 1996 leaders of US managed health care plans met in Mexico City to discuss opportunities for extending their business internationally. The meeting was organised by the American Association of Health Plans and the Academy for International Health Studies. Workshops looked at market opportunities in Israel, Korea, Venezuela, Canada, Mexico, Russia, France, Singapore, Brazil, New Zealand, Australia, Puerto Rico, South Africa and Argentina. What happens in a country is increasingly driven by what is important for business; the United States did not take a hard line with China on human rights because American business did not want to lose markets, but it did take strong action over intellectual property because that was important to

the business community.... The businessmen who run the for-profit managed health care plans in the United States see no reason why they should not follow the path of their colleagues in other businesses and compete globally. Indeed, they may have to. Wall Street expects them to keep growing, which means signing up more people to their plans. And, as one chief executive of a health plan put it, 'We are soon going to run out of people in the United States.' Managed care plans already cover 100 million Americans.... The World Bank is now concentrating on public and primary health care for the poor. It believes in increased private health care for the wealthy in order to release public money for the poor and to raise efficiency and quality in the private sector.... So perhaps managed health care – which has emerged from a country with one of the world's most irrational health care systems – will end up being exported around the world. Just as more and more of us are fed by American fast food chains, so many of us may receive our health care in some way through American managed health care plans. (Smith, R., 'Global competition in health care', *British Medical Journal* 1996; 313: 764–5)

In his own defence, he claims that commercial providers will prove both profitable and more effective than self-employed GPs (Smith, R., 'Viewpoint: new arrangements might finally bring the best primary care to those who need it the most', *British Journal of General Practice* 2006; 56: 361). How he could convince himself that his corporation would do a better job than Bess Barrett, when his corporation had not yet engaged any of the medical staff it would need or consulted the local community in any way, is beyond my comprehension.

[51] Dyer, O., 'Court delays takeover of Derby practice', *British Medical Journal* 2006; 332: 684.

[52] Foster, M., 'Judge holds up PCT private GP contract', *bmaNews*, 25 March 2006.

[53] It had little to fear, however. Cases of this kind have all had good local press coverage, but have been virtually ignored by broadcasters or the national press.

[54] In the East End of London, at least, this seems more or less typical of the costs of tendering for all would-be primary care providers, whether they are experienced GPs already working in the NHS or commercial groups – all must expect to spend at least £30,000 on preparing a bid, none of it reimbursable. In effect, this excludes all but the largest GP groups.

[55] Cole, A., 'Private practice: contracts to allow general practices to be run by private companies were supposed to be a last resort, but is this really the case?', *British Medical Journal* 2008; 336: 1406–7.

[56] The policy of introducing commercial competition into GP care, starting in 2004, was justified by the New Labour government's conviction that this would promote health gain and efficiency. Successive ministers all denied that there was any intention of expanding commercial provision as a policy in its own right. If this were true, one would expect government to have gathered factual data to allow comparisons between GP provision and commercial provision, but in fact no data whatever have been gathered since the policy began through Alternative Provider of Medical Services (APMS) contracts in NHS England (APMS contracts have not been used in Scotland or Wales). So it has been left to the Centre for International Public Health Policy of Edinburgh University and the King's Fund to get data from English Primary Care Trusts under the Freedom of Information Act, with response rates of 93% and 80% respectively. Even these responses were mostly incomplete. Of 49 PCTs responding to the Edinburgh study, only 41 provided data on the value of contracts awarded to commercial providers, justifying this by commercial secrecy. Excluding out-of-hours services, they estimated that just over 1% of the English population were now served by APMS providers (Heins, E., Pollock, A.M., Price, D., 'The commercialization of GP services: a survey of APMS contracts and new GP ownership', *British Journal of General Practice* 2009; 59: 750–3).

[57] Pritchard, L., Munn, F., 'BMA medical students committee annual student finance survey shows that even before introduction of the latest £3,000 tuition fees, average student debt after a five-year medical course is £20,172, and after a six-year course £22,365', *bmaNews*, 24 December 2005.

[58] In 2009 the Department of Health confirmed that up to 16 ISTCs would have to be bought by the NHS over the next two years, at an estimated capital cost of £200m. This was because 'residual value guarantees' were included in the first wave of ISTC contracts, so as to minimise the risks to the private sector providers of accepting five-year contracts to diagnose and treat elective patients. They guaranteed that at the end of the five-year contract, the NHS would buy back the remaining capital assets, valued at the time of the end of the contract. These were additional to guarantees of volume of work. Because the 2007–08 financial crisis made refinancing difficult for private providers, it seemed likely that after repurchase, these assets would be re-leased to them (Gainsbury, S., 'NHS to become a landlord for Private Treatment Centres', *Health Service Journal*, 30 July 2009).

[59] To avoid a loss of £6.5m, Southampton PCT appealed to GPs to refer patients to an ISTC run by Care UK, a commercial provider, whose contract entailed payment by the NHS, whether or not its services were actually used. The Southampton University Hospitals Trust, the original NHS provider, was over-performing in relation to its commercial competitor, the PCT said. Faced with bankruptcy for the PCT, their employer, local GPs reluctantly agreed (Foster, M., 'GPs forced to send patients to ISTC to stop loss of £6.5m', *bmaNews*, 10 October 2009). This is typical of many other such examples.

[60] Nationalisation of all hospitals was a long way to go, and Bevan evidently judged he could not, at that time and in those circumstances, go any further. Through Lord Moran, President of the Royal College of Physicians, he negotiated a compromise with the hospital specialists. He allowed them to work part time in the NHS while continuing in private practice, using NHS resources. He feared that otherwise they would work in their dangerous private nursing homes and neglect their NHS duties (as some still do today). Anticipating that free NHS care would rapidly erode demand for private care, he gave a secret committee of senior consultants full control of substantial additional pensionable income (Distinction Awards) for them to award to those who might otherwise have earned most from private practice, using secret criteria to establish their 'outstanding merit' (Our regular correspondent, 'Foreign letters: London. National Health Service', *JAMA* 1949; 141: 1236, and Lee-Potter, J., '"Honeymoon for medicine" is over, warns chairman of council', *British Medical Journal* 1993; 306: 1073). Bevan famously said that he had choked the consultants' mouths with gold; more importantly, he stuffed their hands with power, giving them access to staff, buildings and equipment they could never have provided themselves, letting them use these resources more or less as they pleased, with only one important exception: they must give care free to everyone who needed it.

[61] Rivett, G., *From Cradle to Grave: Fifty Years of the NHS*, London: King's Fund, 1998. This confirms the view strongly held by George Godber and expressed by him many times.

[62] It seems doubtful whether this view would have been shared by the much larger number of young specialists in training who would soon form most of the hospital medical workforce, but they had little voice and even less inclination to use it: careers depended on identity of views with their seniors.

[63] Productivity (of process, not outcome) was supposed to provide the measure of success for the NHS internal market. Over the 10 years to 2008, according to the King's Fund, productivity (of process) has actually fallen by an average

0.4% a year (Appleby, J., Crawford, R., Emmerson, C., *How Cold Will It Be? Prospects for NHS Funding 2011–2017*, London: King's Fund and Institute for Fiscal Studies, July 2009). We await the response of market advocates who are still saying that the only way to raise efficiency in the NHS is to press on with even more competition and less cooperation, still described as 'reform'.

[64] The Bill legalising Foundation Hospital Trusts was opposed by more Labour MPs than any previous New Labour government measure, including its approval of the attack on Iraq. It obtained a majority only through the votes of most Scottish and Welsh Labour MPs, supporting a measure opposed by both the Scottish Parliament and the Welsh Assembly, and not applied to their own constituents. So far as I know, none has yet explained how they could be loyal both to regional Labour policies to keep the NHS public, and central Labour policies to abandon the NHS to the market.

[65] Colin-Thomé, D., 'Mid-Staffordshire NHS Foundation Trust: a review of lessons learnt for commissioners and performance managers following the Healthcare Commission investigation', The Mid-Staffordshire NHS Foundation Trust Inquiry January 2005–March 2009, 29 April 2009 (Key Documents: www.midstaffsinquiry.com/documents.html).

[66] We have the authority of a Nobel prize-winning economist, leader of the Chicago School, who from the mid-1970s until the global financial crisis of 2007–08 ruled every business school in the world, and kicked both Marx and Keynes apparently permanently into the long grass: 'Few trends could so thoroughly undermine the very foundations of our free society as the acceptance by corporate officials of a social responsibility other than to make as much money for their stockholders as possible' (Friedman, M., Friedman, R.D., *Capitalism and Freedom*, Chicago: University of Chicago Press, 1962, p 133). This principle remains embodied in the laws of world trade, enforced by the World Trade Organisation, the World Bank, and by the courts of almost all trading nations. Companies must justify any act of charity by evidence that, on balance, it is likely to increase its profits. That is the law.

[67] *Daily Telegraph*, 22 August 2007.

[68] The main source for Professor Sikora's claims has been the EUROCARE study, comparing survival figures for cancer in EU countries. The UK registers more than 80% of all cancers diagnosed each year, compared with 28% in Italy, 17% in France and 16% in Spain. In this study, which claimed that cancer cure rates were lower in the UK NHS than in insurance-based systems in the EU in France, Germany, Spain and even Hungary, Germany

was represented by a study including only 1% of its population of 70 million people. The UK contributed over one third of all the cancers considered in the study, though they came from only 12% of the total EU population. Even within those EU countries with registration as complete as in the UK (Austria, Denmark, Finland, Iceland, Norway, Slovenia and Sweden) differences in cancer survival were hard to interpret responsibly, and showed lower UK rates for only a minority of cancers. Claims that UK cancer care has fallen below advanced world standards have not been substantiated, and depend on news media reports of Sikora's claims without regard to more cautious views from cancer epidemiologists.

[69] In 1999, administration accounted for 31% of total health care expenditure in the US, compared with 16.7% in Canada, and probably about 12% in the NHS. Before the NHS was turned towards becoming a business in the early 1980s, administration costs ran at between 4% and 6% of the NHS budget. In the US, between 1969 and 1999, administrative staff grew from 18.2% of the US health care labour force to 27.3%. These figures exclude insurance industry staff (Woolhandler, S., Campbell, T., Himmelstein, D.U., 'Costs of health care administration in the United States and Canada', *New England Medical Journal* 2003; 349: 768–75). Spanish health economists estimated that as a share of GDP, US health care transaction costs were 3.5%, compared with 0.2% in the UK before 'reforms' had got into their stride, a 15-fold difference (Lobo, F., Velasquez, G. (eds), *Medicines and the Economic Environment*, Madrid: Biblioteca Civitas Economia y Empresa, 1998. Review in *Journal of Public Health Policy* 2002; 23: 245–8). This suggests that as commercialisation grows, so do administrative overheads, transaction costs and, of course, profits. Tax-funded public service gives the highest care output for each dollar or pound spent – value for money. In its first decade in office, the New Labour government increased the total NHS workforce in England by 30%, but over the same period its managerial workforce doubled (Shaw, E., *Losing Labour's Soul? New Labour and the Blair Government 1997–2007*, London: Routledge, 2007, p 117).

[70] For example, the main argument used to initiate 'reform' of the NHS in Britain was rising costs and consequent tax burdens on business. In fact the NHS had cost less than health care in any other developed economy. This was partly because successive governments had starved it of funds. UK business was taxed less, business executives paid themselves more, and labour was more flexible than anywhere else except the US. In 1999, according to a survey by *Management Today*, average salaries for chief executives were £404,100 in the US, followed by £394,103 in the UK, £317,698 in France, £263,669 in Australia, £256,932 in Japan, £243,242 in Germany and £216,971 in Sweden. Maximum tax rates were 65% in Japan, 56% in Germany, 55% in Sweden,

54% in Paris, 51% in the US, 47% in Australia and 40% in UK. Redundancy pay for workers was 131% in Japan, 85% in Australia, 42% in Sweden, 29% in the US, 25% in France and 23% in UK (*Guardian*, 28 March 1999). Clearly the UK already accommodated its employers more generously than any other nation except the US, and New Labour has ruthlessly maintained that support ever since. An inquiry chaired by Sir Derek Wanless, a leading businessman, found the NHS had been grossly underfunded for the tasks it had to perform. He estimated a cumulative £267bn shortfall in the NHS compared with average EU investment in health care over the previous 26 years, 1972–98 (*Lancet* 2001; 358: 1971). The arguments about affordability and rising costs were unprincipled. In Sweden, which soon followed Britain with a similar commercialising programme (Nilsson, M., 'Sweden's health reform', *Lancet* 1993; 342: 979, and Walker, A., 'Erosion of Swedish welfare state', *British Medical Journal* 1991; 303: 267), health care costs as a proportion of GDP had actually fallen from 9% in 1982 to 7.8% by 1992 (Gilson, L., 'Health care reform in developing countries', *Lancet* 1993; 342: 800). There, the argument was, first, that every other country was already doing it, and second, that outsourcing and internal competition were bound to give better value for money, so costs might fall even faster. They did not, but having started, commercialisation in Sweden has continued.

[71] The most active organised professional force at that time was the NHS Support Federation, led by Dr Harry Keen, Professor of Medicine at Guy's Hospital, selected as pilot site for the Hospital Trusts first conceived by Thatcher's government and now imposed everywhere by Blair's New Labour government. Harry's repeated attempts to organise a public meeting with Robin Cook, then Labour shadow Minister for Health, all failed, so he finally gave up trying to organise any joint action with the Labour Party, of which he had been a lifelong member. That experience was typical. Even then, Labour leaders were wary of any close alliance with the medical profession. Though they like to attribute this to enduring memories of medical resistance to the NHS in 1948, opposition to doctors (or any other affluent professional group) still provides a populist alternative to tackling serious concentrations of wealth and power.

[72] According to one of the main players in these negotiations, Prime Minister Margaret Thatcher did not share the confidence of her minister, Kenneth Clarke, and suggested the government should back down before it lost public support. Clarke then said that in that event he would resign. This seems to have been enough to tip the balance, but it confirms my belief that the BMA's biggest problem was that it had no clear perspective on what to do with a victory. My informant did not agree.

[73] Shock, M., 'Medicine at the centre of the nation's affairs: doctors and their institutions are failing to adapt to the modern world', *British Medical Journal* 1994; 309: 1730–3.

[74] Like the Munich agreement it so closely resembles, this capitulation seems to have captivated enough of Sir Maurice's audience to suspend critical thought, at least for long enough to disarm collective resistance. A liberal friend distinguished enough to be invited to this great occasion was elated. 'I do wish you could have been there, Julian, you would have been so relieved to hear him. I think we really do have a resolution now to this dreadful situation.' Peace in our time?

[75] From the 1980s onwards, the received wisdom became that doctors primarily served themselves rather than the public interest. Though obviously there was some truth in this, did it contain any more truth in the 1980s than in the 1970s, or come to that, in the 1870s? Typical of this new establishment view was health economist Alan Maynard: '... unless we tackle the doctors, health reforms will fail to deliver ... processes of health care are dominated by clinicians, who merely represent their own vested interests ... [we must] strengthen the role of health managers and economists, who would speak for society at large' ('Taking on the health clinicians: the National Health market', *New Economy* [Institute for Public Policy Research], Autumn 1994). There is no evidence that this shift in trust, from doctors to NHS managers or health economists, ever took place among the general public.

Chapter Six

[1] The now almost universal conflation of fascism and communism into a single category of totalitarianism, a product of the Cold War, ignores this difference, and thus the diametrically opposed aims of those who chose either of these extremes in conflicts in which most of those now making this judgement played no part. However, undeniably, many of the ugliest features of fascism could be found in the behaviour of its most vigorous opponents, and the tone of their propaganda.

[2] For a ripe example of this see Sir James Barr, President of the BMA on the eve of the First World War (Barr, J., 'What are we? What are we doing here? From whence do we come and whither do we go?', *British Medical Journal* 1912; ii: 157–62). Barr led the BMA's campaign against Lloyd George's Insurance Act, in similar eugenic terms; medical care under the Act for losers in society would be, he claimed, a dangerous interference with natural selection of winners, such

as himself (Barr, J., 'Some reasons why the public should oppose the National Insurance Act', *British Medical Journal* 1911; ii: 1713–15).

[3] Though this is true, it is partly an artefact, because before the Nazis, Jews formed a much higher proportion of doctors than they did of the population as a whole, as was true in most of Europe. After the Nuremberg laws, nearly all of them were soon driven out of practice. Their gentile competitors climbed on the bandwagon (Light, D.W., Schuller, A. (eds), *Political Values and Health Care: The German Experience*, Cambridge, MA: MIT Press, 1986).

[4] Burleigh, M., *Death and Deliverance: 'Euthanasia' in Germany 1900–1945*, Cambridge and London: Cambridge University Press and Pan Paperback, 2002.

[5] Paul Martini, pioneer clinical pharmacologist, gave a lecture on 'the conscience of German medicine' to the Society of Internal Medicine in 1948. 'The doctors who sat at Nuremberg', he said, 'were in part criminals and we wish to have nothing to do with their deeds. But they were also in part the product, the flesh and the spirit of the medicine of their time, the medicine of the late nineteenth and twentieth centuries, and not just German medicine' (Shelley, J.H., Baur, M.P., 'Paul Martini: the first clinical pharmacologist?', *Lancet* 1999; 353: 1870–3).

[6] Weindling, P., *Health, Race, and German Politics between National Unification and Nazism, 1870–1945*, New York: Cambridge University Press, 1989.

[7] Armstrong, C., 'Thousands of women sterilised in Sweden without consent', *British Medical Journal* 1997; 315: 563.

[8] Miles, S.H., *Oath Betrayed: Torture, Medical Complicity, and the War on Terror*, New York: Random House, 2000.

[9] This calls to mind Thatcher's view of the New Testament parable of the Good Samaritan (Luke 10). 'No one would remember the good Samaritan', she said to a Conservative Party conference, 'if he had only had good intentions; he had money as well.' She seems not herself to have remembered his actions accurately. Answering the mischievous question 'And who is my neighbour?' (whom I should love as myself), Jesus told the story of a man travelling from Jerusalem to Jericho, who fell among thieves. A priest saw this, but passed by on the other side of the street. A Levite passed by, doing the same. But then a Samaritan came, 'he had compassion on him, and went to him, and bound up his wounds … and set him on his own beast, and brought him to an inn, and took care of him. And the morrow when he departed, he took out two

pence, and gave them to the host, and said unto him, Take care of him; and whatsoever thou spendest more, when I come again, I will repay thee.' There is no suggestion that the Samaritan was ever in danger of having only good intentions. He did all he could himself. Only then did he pay anyone else to care for the man on his behalf. Today, we share this cost through taxes. Those who prefer voluntary charity to income tax are modern equivalents of the priest and the Levite.

[10] *Times Health Supplement*, 11 March 1983, reported under the headline 'Gnat survives sledgehammer'.

[11] Furlong, R., 'Getting tough with "health tourists"', BBC World at One, 29 April 2008.

[12] In 1949, a year after the NHS began, tabloid newspapers floated alarming stories of waste in the new, free NHS, including a tale that foreign seamen were streaming into Liverpool to get free NHS dentures, which then turned up for sale in a Baghdad bazaar. Attlee's cabinet feared this was true, so it set up an inquiry. This revealed a grand total of 10 foreign seamen who had ever seen an NHS dentist in the first year of the service, with no evidence whatever of abuse by any of them, and no NHS dentures in Baghdad (Webster, C., *The Health Services since the War, Vol. 1, Problems of Health Care: The National Health Service before 1957*, London: HMSO, 1988, p 131).

[13] British visitors to Syria or Cuba are treated free in local hospitals if they fall sick or suffer an accident, a level of civilisation we reached in 1948, but have now put behind us.

[14] 'Wherefore putting away lying, speak every man truth unto his neighbour: for we are members one of another' (Ephesians 4: 25). Solidarity does indeed depend upon truthfulness, and recognition that if we want community, we can't choose our neighbours.

[15] At a Chicago Institute of Medicine panel discussion in 1995, *New England Journal of Medicine* editor Arnold Relman reported that for-profit insurance groups were taking 20%–30% of premiums as profits, before paying out for care (Wolinsky, H., 'Ethics in managed care', *Lancet* 1995; 346: 1499).

[16] In 1988, 56% of US doctors said they personally would support an inclusive national health insurance programme, but 74% thought most of their colleagues opposed it (*Harper's Index*, 28 August 2003).

[17] Röntgen refused to patent or copyright his discovery of X-rays. So did: Fleming, Chain and Florey, who developed penicillin; Waksman, who developed streptomycin; Salk, who developed poliomyelitis vaccine; Scribner, who invented venous shunts for kidney dialysis, and innumerable other pioneers of medical science. The race to patent sections of the human genome, and then even some clinical procedures, is a recent development still generally regarded as disgraceful and illegal, even by the US Congress (Gene-Macdaniel, C., 'US could ban patents on medical procedures', *British Medical Journal* 1996; 312: 997). Though between 1981 and 1994, 1,175 patents were granted for human DNA sequences, three-quarters of them to private US or Japanese companies (Thomas, S.M., Davies, A.R.W., Birtwhistle, N.J., Crowther, S.M., Burke, J.F., 'Ownership of the human genome', *Nature* 1996; 380: 387–8), European centres working on the human genome oppose the entire concept of intellectual property in this field. They are supported by some sponsoring multinational pharmaceutical companies who understand the fearful implications of this step for continued advance of science (Berger, A., 'Human genome project to complete ahead of schedule', *British Medical Journal* 1998; 317: 854). Intellectual property is a concept which is intoxicating some parts of the global market while it terrifies others, a struggle whose outcome is unresolved and has implications which are only beginning to be understood (Frow, J., 'Information as gift and commodity', *New Left Review* 1996; 219: 89–108).

[18] This has nothing to do with race, however defined, but everything to do with poverty. The US presents almost all of its public health data in terms of 'race' – black/white/latino – rather than social class, but evidence consistently confirms that income is a better predictor of almost all health-related variables than 'race' (the haemoglobinopathies – sickle cell disease and the like – are rare exceptions).

[19] Since the 1970s, comfort can no longer be taken for granted for a rising proportion even of employed people, even in the most advanced economies. For more than a century, apart from the depression between 1929 and 1940, the US set the global pace for wages, so that most workers eventually came to believe that a steadily rising standard of living was virtually guaranteed everywhere, as long as they followed the same economic and political path. In the 1970s, this growth in affluence came to an end, though the political culture it supported persists, getting angrier as its material base disappears. Corrected for inflation, average hourly wages in the US in 2000 were still 8% lower than their level in 1973, 27 years earlier, and 40 million citizens had no health insurance. In 1970, average household income among the richest 5% was 16 times as much as among the bottom 20%. By 2000 this difference

had increased to 25 times as much. In 1970, average earnings for chief executive officers exceeded average pay in their workforce 39-fold. By 2000, this difference had increased to 1,000-fold (Tilly, C., 'Raw deal for workers: why have U.S. workers experienced a long-term decline in pay, benefits, and working conditions?', *International Journal of Health Services* 2004; 34: 305–11).

[20] Wallace, R., Wallace, D., 'Socioeconomic determinants of health: community marginalisation and the diffusion of disease and disorder in the United States', *British Medical Journal* 1997; 314: 1341–5.

[21] Morris, J.N., Titmuss, R.M., 'Health and social change: I. The recent history of rheumatic heart disease', *The Medical Officer*, 26 August 1944: 69–71.

[22] Few now remember that when Aneurin Bevan was Minister of Health, he was also Minister for Housing. With 20% of British housing stock destroyed or seriously damaged by bombing, in 1948 this was a more pressing need than a new health service, and had corresponding priority. Bevan insisted on building only to the highest (full Parker-Morris) standard, so that council houses constructed before 1952 are for the most part still useful and in good condition. Later council housing reverted to the jerry-built standards considered adequate for the working class by politicians with less anger or conscience. The present government is attempting to eliminate council housing completely, but the need for social housing – particularly in London – is now so great that it is unlikely to succeed.

[23] Morris, J.N., 'Four cheers for prevention', *Proceedings of the Royal Society of Medicine* 1972; 66: 225–32.

[24] Welin, L., Larsson, B., Svardsudd, K. et al, 'Social network and activities in relation to mortality from cardiovascular diseases, cancer and other causes: a 12 year follow up of the study of men born in 1913 and 1923', *Journal of Epidemiology & Community Health* 1992; 46: 127–32.

[25] According to a study by Prof James Davies of the University of Western Ontario in association with the World Institute for Development Economic Research of the United Nations in Helsinki, in the year 2000 the richest 2% of the world population owned 51% of all global assets, while the poorest 50% of the world population owned about 1% of all global assets. All subsequent data indicate that this huge polarisation is increasing as the world economy expands (*Toronto Globe & Mail*, 5 December 2006).

[26] Wilkinson, R.G., Pickett, K.E., 'Income inequality and population health: a review and explanation', *Social Science & Medicine* 2006; 62: 1768–84.

[27] Yamey, G., 'Why does the world still need WHO?', *British Medical Journal* 2002; 325: 1294–8.

[28] Price, D., Pollock, A.M., Shaoul, J., 'How the World Trade Organisation is shaping domestic policies in health care', *Lancet* 1999; 354: 1889–92.

[29] Nair, V.M., 'Health in South Asia: future of Kerala depends on its willingness to learn from past', *British Medical Journal* 2004; 328: 1497, and Jayasinghe, S., 'Health in South Asia: Sri Lanka needs to build on its strengths and gains', *British Medical Journal* 2004; 328: 1497.

[30] This was an important sub-plot in the run-up to referenda on the proposed new Constitution for the European Union. It was better understood in France, which fortunately voted first, than in Britain. Even more than the original Treaty of Rome, part 3 of the proposed new Constitution would have forced hitherto public service institutions into market competition, including multinational commercial providers. Though every EU country has at least one major political party claiming a future socialist society as its aim, this section of the new Constitution would have made anything other than a neoliberal economy illegal. Large majorities against it in referenda in France and the Netherlands have stalled this process for the time being, but the attack will certainly be renewed next time approval is sought for the new Constitution.

[31] Apparently exemption depends on whether health services are classified as economic or non-economic activity, evidently determined not by whether they have a useful product, but whether they operate for profit. Production of pornography, legal prostitution, gambling or advice on legal tax evasion are thus all classed as economic activities, while we have to pretend that the NHS is not. Only services provided without any direct charges (co-payments) can be sure of exemption.

[32] Editorial, 'A manipulated dichotomy in global health policy', *Lancet* 2000; 356: 1923.

[33] Elliott, L., 'Impending crisis in the International Monetary Fund, World Bank, and World Trade Organisations', *Guardian*, 21 May 2003.

[34] *Financial Times*, 15 January 1999.

[35] In the later years of Franklin Roosevelt's New Deal, the US came closer to achieving its own NHS than most people think. Medical co-operatives were developed throughout the rural areas of the US, from 1936 to 1945. In 1938 the *Saturday Evening Post* described the Farm Society Administration (FSA) scheme as a 'gigantic rehearsal for health insurance. It has brought together some 3,000 doctors and more than 100,000 families in twenty-odd states. It has given them a chance to show what would happen if a health insurance law were enacted for them tomorrow.' At its peak in 1942, the FSA had about 650,000 farming people covered by comprehensive health care in 1,200 plans in 42 states, with group prepayments organised jointly between farmers' associations and physicians' county or state associations. Group prepayment had been proposed by the LaFollette Congressional Committee on Costs of Medical Care, founded in 1927 and reporting in 1932 in *Medical Care for the American People: The Final Report of the Committee on Costs of Medical Care.* The report noted that medical resources were not 'distributed according to needs, but rather according to real or supposed ability of patients to pay for services'. The American Medical Association described the report as an 'incitement to revolution'. In 1945 it would have been extended to a national health insurance plan similar to those in other developed economies, through the Wagner-Murray-Dingell Bill, supported by President Truman, but in 1946 Congress ended all the New Deal legislation supporting the programme. Drs Fred Mott and Milton Roemer, who had headed the FSA programme, moved to Canada to develop the comprehensive health insurance programme in Saskatchewan, which laid foundations for Canada's present single-payer model for all Canadian health care (Grey, M.R., *New Deal Medicine: The Rural Health Programs of the Farm Security Administration*, Baltimore, MD: Johns Hopkins University Press, 1999).

[36] Obviously, in this context, property means wealth as capital, not as objects for personal use, though a wheelbarrow or a car can come into either of these categories. For a large majority of people in developed economies, ownership of capital is almost or completely limited to ownership of their own home, which has both a personal use-value and a market value. This has obvious implications for politicians eager to recruit as many people as possible to the sound views of property owners, from 'two hectares and a cow' in the days of Thiers, to Margaret Thatcher's populist capitalism in the 1980s. By introducing her 'right to buy' policy for tenants of social housing, she hoped to extend the ideology of people who live from what they own to a large proportion of people who live from what they do. Houses were sold to tenants at prices far below their market value. This was followed by shares in previously nationalised industries available at similar knock-down prices. A generation of workers, formerly dependable Labour voters, became

more receptive to the Conservative message. New Labour has followed the same course, accepting an end to all socially provided housing, as well as to nationalised industries and public utilities. The number of officially recognised homeless families in Britain consequently rose from 53,000 in 1978 to 287,000 by 1993. Fortunes were made by estate agents, banks and speculative builders. The generation which profited from this looting of public property was left to wonder how it could help its children to pay the now astronomical price of getting a roof over their heads (Victor, C.R., 'The health of homeless people in Britain: a review', *European Journal of Public Health* 1997; 7: 398–404, and OPCS report, *The Health of Our Children*, London: HMSO, 1995). The Thatcher legacy includes transformation of houses from consumer commodities, places to live, into speculative investments, places to develop and sell profitably. As she intended, this has been socially divisive and politically confusing. It has promoted growth of a third social category, people who live both from what they own and from what they do, with minds divided accordingly. Nevertheless, they must ultimately choose between these bases for their own lives.

This important story is not yet concluded. Speculative inflation of house values has continued since the 1970s, providing a basis for borrowing that supports rising consumer spending even where real wages are falling, as in the US. US national house prices in 2006, when the first edition of this book appeared, were still rising by 15% annually. Total value of house property in OECD countries had more than doubled over the past five years, from $30bn to $70bn, more than equal to their entire annual output of services and manufactures; in the words of the *Economist* (June 2005), 'Never before have real house prices risen so fast for so long in so many countries'. That 2006 edition included the following forecast: 'As rising house prices are almost entirely speculative and represent little material production, this is a bubble comparable to speculation preceding the US market collapse of 1929–33, which led to a world crisis of capitalism, fascism, and the Second World War. There is today a growing divergence between real economies producing use-value, and notional economies apparently creating wealth, much of which could prove illusory, and the brunt of this will be felt by workers who accepted the illusion that they had become successful capitalists.' Events in 2007–08 seem to have confirmed that forecast.

[37] Zweig, M., *The Working Class Majority: America's Best Kept Secret*, New York: IRL Press, 2001.

[38] This seems to be a long-term trend in all fully mature industrial economies. According to the *Economist*, 45% of all the profits made by the 500 wealthiest

US companies now come from the financial sector rather than manufacture or non-financial services.

[39] According to the BBC, in July 2000 her personal fortune amounted to £1.9bn, ranking her 19th in the world list.

[40] Sir Fred Goodwin, Chief Executive of the Royal Bank of Scotland (RBS), was named Forbes Businessman of the year in 2002, the ultimate accolade in the international business world. In January 2009 we learned that his bank had lost £28bn, the highest of any UK company in the current crisis. RBS shares fell by two-thirds in one night, and the bank's estimated total value fell from £50bn to £5bn. The New Labour government saved the bank with £20bn of public money, and nominally took control, but with the stated intention of returning it to the private sector as soon as possible. Meanwhile, it allowed Sir Fred to receive £4.2m over his last year at work, and to retire at age 55 with an annual pension of £579,000 (Hattenstone, S., *Guardian*, 24 January 2009).

[41] Seager, A., 'Bank crisis will burden a generation, says King', *Guardian*, 21 October 2009.

[42] More than twice as many, 49,000 such bankers lost their jobs after the crash, so the £6bn in bonuses expected in 2009 was substantially less than the £10bn they got in 2007, the last boom year (Treanor, J., 'City bonuses to soar by half to £6bn', *Guardian*, 21 October 2009).

[43] Smith, D., Goodman, M., Marlow, B., Walsh, K., 'Hammering the City: Lord Turner talks tough', *Sunday Times*, 30 August 2009.

[44] At the end of the Second World War, 30% of US jobs required educated people; by 2000 this proportion had risen to about 70%. Half of all new jobs, and 35% of all jobs, now need people with higher education. At least within one's own sphere of work, the habit of honesty has become priceless, together with the ability to solve problems without answers at the back of the book (Anderson, W.E.K., 'Green College lecture: Responsibility of the educator', *British Medical Journal* 1989; 298: 1660–1).

[45] Study of voting by social class, using detailed categories for turnout, shows no clear decline in cohesion of voting by the industrial working class since the 1930s in either Britain or France. The process of *embourgeoisement*, through which material affluence is supposed to make workers reallocate themselves to a middle class, seems confined to the US (Weakliem, D.L., Heath, A., *The Secret Life of Class Voting: Britain, France and the United States since the 1930s*, Centre

for Research Into Elections and Social Trends, Working Paper 31, Glasgow: University of Strathclyde, February 1995). Even there, the process is far less complete than most media reporting implies. Commenting on the British general election in 2001, Prof Greg Philo of the Glasgow University Media Group thought the result reflected changes in class structure since Thatcher's deregulation measures in the 1980s (*Guardian*, 13 June 2001). The top 10% of population now earned as much as the bottom 50% put together, and 20 million adults had only a state pension. This meant that at least two-thirds of the population had to rely on the public sector, including many of the traditional middle class, who were now faced with the industrialisation of their work, as 'safe' occupations in banking and insurance turned into low-paid call-centre jobs. This was why health and education became the main concerns of the electorate, and why New Labour regained a 'natural' majority. He believed this could be sustained only by a wealth tax, with currency controls to prevent flight of capital. As a new party of big business, New Labour cannot provide such a tax or controls, so if it wants to regain its natural majority, the Labour Party will have to revert to its former compromises.

[46] Market failure is not possible for any essential public service. All promises that outsourcing, public-private partnerships or privatisation can transfer risks from taxpayers (the population as a whole) to private investors are therefore false. Many examples confirm this. In the 1980s, in the first wave of privatisation of care homes for the elderly, about 85% of provision was shifted into the private sector. As house prices rocketed in the 1990s, many care homes, particularly in the wealthiest part of the UK, the south-east of England, acquired greater value as property than as a profitable service. As the aim of the private sector is profit, they were naturally sold, and the old people they were supposed to be caring for were tipped out, to find somewhere else to live. For privately owned public services to be abandoned, they need not reach bankruptcy, they just have to seem less profitable than some other way to make money. Expectations for profitability of US and other transnational corporations from investment in Latin American and European public health care services were often too optimistic, so whole nations which had shifted responsibility to transnational corporations found themselves still responsible for whatever seemed least profitable (Jasso-Aguilar, R., Waitzkin, H., Landwehr, A., 'Multinational corporations and health care in the United States and Latin America: strategies, actions and effects', in Mackintosh, M., Koivusalo, M. (eds), *Commercialisation of Health Care: Global and Local Dynamics and Policy Responses*, London: Palgrave Macmillan United Nations Research Institute for Social Development, 2005, pp 38–50).

Chapter Seven

[1] Despite hypercritical media coverage for the past decade at least, the NHS is still also more popular than care systems which remained more or less market-driven, most notably in the US. Americans do not love the non-system they have, but enough of them have been made to fear change of any kind to stifle the changes a majority voted for in 2009, preferring devils they know.

[2]   O traveler, there is no path
   Paths are made by walking.
        Antonio Machado (1875–1939)

[3] Before the NHS, the workload in a South Wales mining practice was back-breaking, with up to 70 home visits a day and 100 patients attending each morning and evening surgery (Levers, A.H., 'The GP at the crossroads', *Lancet* 1950; I: 1369, echoing a similar letter from A. Sanjana in the *Lancet* 1950; I: 1201). When I was a GP locum in the Rhondda Fach in the summer of 1961 I had to cope with about 60 patients at each morning and evening surgery, ending around 9pm, with about 25 home visits between them and night duty to follow. Relatively few of these patients had acute health problems susceptible to cure. As a contribution to health gain, almost all of this work was futile, except as support for morale and access to benefits (which for the most part were very necessary). Obviously most doctors compelled to work in this way perceived patients' demands as much larger than their needs, as medical students had been taught to understand them. A brilliant piece of research in Newcastle confirmed this, showing that GPs in a deprived inner city area thought their consultation rate was two to three times more than normal for such an area. In fact it was about average, and so was their average consultation time at 5–6.5 minutes. Subjectively estimated workload was closely associated with high rates of consultation by consulters, but this was balanced by an unusually high proportion of non-consulters (Bhopal, J.S., Bhopal, R.S., 'Perceived versus actual consultation patterns in an inner city practice', *Journal of the Royal College of General Practitioners* 1989; 39: 156-7). Doctors cannot perceive registered patients who do not consult, unless they go out of their way to discover them. Few doctors who are already overworked can do that, even if they want to.

[4] For example, it has hugely accelerated development of cars, and road networks to support them, but it has impeded development of rational and sustainable mobility for entire populations, by subordinating all social pathways towards greater personal mobility to the production, sale and use of cars.

[5] That was what I found in my own practice, and every colleague I know who subjected their work to similar objective study found similar shortcomings

(Hart, J.T., 'Measurement of omission', *BMJ* 1982; 284:1686-9). Phoney research reveals itself by the perfection of its claims. People who have undertaken years of hard grind in the front-lines of care know that perfect delivery of medical science to any whole population is always a long way off, and anyone who claims already to have arrived as soon as they start must be extremely suspect.

[6] Education is supremely important, but it is a great mistake to suppose that uneducated people are necessarily less able to think for themselves. In 1920, speaking of his constituents in Bermondsey, Dr Shapurji Saklatvala wrote the following aphorism: 'It is much easier to deceive people who read but cannot think, than people who think but cannot read' (Benn, C., *Keir Hardie*, London: Hutchinson, 1992: p 394). He was the UK's first Communist MP, out of a cumulative total of three.

[7] Irvin, G., Byrne, D., Murphy, R., Reed, H., Ruane, S., *In Place of Cuts: Tax Reforms to Build a Fairer Society*, www.compassonline.org.uk, accessed 1 January 2010.

[8] National output grew by 25%, almost all in the state sector, which accounted for more than half of all expenditure by 1943. The cost of living was stable from 1941 because of strict price controls. There were rising living standards for poorer people, and full employment. Despite 360,000 war deaths, the total population grew by 3% (*Fighting with Figures: A Statistical Digest of the Second World War*, London: HMSO, 1995).

[9] Hart, J.T., 'The teaching of medical history and education for change' (Gale Memorial Lecture), *Social History of Medicine* 1989; 2: 391-8.

[10] Calder, N., *The People's War: Britain 1939–1945*, London: Pimlico, 1969. Later books on the same theme may be more fully documented, as the edges of official secrecy roll back, but unlike Nigel Calder, their authors have no personal experience of those times, in my opinion a vital ingredient, if you can get it. Of course, the people's war was not the only war. For Winston Churchill, it was above all a war for the survival of the British Empire. His stance as defender of the Empire and its ruling class, while still ignorant of the lives of most working people, was well understood even by many officers, and by a large majority of enlisted lower ranks. The 1945 Labour landslide astonished almost all politicians and journalists, but was no surprise to service men and women or their families. They had redefined the nature of patriotism.

[11] Though these rigidities have never been fully restored, since the 1980s UK culture has become risk-averse as never before. Every responsible decision must apparently ensure that when anything goes wrong, responsibility will lie elsewhere. No school outing can be organised without some preliminary scouting party to search out every conceivable contingency, and nothing can be allowed to happen without insurance, anticipated and paid for. The stultifying effect on imagination has been catastrophic for teaching, and may eventually be so for clinical medicine if we continue to follow the US path of contingency lawyering. This litigious nightmare has been a predictable product of making all relationships follow a similar basic transactional pattern, as if teachers were selling education to their students, and doctors were selling clinical decisions to patients, with everyone entitled to sue if things don't work out exactly as expected. Human institutions need human laws.

[12] How far were these spaces ever really open to imagination? No further than bureaucrats at all levels would allow. Seldom was that far, most often it was not at all, and that applied as much to the NHS as to any other welfare institution. However, huge possibilities were visible, and these dominated progressive thought at least until 1985. They were then defeated by the outcome of the miners' strike, ending an era of political and social thought that had lasted roughly 100 years in the UK, rather longer elsewhere in Europe. In the new context of a knowledge-based economy, they will eventually return..

[13] Tett, G., *Fools' Gold*, New York: Little, Brown, 2009.

[14] Letter to *Guardian*, 8 September 2009.

Index of names

Index of subjects

Lightning Source UK Ltd.
Milton Keynes UK
UKHW020108280319
340051UK00004B/175/P

9 781847 427823